Primary Care for Older Adults

Michael Wasserman • James Riopelle

Editors

Primary Care for Older Adults

Models and Challenges

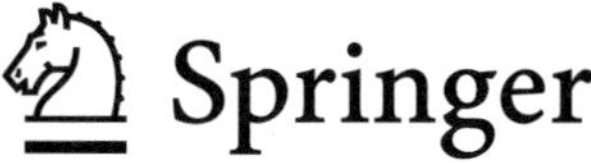 Springer

Editors
Michael Wasserman
Rockport Healthcare Services
Los Angeles, CA
USA

James Riopelle
Physician Consultant Institute
Denver, CO
USA

ISBN 978-3-319-61327-7   ISBN 978-3-319-61329-1   (eBook)
DOI 10.1007/978-3-319-61329-1

Library of Congress Control Number: 2017955834

This Springer imprint is published by Springer Nature
The registered company is Springer International Publishing AG
The registered company address is: Gewerbestrasse 11, 6330 Cham, Switzerland

Preface

The Challenge of Primary Care for Older Adults

As a fourth year medical student at the University of Texas, Medical Branch, in 1984, I wrote a paper on whether geriatrics should be a primary care or consultative discipline. Over 30 years has passed, and I have been blessed with opportunities to experience the field of geriatrics from a variety of vantage points. I recount some of these in the first chapter, "Primary Care in the United States Today." One thing is clear, that is, the baby boomer generation is transforming the demographic makeup of our society. Annual Medicare expenditures presently exceed $650 billion. It is only a matter of time before this number exceeds a trillion dollars. Medicaid spending is close behind. A generally underappreciated fact is that a large portion of the Medicaid budget goes toward paying for long-term care services for older adults. The need for long-term care services is directly associated with a person's health. How we address primary care for older adults is not only an issue for the individuals seeking such care but a critical question for our society to tackle in terms of how we are going to pay for it.

The field of geriatric medicine has been growing, with a surge in the evidence-based literature around the care of older adults. A growing body of literature has questioned the use of antipsychotic medication in older adults with dementia [1]. The Centers for Medicare and Medicaid (CMS) have championed the National Partnership for Dementia Care, which has targeted the inappropriate use of antipsychotic medications in the long-term care setting [2]. The ramifications of efforts such as this are significant. A recent study out of Great Britain has questioned aggressive treatment of cholesterol, blood sugar, and blood pressure in elderly diabetics [3]. Sharing this knowledge with a workforce that has been trained primarily to treat a younger population is one of our country's greatest challenges. We presently suffer from significant workforce issues in the field of geriatrics. The number of board-certified geriatricians is presently under 7000 and is going down every year [4].

How we address the primary care healthcare needs of older adults will have ramifications on our country for many years to come. While the issues of how we train our workforce to care for older adults is beyond the scope of this book, the reader will find insights into how we can work within the construct of our existing workforce to provide quality care to older adults. We have been fortunate to engage a broad cross section of clinicians who care for older adults across the continuum. By definition, the field of geriatrics requires an interdisciplinary approach. Within these pages, the reader will find expertise not only from geriatricians but from nurse practitioners, physician assistants, pharmacists, and practice managers.

I regularly opine that the geriatric approach to care, as I like to call it, is the "secret sauce" necessary to bring cost-effective, high-quality care to older individuals. You will find this to be a constant theme throughout this book. We are not proposing a single solution to how primary care is delivered, nor would we want to. The spirit of exploration and the ongoing search for quality requires us to try different approaches. With that said, the geriatric approach certainly appears to be a necessary "constant" in the various methodologies espoused in this book.

I recently became aware of the concept of cargo cult science, put forth by Dr. Richard Feynman in his 1974 Cal Tech Commencement address.

> In the South Seas there is a Cargo Cult of people. During the war they saw airplanes land with lots of good materials, and they want the same thing to happen now. So they've arranged to make things like runways, to put fires along the sides of the runways, to make a wooden hut for a man to sit in, with two wooden pieces on his head like headphones and bars of bamboo sticking out like antennas—he's the controller—and they wait for the airplanes to land. They're doing everything right. The form is perfect. It looks exactly the way it looked before. But it doesn't work. No airplanes land. So I call these things Cargo Cult Science, because they follow all the apparent precepts and forms of scientific investigation, but they're missing something essential, because the planes don't land [5].

How is this relevant to effectively delivery primary care to older adults? It is relevant because there seems to be a belief that specific structural models of care are all that is necessary to enhance the delivery of care to older adults. Care coordination models are commonly touted as the solution, although the evidence is quite lacking [6]. I would suggest that without including the "secret sauce," which is the geriatric approach to care, we are just building our care models out of wood and bamboo sticks, which is why the planes don't come. Within the pages of this book, the reader will find how the geriatric approach to care has been integrated into a variety of care models and clinical disciplines.

George Santayana said, "those who cannot remember the past are condemned to repeat it." Throughout this book are examples of successful models of care and insight into what has made these models successful. Primary care isn't the same thing to each individual. Nor is it always the same thing to each population. Hopefully, exposure to a variety of care models along the entire continuum of care will give the reader a starting point from which to evaluate effective approaches for their practice or community.

Los Angeles, CA, USA   Michael Wasserman, MD, CMD
Denver, CO, USA   James Riopelle, MD

Acknowledgments

A few years ago, I read a "hindsight" article in the *Journal of the American Geriatrics Society* by Dr. Gene Stollerman [7]. Dr. Stollerman was one of the leading figures during the early development of geriatric medicine in the United States. I was able to meet with him before he passed away, and he encouraged me to focus my "next chapter" in life on my passion to improve how we as a society care for older adults. I hope that this book will contribute to the work that Dr. Stollerman and others started many years ago in advancing the cause of improving care for older adults.

I was fortunate to "come of age" as a geriatrician under the leadership and mentorship of some of the most prominent people in the field. It gives me great pleasure to recognize and thank Drs. Joe Ouslander, Dan Osterweil, John Morley, Al Sui, Tom Yoshikawa, Mark Beers, David Reuben, Larry Rubinstein, John Beck, Jim Davis, Charles Marshall, Mark Levinstein, Derek Princely, Dave Solomon, and John Burton. I'd like to thank Dr. Tom Cole for adding to my understanding of healthcare policy as a medical student. I also want to thank Paul Starr, whom I've never met, but whose book, *The Social Transformation of American Medicine*, inspired many of my views on healthcare policy.

I want to thank Dr. Caroline Braun for coming up with the concept for this book. It's been over 20 years since Drs. Braun, Cheryl Phillips, Adrienne Mims, Steve Phillips, and I founded the American Geriatrics Society's Managed Care Task Force, which ultimately morphed into the Health Systems Committee. The AGS has been my society "home" for almost 30 years. There are countless names of people whom I have learned from over the years through my association with AGS and AMDA. We make each other better through our ongoing search for the "truth."

I would like to thank my coeditor, friend, and mentor, Jim Riopelle. You taught me most of what I know about managed care and business. To Raymond Delisle, my friend, mentor, and patient, I only wish you were still around to give me your sage advice and support. To Jim Graham, who taught me that we must understand the finance side of healthcare in order to deliver quality care. To Susan Johnson, who demonstrated the importance of having someone at your side making sure the wheels are turning properly. To Shelly Thomas, who taught me if you don't code, bill, and collect properly, you can't keep the doors open. To Don Murphy, one of the greatest healthcare visionaries I've ever worked with, for always challenging me to find ways to make our dreams happen.

I'd also like to thank Springer Publishing, for recognizing the growing need for geriatric-related content.

Last, and certainly not least, I thank my wife, Sherri. As a fourth year medical student, I came home one day talking about the disease rather than the person. You set me straight that very day, and I have been focusing on a person-centered approach to patient care ever since. You also supported me in following my dreams and focusing on my passion for older adults. Similarly, my children, Raishel and Justine, did not see me as much growing up due to this passion (and a workaholic nature), but have let me know that they value my commitment to older adults. Ultimately, I must dedicate this book to my grandson, Bailey, who will see the dawn of the twenty-second century as an 85-year-old. I hope that we will have finally worked out all the kinks in how we deliver primary care to older adults by then!

References

1. Office of Inspector General, Report (OEI-07-08-00150) Medicare Atypical Antipsychotic Drug Claims for Elderly Nursing Home Residents. http://oig.hhs.gov/oei/reports/oei-07-08-00150.asp.
2. https://www.cms.gov/Medicare/Provider-Enrollment-and-Certification/SurveyCertificationGenInfo/National-Partnership-to-Improve-Dementia-Care-in-Nursing-Homes.html.
3. Hamada S, et al. Mortality in individuals age 80 and older with type 2 diabetes mellitus in relation to glycosylated hemoglobin, blood pressure, and total cholesterol. J Am Geriatr Soc. 2016;64:1425–31.
4. Wasserman M. Geriatric and primary care workforce development. In: Powers JS, editor. Healthcare Changes and the Affordable Care Act. http://dx.doi.org/10.1007/978-3-319-09510-3_6. Springer. P. 99–115.
5. Feynman R. Cargo Cult Science. http://calteches.library.caltech.edu/51/2/CargoCult.htm.
6. Wasserman M. Care management: from channeling to grace. In: Powers JS, editor. Healthcare Changes and the Affordable Care Act. http://dx.doi.org/10.1007/978-3-319-09510-3_8. Springer. P. 133–52.
7. Stollerman GH. Geriatrics: a perspective of hindsight. J Am Geriatr Soc. 2013;61:151–4.

Contents

Contributors

Steven Atkinson, PA-C, MS Twin Cities Physicians, Minneapolis, MN, USA

Debra Bakerjian, PhD, APRN, FAAN, FAANP Betty Irene Moore School of Nursing, University of CA, Davis, CA, USA

Peter Boling, MD Geriatrics and Long Term Care, Georgetown University School of Medicine, Washington, DC, USA

Patrick P. Coll, MD, AGSF, CMD Center on Aging, UConn Health, Farmington, CT, USA

Julia Dolejs, MSN, RN, APRN, FNP-BC R. L. Roudebush VAMC, Indianapolis, IN, USA

Terry E. Hill, MD Hill Physicians Medical Group, San Ramon, CA, USA

Janice Hoffman, Pharm.D, CGP, FASCP Western University of Health Sciences, College of Pharmacy, Pomona, CA, USA

Peter A. Hollmann, MD University Medicine-Geriatrics, Warren Alpert Medical School, Brown University, Providence, RI, USA

Bruce Kinosian, MD Geriatrics and Long Term Care, Georgetown University School of Medicine, Washington, DC, USA

Jason F. Lee, MD, MPH UCLA Health, Los Angeles, CA, USA

Magda Lenartowicz, MD, (IM/Geriatrics) Comprehensive Senior Care Program, Encino Hospital Medical Center and Sherman Oaks Hospital, Encino, CA, USA

Justine May, MSW, LCSW R. L. Roudebush VAMC, Indianapolis, IN, USA

Jeremy V. Phillips Geriatric Specialty Care, Reno, NV, USA

Steven L. Phillips, MD Geriatric Specialty Care, Reno, NV, USA

James Riopelle, MD Physician Consultant Institute, Denver, CO, USA

Cathy C. Schubert, MD Indiana University School of Medicine, Indianapolis, IN, USA

R. L. Roudebush VAMC, Indianapolis, IN, USA

George Taler, MD Geriatrics and Long Term Care, Georgetown University School of Medicine, Washington, DC, USA

Shelly Thomas Rocky Mountain Senior Care, Golden Colorado, A member of the American Academy of Professional Coders, NY, USA

Michael Wasserman, MD, CMD Rockport Healthcare Services, Los Angeles, CA, USA

Robert A. Zorowitz, MD, MBA, FACP, AGSF, CMD Optum, Inc., New York, NY, USA

Introduction: Primary Care in the United States Today

Michael Wasserman and James Riopelle

A recent publication by the John A. Hartford Foundation opened with the following statement: "Reform efforts, such as the patient-centered medical home (PCMH) model, are a promising template for better primary care. However, national and local definitions of PCMHs have little or no focus on geriatric expertise, including advance care planning, functional status, or comprehensive assessments and interventions for older or medically complex patients and their caregivers" [1]. There is no question about the declining number of primary care physicians in the United States. There is also no question about the increasing number of older adults and the geriatric imperative that the baby boomer generation has brought about. Many geriatricians are used to being told by internists and family physicians alike that they practice geriatrics because many of their patients are old. Where does this leave geriatrics in relation to the primary care challenges that we are facing today?

Is geriatrics a primary care specialty or subspecialty? This is a question that has been asked for the past few decades. As a young geriatrician in the 1990s, it was a question that I (Michael Wasserman) encountered in various practice settings. We developed a geriatric consult clinic at Kaiser Permanente in 1989 in order to share geriatric medical expertise with primary care physicians. In the 1990s, GeriMed of America managed hospital-based senior clinics and then opened their own in an effort to deliver a primary care-based model for older adults. There have clearly been various approaches to the delivery of primary care to older adults in the past few decades. The Affordable Care Act endeavored to promote a variety of primary care models and approaches. It even included a 10% reimbursement bonus to primary care physicians for 5 years.

M. Wasserman, MD, CMD (✉)
Rockport Healthcare Services, Los Angeles, CA, USA
e-mail: wassdoc@aol.com

J. Riopelle, MD
Physician Consultant Institute, Denver, CO, USA

© Springer International Publishing AG 2018
M. Wasserman, J. Riopelle (eds.), *Primary Care for Older Adults*,
DOI 10.1007/978-3-319-61329-1_1

It is heartening that the Hartford Foundation paper attempts to shine a spotlight on the paucity of geriatric expertise that exists in primary care today. The lack of geriatric competencies in the physician workforce and primary care workforce in particular begs the question of how to "geriatricize" primary care. This brings us to the focus of this book.

Let's begin by stating what this book is not about. It is not meant to be a treatise on the history of primary care. It is not even meant to focus on primary care methods and programs as a whole. The baby boomers have begun to "age in" at a rate of roughly 10,000 per day.[1] We will leave a discussion regarding primary care for the pediatric and commercial population to others. Instead, we will focus on the population over 65 and the need for, and importance of, more effective primary care services for this growing population. The most rapidly growing demographic in the United States are those 85 and older, with a projected increase from 5.7 million in 2011 to 14.1 million in 2040.[2] In 2011, Medicare beneficiaries over the age of 80 comprised one third of all Medicare spending while representing 24% of the Medicare population.[3]

While projections vary, there is no question that there will be a significant shortfall of primary care physicians in the coming years.[4] This creates a perfect storm. Anyone with knowledge of the CPT coding system knows that reimbursement decreases with the number of problems and length of visits. This puts a premium on trying to see the most patients in the course of a day, which suits itself toward younger individuals with single problems. That does not describe the older population. A study in 2002 demonstrated how primary care physicians found caring for elderly patients to be difficult [2]. Older adults require more time and thus require a greater number of physician full-time equivalents (FTEs) for similar numbers of patients.

In 1966, the Folsom report stated: "Every individual should have a personal physician who is the central point for integration and continuity of all medical services to his patient. Such physician will emphasize the practice of preventive medicine … He will be aware of the many and varied social, emotional and environmental factors that influence the health of his patient and his family … His concern will be for the patient as a whole, and his relationship with the patient must be a continuity one" [3]. These hallmarks of primary care are also key elements of a geriatric approach to care.

Primary care was defined by the World Health Organization in 1978 as "essential healthcare based on practical, scientifically sound, and socially acceptable methods and technology made universally accessible to individuals and families in the community by means acceptable to them and at a cost that the community and the

---

[1] https://www.ssa.gov/pressoffice/pr/babyboomerfiles-pr.htm.

[2] http://www.aoa.gov/Aging_Statistics/Profile/2012/docs/2012profile.pdf.

[3] http://kff.org/report-section/the-rising-cost-of-living-longer-section-1-medicare-per-capita-spending-by-age-among-traditional-medicare-beneficiaries-over-age-65-2011/.

[4] https://www.aamc.org/download/426260/data/physiciansupplyanddemandthrough2025keyfindings.pdf.

country can afford to maintain at every stage of their development in a spirit of self-reliance and self-determination. It forms an integral part of both the country's health system (of which it is the central function) and a main focus of the overall social and economic development of the community. It is the first level of contact for individuals, the family, and the community with the national health system, bringing healthcare as close as possible to where people live and work, and constitutes the first element of a continuing healthcare process" [4, 5]. How do these essential elements of primary care mesh with the principles and practice of geriatric medicine?

In 2010, Robert Phillips and Andrew Bazemore described the history and status of primary care in the United States and around the world [6]. They concluded that "the United States has fallen behind other developed and developing countries that share a common focus on, and dedication to, to primary care."[5] It is unclear what the subsequent years have brought in terms of primary care workforce development. However, a number of primary care-based initiatives have come forward in the past several years, many of which are topics in this book.

In 2012, the Center for Medicare & Medicaid Innovation (CMMI) of the Centers for Medicare & Medicaid Services (CMS) began the Comprehensive Primary Care (CPC) initiative. This collaborative endeavor between CMS and other private and public payers aimed to improve primary care delivery. They focused on helping medical practices implement five key functions in their delivery of care: (1) access and continuity, (2) planned care for chronic conditions and preventive care, (3) risk-stratified care management, (4) patient and caregiver engagement, and (5) coordination of care across the medical neighborhood [7]. In the first 2 years of the program, there have been some positive results, but there has yet to be demonstrated any net savings to the Medicare program, after deducting the cost of providing for additional case management services. This is consistent with previous initiatives funded by CMS evaluating case management and care coordination models of care [8].

There continues to be hope that patient-centered medical home models can improve the care of older adults in a cost-effective manner. The John A. Hartford Foundation paper outlined what they believe to be important attributes in making patient-centered medical homes senior friendly. These include a focus on patient-centered care, coordinated care, accessible services, and a commitment to quality and safety [1]. The most problematic aspect of impacting primary care in older adults may have more to do with a lack of adequate expertise in geriatric medicine among the clinicians in the healthcare workforce. This has been described in detail in a previous publication on the importance of integrating a geriatric medical approach within various delivery models [9].

This book will view the geriatric primary care challenge from a variety of vantage points. We will look at some of the more robust initiatives that have been set forward in the past several years, with a particular focus on the patient-centered medical home. The concept of population health has also taken on a significant part of the primary care discussion, and this will be looked at from both a general and program-oriented prospective. We will also look at approaches to impacting more

---

[5] ibid.

traditional primary care practices. Finally, there will be a view from the provider perspective, as the opportunity to involve a wider variety of clinicians throughout the continuum of care has come about.

It is our hope that the relevance of older adults in the primary care discussion will be made very obvious throughout the course of this book. That is not nearly enough, however, in a healthcare market that has a significant deficit in geriatric clinical competencies. Every chapter in this book shines a light on developing systems of care that are ingrained with a geriatric approach. If we are to significantly impact the delivery of primary care to older adults in the coming decades, we ignore this at our peril.

References

1. Dorr D, et al. Patient-centered medical homes and the care of older adults. New York: John A. Hartford Foundation; 2016.
2. Adams W. Primary care for elderly people: why do doctors find it so hard. Gerontologist. 2002;42(6):835842.
3. Folsom MB, National Commission on Community Health Services. Health is a community affair. Cambridge, MA: Harvard University Press; 1966. p. 26.
4. World Health Organization (WHO). Primary health care. Geneva, Switzerland: WHO; 1978.
5. Shi L. The impact of primary care: a focused review. Scientifica. 2012:432892. 22 pages. doi:10.6064/2012/432892.
6. Phillips RL Jr, Bazemore AW. Primary care and why it matters for U.S. Health System Reform. Health Aff. 2010;29(5):806–10. doi:10.1377/hlthaff.2010.0020.
7. Peikes D, et al. Evaluation of the comprehensive primary care initiative: second annual report. April 2016.
8. Schore J, et al. Fourth report to congress on the evaluation mathematica policy research of the Medicare coordinated care demonstration. March 2011.
9. Wasserman M. Care management: from channeling to grace. In: Powers JS, editor. Healthcare changes and the affordable care act. Berlin, Germany: Springer International Publishing. p. 133–52. doi:10.1007/978-3-319-09510-3_8.

Geriatric Consultative Models in Primary Care

2

Magda Lenartowicz

Geriatric consultants are not a new invention. This is essentially the way that many geriatric medicine pioneers, such as the British physician Dr. Marjory Warren, practiced at the beginning of the twentieth century. Although it was Dr. Ignatz Nascher who coined the term "geriatrics" in the USA in 1909, Dr. Warren instituted the first geriatric medicine ward akin to what we would think of today, complete with comprehensive assessments, focus on early mobility, and coordinated discharge planning [1]. Dr. Warren was luckily also a prolific writer and researcher, becoming the first geriatrician to publish her unit's outcome statistics, [2] and thus firmly establishing the key role of evidence-based practice within geriatric medicine.

The British tradition of geriatrics as a subspecialty arrived in Canada along with some of the specialty's early adopters. Geriatric medicine specialists in Canada are all essentially geriatric hospitalists and have been ever since the specialty was enshrined by the Royal College in Canada in 1977, limiting entry only to those trained in internal medicine (this decision was not without its detractors). Geriatric physicians thus remain mostly as consultants at large academic hospitals, or medical managers of ACE units and specialty clinics, which is likely the most judicious use of their rather small numbers. Currently there are only 261 geriatric specialists in Canada, which is approximately 0.7 per 100,000 people, with 40% of these MDs being over the age of 55 [3].

American geriatrics really took off during the 1960s, with the first geriatric fellowship program in the USA being established in 1966. In contrast to its Canadian and UK counterparts, however, US geriatric medicine developed into a mostly primary specialty, which put it in somewhat of a double bind, in being a primary specialty *and* working with a population that has been traditionally overlooked. This is

M. Lenartowicz, MD, (IM/Geriatrics)
Comprehensive Senior Care Program,
Encino Hospital Medical Center and Sherman Oaks Hospital, Encino, CA, USA
e-mail: mlenartowicz@gmail.com

© Springer International Publishing AG 2018
M. Wasserman, J. Riopelle (eds.), *Primary Care for Older Adults*,
DOI 10.1007/978-3-319-61329-1_2

likely a contributing factor to the reality that recruitment into geriatrics has not been easy—in 2016 geriatric fellowships across the country only filled 50% of available spots, and 100/137 programs went unfilled altogether [4]. In addition, the volume-driven fee-for-service system, mostly based on Medicare payments, has made the practice of primary care geriatrics a formidable task. It has proven difficult to sustain a geriatric private practice (primary or otherwise) since comprehensive geriatric assessments take time, and multidisciplinary teams are expensive. The US Medicare and private insurance payment systems lack the type of specialized reimbursements available to Ontario (Canada) geriatricians, for example, where an initial consult visit with a geriatrician ($175) is reimbursed differently than a 75-min or 90-min CGA (reimbursed at $300 and $365 Canadian, respectively) [5]. In addition, the 90-min CGA can be claimed for all patients with dementia, regardless of age. In comparison, based on Medicare reimbursement thus far, the most complex new patient visit (60 min) is approximately $200 US, and no special reimbursement is available for CGAs. Follow-up visits are reimbursed at a lower rate in both countries, but geriatricians in Ontario do get payment for providing phone-based support to caregivers of persons with cognitive impairment, as well as for specialized telehealth visits. In contrast, Medicare requires that services be delivered face-to-face, thus making it difficult to justify the prolonged time that many geriatricians spend on the phone or with caregivers. These facts make it a little less surprising that when combined with entrenched societal ageism and complexity of geriatric patients, the (comparatively) middling compensation does not entice young residents with astronomical student loans to pursue this path. This is reinforced by the argument that the low interest also stems from a lack of definition for the specialty, and the fact that the practice of geriatrics can be seen as an approach rather than a special skill, which then leads to the perception of a lack of "prestige" and respect afforded other specialists. Combined with the pay, these factors may contribute to the fact that, despite reports of geriatricians being some of the most content physicians out there [6, 7], the low interest in the specialty has not thus far improved.

As a result, Dr. Warren's call to increase training of geriatric specialists *as well as* improve geriatrics education among all physicians is still the same argument being made today. It seems that despite making great strides in terms of establishing itself as a specialty, and prolific academic research on the topic, geriatrics still appears uncertain of its rightful place within the medical field. This is not a new problem but a persistent one since the time geriatrics was developed as a separate field, with detractors accusing geriatricians of not being able to "make it" in another specialty. Both patients and other physicians still often do not understand what a geriatrician actually does, and physicians who practice geriatric medicine, but have no extra training in geriatrics, are viewed on the same level as boarded geriatricians.[1] Yet it is important to note that few would dare, in this litigious society, call themselves cardiologists just because they deal with heart failure. This frustrating reality has even been demonstrated in literature, where a 2013 survey from Johns Hopkins reported the same findings that many geriatricians encounter in their daily

---

[1] The caveat being that this excludes physicians who were grandfathered into the specialty.

work, including a "shocking lack of public awareness of our field" and the inexplicable tendency to conflate the term Geriatrician with "nutritionist" [8]. Not only does this not endear the specialty to new grads, but why would patients want to switch from their primary physician to a primary care geriatrician if they do not have any idea what benefit this type of care would provide (nor why they should if they have a good relationship with their original primary)?

The reality is that geriatrics *does* have a specific scope of practice, which becomes diluted when pursued solely as a primary care service. Geriatricians as a group have tried to become too many things to too many people, spreading themselves too thin in the end and moving too far away from the focused work of people like Marjory Warren. Primary care physicians who are not geriatricians are perfectly capable of managing the myriad chronic care conditions that afflict our society, in both the old and the young. Where geriatric expertise becomes key are those who are cognitively impaired, frail, falling, in need of transition, or overmedicated, where the geriatric minutiae of aging pathophysiology and medication interactions can make a world of difference. I argue that in order to manage the increasing numbers of people living well into their 80s and 90s, and to more firmly establish geriatrics as a specialty, we need to move away from primary practice and toward a more consultative-based or, even more boldly, a co-management approach.

Consultative models are in fact already present in a wide variety of settings in the USA. Many are based within academic centers and large health systems, although community hospitals are also becoming interested in this model of care. Increasing numbers of adults over the age of 75, few evidence-based guidelines for the management of chronic diseases in seniors, the prevalence of cognitive impairment, and changes in reimbursement that focus on transitional care are just a few of the reasons geriatricians are starting to become an attractive investment. Geriatric specialty care is also commonly tied to clinics specializing in the management of cognitive impairment, for example, as the broad expertise that geriatricians can provide is especially relevant in the care of adults with dementia [9]. Another type of specialty clinic involves assessing adults with multiple falls, often in concert with orthopedists or physical medicine and rehabilitation physicians, as a way of mitigating the monetary and societal costs of high mortality and morbidity in these patients. Geriatricians also staff many Chronic and Transitional Care clinics, set up to help prevent readmissions in increasingly older adults with multiple illnesses. In addition, Medicare has begun to recognize and address the importance of assessment and care planning for chronically ill patients, and new reimbursement codes will hopefully allow geriatricians to bill for the specialized, but often time-consuming, care that they routinely provide.

Geriatric consultants most commonly work in interdisciplinary settings, from geriatric surgical teams that include a geriatrician, geropsychiatrist, surgeon, or surgical NP to geriatric specialty clinics that often include a geriatrician, a mental health provider, as well as key Allied Health Partners including occupational and physical therapies, speech therapy, nutrition, and pharmacy. The involvement of geriatricians in perioperative care has worked so well, in fact, that is has been enshrined in the National Surgical Quality Improvement Program

(NSQIP)/American Geriatrics Society (AGS) Guidelines for the Optimal Perioperative Care of the Geriatric Patient [10]. Promising evidence for improved outcomes in older trauma patients who undergo proactive geriatric assessments has also led to the development of the ACS/TQIP Geriatric Trauma Management Guidelines [11]. This interdisciplinary milieu is in fact the exact format within which geriatric care is most likely to show benefit, as the comprehensive geriatric model is a truly holistic, detail-heavy assessment that requires excellent team coordination and communication. These types of evaluations are really only possible based on the expertise of several specialties, and there is good evidence of their utility. A 2011 Cochrane review concluded that comprehensive geriatric assessments performed in hospitals improved mortality, decreased discharges to long-term care facilities, and appeared protective against deterioration in patients' cognitive function [12]. Surgical specialties, oncology, and cardiology have been reporting improved outcomes with this type of approach as well [13–16], and shortened versions of the CGA are being developed to focus in on specific issues, such as predicting mortality following hospitalizations in older adults with heart disease [17].

So why is it that surgical specialties have embraced the co-management or consultation model, yet most primary care physicians and internists have not? This goes back to the perception of value and the persistent conflict between the ideas of "geriatricized" medicine and geriatric specialists, whose scope of practice is erroneously perceived as too broadly overlapping with that of other physicians. It is not well understood that geriatricians practice within a very specific model that looks at medical problems *as related to* function, mobility, and cognition, rather than a focus on a specific disease process, with the goal of identifying *unmet needs* that are not a part of the standard medical assessment. Yes, other modern physicians may practice in this holistic way, but geriatricians apply this approach to every single patient, rather than only those perceived as needing this type of care. A geriatric specialist coalesces a multiplicity of specialties and approaches into an assessment that can only enhance, rather than detract from, the busy practice of today's primary care physician.

Hence, let me challenge the idea that primary care physicians would find no use in working with a geriatric consultant. In fact, geriatricians are experts in interdisciplinary communication and maintaining continuity of care, as well as ensuring close communication with direct care providers. Within both private insurance networks and novel payment models introduced by Medicare, the utilization of geriatric consultants opens up an opportunity for co-management and eases the path toward meeting ever-steeper quality indicators. Some pertinent quality measures here include the staging, assessment, and management of dementia, medication reconciliation and high-risk medication assessment, incontinence assessment and plans of care, functional assessment for adults >65 with heart failure, and fall risk assessments.

The interdisciplinary nature of most geriatric clinics means that dementia care plans, functional assessments, and medication reconciliations can be done efficiently, giving the primary care provider ready access to PT, OT, SLP, or home care services through the geriatric specialist. This not only helps to maintain excellent patient experience but enhances the primary physician's 360°

knowledge of his or her patient, in essence *sharing* the time required to obtain this information. Geriatric consultants or co-managers can also help with chronic care management of complex, elderly people to whom current guidelines are not readily applicable (resulting from the lack of robust studies inclusive of the 80+ crowd). Geriatricians are also well versed in end-of-life counseling and palliative care approaches to the older adult, assisting with conversations that can be difficult to have in a busy primary practice. Finally, hospital-based geriatric consultants can help provide continuity of care if a patient is admitted, facilitating the transitions of care necessary to ensure a smoother experience for both the patient and her family/ caregivers.

This naturally leads into a discussion of how acute care/inpatient geriatric models can also provide significant value to the primary physician and the hospitalist. The world of medicine has certainly changed, and increasingly fewer primary physicians see their patients in hospital or follow them to tertiary care centers. Today's inpatient wards are also notoriously overflowing, and many hospitalists juggle a large list of patients, the majority of whom tend to fit the "geriatric" label. In 2012 over 30% of hospital admissions involved patients over the age of 65, with an average length of stay of 5 days [18], which is longer than their younger counterparts. In addition to primary care physicians no longer following patients into acute care settings, hospitalist models vary widely in their scheduling patterns, meaning that continuity of care may not always be achievable. It is also sometimes necessary to prioritize the acutely ill patient over an older adult with a deceptively less emergent issue, such as delirium, and the involvement of a geriatric specialist may help mitigate the significant adverse effects that syndromes like delirium can have on both function and post-discharge mortality.

The ideal format for the delivery of inpatient geriatric care is not yet clear, although it is true that the analyses available thus far suggest dedicated geriatric wards, or Acute Care of the Elderly (ACE) units, rather than consultative teams, offer more measurable benefit, such as fewer falls, shorter length of stay, decreased cost of care, and less delirium [19]. It has been difficult to truly compare inpatient consultative services, however, since the frequency with which recommendations are implemented and the structure of the consultative teams tend to be quite varied. A tantalizing explanation offered by Calkins et al. (1999) is also a tricky one and posits that whereas other consulting specialties can leave concrete and specific recommendations, geriatric suggestions often require the primary provider to "change their approach," so that the care recommended is performed in a specific way, often requiring a global, rather than just an individual, effort [20]. An example of this would perhaps be the institutional implementation of a non-pharmacological sleep protocol before a sleep aid is actually given to an older patient, as a result of the geriatric team consistently recommending this via consultation. This means that many geriatric recommendations go beyond a suggested lab or change in medication and can affect not just the actions of the primary physician but also nursing and ancillary staff. Simply put, they appear harder to implement.

Yet there are few studies so far that have looked at a standardized, validated, acute-focused geriatric assessment that could be utilized by geriatric consultation teams to communicate with both hospitalist and primary care providers in a systematic fashion. The development of such an assessment, focusing on four axes—cognition, function, mobility, and medication reconciliation—may one day provide a standardized way to provide clear recommendations and consistent communication with primary physicians. Regardless of its ultimate form, the key to useful inpatient consultation models should most definitely be targeted co-management rather than general consultation, focusing on function, mobility, cognition (delirium), and discharge planning, as well as suggestions for care that take into consideration pathophysiological changes of aging, and the resulting atypical presentations of acute illnesses.

Many primary providers have also likely discovered that over the past few years, non-medical "geriatric consultation" business models, focused on helping families and older adults to decide "what's next" when issues such as falls, frailty, and cognitive impairment arise, have proliferated. Individuals who run these businesses have a wide variety of training, from no special education at all to geriatric MSWs and RN-PhDs. As a result their services vary quite widely, from transitional care support to advocacy and assistance with legal issues. There is in fact a national association called the Aging Life Care Association, which unites geriatric care managers/professionals under one umbrella. There are also many private companies who offer support and guidance to help "place" older adults in various assisted living situations. These companies usually do not charge the client, but are rather paid by the facilities in which their client ends up, usually taking a percentage of one or several months' rent. With the business world's realization that "senior" business is lucrative business, there is also an opportunity for the geriatrician to serve as a navigator that helps patients and their primary providers survive those murky waters of various support services. In fact, a good geriatric co-management model would include care managers who can support chronic care with the goal of preventing readmissions and delaying the need to live in a care facility for as long as possible. Funnily enough, many of the extra services offered out there can be arranged easily enough within the walls of a geriatric consultant's office.

So while some argue that instead of training geriatric specialists, aspects of the care of older adults specific to each field should be instilled during residency and medicine "geriatricized," I posit that this is happening anyways with the aging of the baby boomers, and most physicians will (and do) know *something* about geriatric medicine. Whether this happens "on the job" or with formal education may become less relevant with increasing need, although I am a strong proponent for mandatory geriatric training modules for all physicians. However, in this world of changing priorities among those who fund medicine, on quality vs. quantity and chronic vs. acute care, I argue that geriatric subspecialists can play a unique and important role in not only helping other physicians manage complex, frail, and often very work-intensive patients, but assisting those patients in navigating the increasingly complex world of chronic care medicine. The truth is that co-management is *already* becoming increasingly attractive to surgeons, as well as subspecialists, including cardiologists and oncologists, and primary providers should benefit from this as well. There are multiple formats that can support geriatric primary co-management, including multidisciplinary geriatric specialty clinics, geriatric inpatient teams, and even group practices that include primary physicians working alongside a geriatrician, as well as a few key subspecialists such as cardiology or nephrology. Geriatric eMedicine and telehealth visits, in conjunction with regular primary care office visits, are also starting to become an indispensible tool to care for the homebound and less mobile patients (and hopefully reimbursement will catch up with services that have been available for many years now).

I strongly believe that it is incumbent upon the geriatric profession to band together and continue educating both other physicians and the public. With vigorous outreach, this type of care can become more attractive to patients who are lucky enough to find a primary co-management model, as it gives them options and increased access to their physicians. In the end, primary care of older adults is a challenging area of practice, requiring a degree of mental flexibility, and an active interest in the lives of patients beyond the "medical problem." Yet it is also extremely rewarding, and the effects of small changes in the medications, environment, or social situation can quickly show visible results. At a time of a growing senior population, changing payment models and increasingly complex chronic care, patients, their families, as well as their primary physicians can find geriatric consultants of great value in adding quality to those crucial years of life.

References

1. Barton A, Mulley G. History of medicine: history of the development of geriatric medicine in the UK. Postgrad Med J. 2003;79:229–34. doi:10.1136/pmj.79.930.229.
2. Denham MJ. Dr Marjory Warren CBE MRCS LRCP (1897–1960): the mother of British geriatric medicine. J Med Biogr. 2011;19(3):105–10.
3. Canadian Medical Association. Geriatric Medicine Profile. https://www.cma.ca/Assets/assets-library/document/en/advocacy/Geriatric-e.pdf. Accessed 5 Nov 2016.
4. National Resident Matching Program. Results and Data: Specialties Matching Service, 2016 Appointment Year. 2016. http://www.nrmp.org/wp-content/uploads/2016/03/Results-and-Data-SMS-2016_Final.pdf. Accessed 18 Oct 2016.
5. Ontario Ministry of Health and Long Term Care. Schedule of Benefits: Physician Services Under the Health Insurance Act. 2015. http://www.health.gov.on.ca/en/pro/programs/ohip/sob/physserv/sob_master11062015.pdf. Accessed 5 Nov 2016.
6. Leigh JP, Kravitz RL, Schembri M, Samuels SJ, Mobley S. Physician career satisfaction across specialties. Arch Intern Med. 2002;162:1577–84.
7. Leigh JP, Tancredi DJ, Kravitz RL. Physician career satisfaction within specialties. BMC Health Serv Res. 2009;9:166. doi:10.1186/1472-6963-9-166.
8. Campbell JY, Durso SC, Brandt LE, Finucane TE, Abadir PM. The unknown profession: a geriatrician. J Am Geriatr Soc. 2013;61(3) doi:10.1111/jgs.12115.
9. Kadowaki L, Chow H, Metcalfe S, Friesen K. Innovative model of interprofessional geriatric consultation: specialized seniors clinics. Healthc Q. 2014;17(3):55–60.
10. American College of Surgeons. Optimal Perioperative Care of the Geriatric Patient: Best Practices Guideline from ACS NSQIP/American Geriatrics Society. 2012. https://www.facs.org/~/media/files/quality%20programs/geriatric/acs%20nsqip%20geriatric%202016%20guidelines.ashx. Accessed 15 Oct 2016.

11. American College of Surgeons. ACS/TQIP Trauma Quality Improvement Program. ACS/ TQIP Geriatric Trauma Management Guidelines. https://www.facs.org/~/media/files/quality%20programs/trauma/tqip/geriatric%20guide%20tqip.ashx. Accessed 15 Oct 2016.
12. Ellis G, Whitehead MA, O'Neill D, Langhorne P, Robinson D. Comprehensive geriatric assessment for older adults admitted to hospital. Cochrane Database Syst Rev. 2011;(7). Art. No.: CD006211. doi:10.1002/14651858.CD006211.pub2.
13. Parks RM, Hall L, Tang SW, et al. The potential value of comprehensive geriatric assessment in evaluating older women with primary operable breast cancer undergoing surgery or non-operative treatment – a pilot study. J Geriatr Oncol. 2015;6(1):46–51. doi:10.1016/j. jgo.2014.09.180.
14. Indrakusuma R, Dunker MS, Peetoom JJ, Schreurs WH. Evaluation of preoperative geriatric assessment of elderly patients with colorectal carcinoma. A retrospective study. Eur J Surg Oncol. 2015;41(1):21–7. doi:10.1016/j.ejso.2014.09.005. Epub 2014 Sep 18
15. Adunsky A, Lusky A, Arad M, Heruti RJ. A comparative study of rehabilitation outcomes of elderly hip fracture patients: the advantage of a comprehensive orthogeriatric approach. J Gerontol A Biol Sci Med Sci. 2003;58(6):542–7.
16. Owusu C, Berger NA. Comprehensive geriatric assessment in the older cancer patient: coming of age in clinical cancer care. Clin Pract (Lond). 2014;11(6):749–62.
17. Rodriguez-Pascual C, Paredes-Galan E, Vilches-Moraga A, et al. Comprehensive geriatric assessment and 2-year mortality in elderly patients hospitalized for heart failure. Circ Cardiovasc Qual Outcomes. 2014;7:251–8.
18. Weiss AJ, Elixhauser A. Overview of Hospital Stays in the United States, 2012. Agency for Healthcare Research and Quality, Healthcare Cost and Utilization Project, Statistical Brief #180. 2014. http://www.hcup-us.ahrq.gov/reports/statbriefs/sb180-Hospitalizations-United-States-2012.pdf. Accessed 15 Oct 2016.
19. Fox MT, Persaud M, Maimets I, et al. Effectiveness of acute geriatric unit care using acute care for elders components: a systematic review and meta-analysis. J Am Geriatr Soc. 2012;60(12):2237–45.
20. Calkins E, Naughton BJ. Care of older people in the hospital – geriatric consultation. In: Calkins E, Boult C, Wagner EH, Pacala JT, editors. New ways to care for older people: building systems based on evidence. New York: Springer; 1999. p. 106–8.

GRACE Team Care Model

Cathy C. Schubert, Julia Dolejs, and Justine May

Delivering high-quality, coordinated medical care to older adults, many of whom have multiple medical and psychosocial comorbidities, is challenging, whether one is the patient, the clinician, or the healthcare system. Interdisciplinary teams providing in-home geriatric assessment and ongoing care management, such as Geriatric Resources for the Assessment and Care of Elders (GRACE), are one solution to the challenges of caring for this patient population.

Current Issues and Challenges in the Care of Complex, High-Risk Older Adults

Perspective of the Patient

As they age, our patients frequently accumulate multiple chronic medical conditions (multimorbidity) such as diabetes mellitus, coronary and vascular atherosclerosis, chronic obstructive pulmonary disease, and chronic renal insufficiency. As a result, an older adult will often see multiple medical providers as part of the management of these myriad comorbid conditions. In a given year, the average Medicare beneficiary sees seven different outpatient providers (two primary care providers and five specialists) from four different practices; for older adults with multimorbidity, that number is even higher [1]. Adding in a major transition of care, such as a

C.C. Schubert, MD (✉)
Indiana University School of Medicine, Indianapolis, IN, USA

R. L. Roudebush VAMC, Indianapolis, IN, USA
e-mail: caschube@iu.edu

J. Dolejs, MSN, RN, APRN, FNP-BC • J. May, MSW, LCSW
R. L. Roudebush VAMC, Indianapolis, IN, USA
e-mail: Julia.Dolejs@va.gov; Justine.May@va.gov

© Springer International Publishing AG 2018
M. Wasserman, J. Riopelle (eds.), *Primary Care for Older Adults*,
DOI 10.1007/978-3-319-61329-1_3

hospitalization or a subacute rehabilitation facility stay, can cause even more complexity in the older adult's case and increase the risk of complications, including medication errors, poor communication between providers and settings, and lack of appropriate or missed outpatient follow-up. Thus, treatment of multimorbidity can lead to complex, complicated management regimens that may include multiple medications, dietary restrictions, frequent medical appointments, and lifestyle changes, which sets the stage where an older adult may struggle with compliance and maintaining health.

Low health literacy can be a significant and often unrecognized impediment for older adults and their compliance with care instructions. Health literacy is described as the individual's ability to access, process, and understand basic health information and health services. It involves the complex interaction of reading, listening to, and interpreting health information, making decisions based on that information, and then communicating those choices to healthcare providers and caregivers. Of adults in the United States over the age of 60, 71% have difficulty understanding and utilizing print materials; 80% have difficulty completing forms or using charts for information; and 68% struggle to interpret numbers and to perform calculations [2]. Thus, instructions that seem simple to clinicians may actually be daunting or even overwhelming to older patients who have a hard time grasping the concepts and then developing the plan for integrating them into their daily routines.

In addition to the health literacy issues, older adults may also have underlying geriatric syndromes that impact their ability to manage their health and chronic comorbid conditions. Cognitive impairment, which often is not detected in primary care until the severe stages of dementia [3], compounds the issues with compliance by making it difficult for the older adult to remember instructions, appointments, and medication regimens. Depression also has a negative impact on health in chronic medical illness, being associated with higher symptom burden and functional decline, poor compliance with self-care and lifestyle changes, and increased medical costs and risk of morbidity and mortality [4]. Functional impairments such as difficulty walking, hearing loss, or visual impairment are also common in older adults, especially among those with frailty. Such impairments make it more difficult for the older adult to access medical care because of limited handicapped-accessible transportation options, many medical facilities not being geriatric-friendly in their layout and design, and clinicians being untrained or poorly equipped in how to accommodate such functional impairments during their care of the older adult.

Social concerns and unmet psychosocial needs can impede care of medical illness and patient self-management as well, particularly among the frail elderly and those with low incomes who may struggle even to afford the care they need. Even with Medicare and other insurance support, costs of care, such as for some medications and transportation to and from appointments, continue to be out-of-pocket expenses for the patient, and they may not be able to afford or find the appropriate foods for their prescribed diets. If they are no longer able to drive and either cannot navigate public transportation or cannot afford available transportation options, older adults may miss clinical appointments, be unable to access a pharmacy to obtain their medications, and become increasingly socially isolated. If the patient is physically frail and requires assistance with instrumental activities of daily living (IADLs) and/or basic activities of daily living (ADLs), obtaining such assistance in the home environment is often exorbitantly expensive. Sometimes, older adults have family or friends who can take on a caregiving role and assist with these needs. For those who are socially isolated, however, they may need help but have nowhere to turn to obtain it. In such cases, the older adult may enter a steady downward spiral of physical decline that often leads to emergency room visits, acute hospitalizations, and eventually institutionalization.

When an older adult's care is medically complex and there is a caregiver involved, the burden of multimorbidity and functional decline broadens and expands to impact more than just the patient. For example, multiple and frequent clinic appointments with various providers may require the caregiver to take time off from work, compounding the already present stress of helping the patient get ready for the appointment, providing the transportation, and then assisting the older adult with any changes to the treatment regimen after the appointment. Geriatric syndromes such as dementia, depression, frailty, and falls increase the burden of caregiving as well. In some cases, the caregiver may have medical illness and care needs of his own also, such as when an elderly spouse is caregiver for his frail wife. In such fragile medical and psychosocial situations, both the caregiver and the patient are at high risk for functional decline, worsening morbidity, and other adverse outcomes.

In its seminal 2001 report "Crossing the Quality Chasm: A New Health System for the 21st Century [12]," the Institute of Medicine (now called the National Academy of Medicine) described patient-centered care as "respectful of and responsive to individual patient preferences, needs, and values and that ensures that patient values guide all clinical decisions." Unfortunately, in busy clinical settings that make up today's modern healthcare systems, conversations about personal values, care preferences, and goals, which are often time-consuming, tend to fall by the wayside until a time of medical crisis, such as admission to the medical intensive care unit (MICU) with life-threatening illness. Perhaps this ongoing lack of patient-centered care was part of the motivation behind the American Geriatrics Society's 2016 update [13] on this issue, where they describe person-centered care as when "… the individuals' values and preferences are elicited and … guide all aspects of their health care, supporting their realistic health and life goals." Having such discussions with older adults with complex medical conditions and functional impairment *before* a medical crisis is of paramount importance for ensuring the older adult receives the amount and quality of care she wants while avoiding potential harms of unwanted or futile treatment.

Perspective of Providers and the Health System

Older adults with multiple comorbid medical and psychosocial conditions present myriad challenges for providers, staff, and health systems. Multimorbidity is associated with many adverse outcomes, including greater use of healthcare resources, higher risk of adverse effects of treatment, poorer quality of life for the patient, and higher rates of disability, institutionalization, and death.

Most health professionals are taught to manage a specific disease entity or a single organ system at a time, and they receive little education in the comprehensive management of patients who have multiple medical conditions that are interplaying and interacting to impact that patient's health. Being confronted with an older adult with multimorbidity during what is supposed to be a brief outpatient clinic visit is often overwhelming and frustrating for clinicians.

Additionally, while many chronic diseases have specific clinical practice guidelines that have been developed for each single disease, those guidelines for care do not take into account how management may need to change in the face of other chronic medical conditions or of geriatric syndromes such as frailty, incontinence, or dementia [5]. This increases the risk for harm to the older adult during treatment. To complicate matters further, many well-meaning health systems and insurance providers have implemented quality measures by which providers' performance is judged according to their patients' outcomes per these published disease guidelines (e.g., achieving hemoglobin a1c of less than 7.0% in type 2 diabetes). Often, these quality measures do not take into account individual patient characteristics such as frailty, multimorbidity, or advanced age and can result in harm to the older adult. If such performance measures are not met, though, clinicians may face retribution, such as loss of income. Unfortunately, such a situation can lead to harm, either to the patient if the guidelines are stringently followed or to the provider if the performance measures are not met.

Providers and health systems continue to struggle with coordination and integration between primary and specialty care and inpatient and outpatient visits, even when electronic health records are in place. For every 100 Medicare beneficiaries a primary care provider manages, she typically coordinates care with 99 additional physicians from 53 different practices. Based on Medicare population data, about a third of those beneficiaries are those older or disabled adults who have four or more chronic medical conditions and thus would benefit the most from ongoing care coordination. For that subset of patients alone, however, the primary care provider interacts with an average of 86 physicians in 36 practices [1], making efficient, effective care coordination in primary care by the clinician alone an impossible task.

Just as with patients themselves, low health literacy presents challenges to clinicians and health systems, especially those caring for underserved populations who are living at or below the poverty level. At the individual level, low health literacy is associated with decreased ability to take medications correctly, less use of preventive care, and higher risk of needing emergency room visits and hospitalizations. From the wider standpoint of health systems and population health, it is linked to greater healthcare service utilization, higher risk of poor outcomes, greater risk of hospitalization and higher costs for that inpatient care, and higher mortality rates [2].

When older adults with the complexity of multimorbidity and geriatric syndromes encounter the healthcare system, be it a simple doctor's visit or an acute hospitalization, they are at higher risk for negative outcomes such as adverse drug reactions, polypharmacy, delirium, functional decline, and falls. These negative outcomes contribute to higher rates of acute care utilization, prolonged hospitalizations, and higher care costs because of a higher density of medical staff needed to provide their care over a longer length of stay. Poorly structured transitions of care serve to compound these issues because of ineffective communication between sites of care, increased possibility of errors and omissions in care because of its complexity, duplicated tests and studies, and missed opportunities for outpatient follow-up. From a clinician and health system perspective, older adults with multimorbidity are high-risk, high-cost patients for whom to provide care.

An area of particular concern and struggle for clinicians and health systems is when an older adult's social concerns become impediments to medical care and self-management. When the patient is on a low or fixed income, she may not be able to afford her prescriptions or the appropriate foods for a healthy diet. If he can no longer drive due to illness or geriatric issues such as vision loss or dementia, the older adult may miss doctor's appointments, be unable to obtain medications or food, or become depressed due to loss of social interaction. Transportation may be a particular problem in rural areas or in urban areas that lack options for public transportation. A particularly challenging situation occurs when an older adult is in need of social supports but has no one available to provide it. As mentioned above, hiring paid caregivers to provide assistance with IADLs and ADLs in the home is expensive to the point of being beyond what most families on fixed incomes can afford. In many cases, institutionalization and applying for Medicaid benefits becomes the only financially viable option for many older adults, which is unfortunate since remaining in their homes and communities is an important goal for many.

Geriatric Resources for Assessment and Care of Elders: The GRACE Model

To adequately address the medical and psychosocial needs of complex older adults with multimorbidity, we need innovative models of care that utilize input from providers with geriatric expertise. As such clinicians are in short supply, however, such new models must also efficiently leverage what geriatric expertise is available in a health system so that as many older adults benefit as possible.

Geriatric Resources for Assessment and Care of Elders (GRACE) Team Care collaborates with primary care providers and the patient-centered medical home to provide in-home geriatric care management focusing on geriatric syndromes and psychosocial issues commonly found in older adults that are often difficult to address adequately in primary care. By utilizing an interdisciplinary team that includes a geriatrician, advanced practice nurse, social worker, pharmacist, and a mental health liaison, GRACE is able to assess and address medical and social concerns concomitantly and effectively using home-based comprehensive geriatric assessment and ongoing, protocol-driven care management. Because GRACE is integrated with primary care and the medical home, implementation of the plan of care for the older adult's geriatric and psychosocial issues is collaborative, efficient, and effective.

Key Components of GRACE

At the heart of the GRACE model is the GRACE Support Team, which is composed of an advanced practice nurse (APN) and a licensed clinical social worker (SW). Both have clinical backgrounds and training in geriatrics, and both are employed by the healthcare system. The intervention [10] begins with the GRACE Support Team conducting an in-home comprehensive geriatric assessment that includes a medical and psychosocial history, medication reconciliation, functional assessment, review of social support, review of any existing advanced directives, a home safety assessment, and screening for caregiver stress. The visit continues with a physical examination, including a focus on orthostatic vital signs and screening for geriatric syndromes such as vision and hearing loss, gait and balance impairments, depression, and cognitive impairment. The APN and the SW collaborate throughout the assessment, discerning and exploring the medical and psychosocial issues together in concert. That the assessment is conducted within the patient's home allows for a unique, valuable, and highly informative glimpse of the patient's daily life and function that is otherwise impossible to achieve within the confines of an office or inpatient visit.

Within a week of the in-home comprehensive assessment, the GRACE Support Team meets with the larger GRACE interdisciplinary team composed of the APN and SW, geriatrician, pharmacist, and mental health liaison, all of whom are also employed by the health system. During this meeting, the APN and SW summarize the pertinent positives of the case found during the in-home assessment, and the interdisciplinary GRACE Team develops a patient-centric, individualized care plan utilizing the 12 GRACE protocols as appropriate to the case (Fig. 3.1). These 12 protocol conditions were initially chosen by primary care providers and opinion leaders in geriatrics within the Eskenazi Health system, the safety net health system located in Indianapolis, Indiana, where GRACE was first developed as a randomized clinical trial. For each condition, the GRACE protocols specify recommendations for evaluation and management that are based on published practice guidelines [6, 7]. All patients receive the medication management, health maintenance, and advanced care planning protocols, while the other protocols are activated only when appropriate to the individual patient. Each protocol contains evaluation and management suggestions specific to the condition, some of which are meant for the Support Team to implement themselves on a routine basis, while others they review with the primary care provider and then implement with the provider's approval. For example, routine team interventions for the difficulty walking/falls protocol include monitor orthostatic vital signs, provide education on falls prevention, and encourage exercise for balance and strengthening. Suggestions that the team would discuss with the primary care provider might be checking thyroid function, vitamin B12 level, and a vitamin D level and considering referral for physical therapy.

With the patient-centric, individualized care plan in hand, the GRACE APN and SW discuss the recommendations with the primary care provider and medical home team. Such communication can be accomplished via face-to-face meeting,

Fig. 3.1 GRACE Protocols for common geriatric conditions

GRACE Protocols

1. Difficulty walking/falls

2. Depression

3. Cognitive Impairment

4. Incontinence

5. Malnutrition/Weight Loss

6. Visual Impairment

7. Hearing Impairment

8. Chronic Pain

9. Caregiver Burden

10. Medication Management

11. Health Maintenance

12. Advanced Care Planning

phone call, encrypted e-mail, or using the health system's electronic health record. In collaboration with the primary care provider, the GRACE Support Team then implements the care plan, with the first step being a follow-up home visit to discuss the recommendations with the patient and ensure that the plan of care is consistent with the patient's goals. During this follow-up visit, the team provides literacy-level-appropriate education to the patient and caregiver for the corresponding activated GRACE protocols, including encouraging the patient in goal setting and self-care activities for her own health. Another important part of the follow-up visit and care going forward is linking the patient with appropriate existing health-system and community-based resources and services, such as the local Area Agency on Aging, transportation services for the disabled, programs for those with impaired vision or hearing, low-cost dental services, Senior Law assistance, the Alzheimer's Association, and senior centers. Finally, patients and their caregivers are provided with the contact information for the GRACE Team so that they have a direct phone number to reach their GRACE providers during business hours. The GRACE Team stresses to patients and caregivers the importance of calling GRACE if feeling ill, if they have questions about their healthcare or medications, or if they are hospitalized or seen in the emergency department outside of their primary healthcare system.

After the follow-up educational visit, GRACE remains involved with the patient for ongoing geriatric care management. Each GRACE Support Team dyad of APN and SW can manage a census of 80–110 patients, with the actual number being dependent on factors such as geographic reach of the program and population acuity and complexity. At a minimum, every GRACE patient receives one phone contact per month from either the APN or SW. The purpose of the monthly contact is to ensure proactive follow-up with the treatment plan and to check in if the patient or caregiver has new issues or concerns. All patients also receive an annual comprehensive geriatric assessment and follow-up educational visit to assess for any changes in their geriatric or psychosocial issues and to evaluate for any new problems that may have developed. Beyond these minimum contacts, further encounters with the patient occur as needed to implement the care plan. In addition, the GRACE Support Team visits the home and discusses the case with the interdisciplinary team again after any acute hospitalizations or other major transitions of care, such as a stay in a subacute rehabilitation facility. In this manner, GRACE facilitates coordination of care across providers and sites of care as much as possible and helps the patient maintain contact with the primary care provider and medical home.

Outcomes of the GRACE Model

Perspective of the Patient

In the original randomized controlled trial of GRACE, the older adults in the intervention arm reported improved general health, vitality, social functioning, and mental health on the Medical Outcomes 36-Item Short-Form (SF-36) scale after being enrolled in the program for 2 years. The quality of their geriatric care improved as well compared to the control group, as the patients enrolled in GRACE were more likely to be assessed and treated for geriatric syndromes including difficulty walking/falls, urinary incontinence, depression, vision impairment, and hearing impairment [8]. In our experience, older adults and their caregivers appreciate the holistic nature of the care offered by the GRACE model, particularly that their individual goals of care are assessed and honored and that their psychosocial concerns are being addressed along with their medical illnesses (Fig. 3.2).

"The GRACE team is a blessing! During the time the team came to our home, they were professional yet caring and made a huge difference for us. When a chronically ill patient's family calls with concerns, send a GRACE team out to the home ASAP!"

"I am amazed at how you guys keep track of me. GRACE is wonderful, and I surely do appreciate you guys!"

"The GRACE team saved my husband's life and my sanity. I had hit rock bottom when the team came to our home and didn't know how we were going to continue like this. GRACE was absolutely superb in getting his medications properly managed and helping me access the services I needed to care for him. Thank you from the bottom of my heart for giving me my husband back."

Fig. 3.2 Examples of satisfaction feedback from patients and families about GRACE

Perspective of Providers and the Health System

GRACE is a natural fit with the concepts of the medical home model for primary care that many healthcare systems are enacting. While not every older adult needs a proactive, in-home care management program such as GRACE, health systems and providers can reap significant benefits by having a GRACE program for their complex older adults with multimorbidity, especially those who are at high risk for hospitalizations and functional decline. In fact, GRACE has been shown to reduce emergency department visits, hospitalizations, 30-day readmissions, and total inpatient bed days of care in high-risk patients [8, 9]. At the same time, older adults enrolled in a GRACE program have improved continuity of care, including being more likely to maintain an established primary care provider, to obtain posthospital follow-up visits in primary care, and to have an updated and accurate medication list. GRACE patients are also more likely to receive needed preventive care, such as immunizations and age-appropriate cancer screening, and they are more likely to have engaged in advanced care planning, such as completing a living will and naming a healthcare representative [8].

Geriatricians and healthcare providers with geriatric expertise are in short supply, so their time must be carefully and efficiently leveraged so that they can positively impact as many older adults as possible. In our experience, once a GRACE program is established within a health system and is operating at full capacity with two or three GRACE Support Teams, the geriatrician's time commitment is primarily the 2 to 3 h per week that are devoted to the weekly interdisciplinary team meetings. Because of the team structure of GRACE, however, that small time commitment benefits many older adults, usually several hundred per year depending on the size of the program and far more than the geriatrician would ever have been able to help via individual face-to-face visits. In addition, we have also noticed providers in our health system beginning to implement some of GRACE's typical geriatric recommendations in their patients who are not enrolled in the program, such as screening for depression and checking vitamin D levels in older adults with falls. Such "geriatricizing" of primary care and other providers can thus further broaden the reach of the limited supply of specialists in geriatrics and begins to benefit the health system as a whole.

In the initial randomized controlled trial of GRACE, primary care physicians whose patients received the intervention were surveyed for their satisfaction with the program. These physicians were much more satisfied with the resources provided by GRACE compared with usual care, and many rated the amount of care provided by the GRACE Support Team as "just right" (Fig. 3.3).

"GRACE is absolutely so helpful, and we are thankful for all the assistance."

"Thank goodness GRACE is involved with this patient!"

Fig. 3.3 Examples of satisfaction feedback from providers about GRACE

Lessons Learned from GRACE Implementation

Factors for Success

GRACE has been successfully implemented in over 20 different health organizations in five states, including Accountable Care Organizations (ACOs), Medicare Advantage Plans, and Veterans Affairs Medical Centers. Factors that contributed to these successes at the health system level include early engagement of system leadership and providing regular updates on implementation progress and positive outcomes for patients, providers, and the health system; clearly communicating from the outset the anticipated return on investment, costs, and savings to the system; and being a model of care that can be adapted to fit the health system's local needs, goals, and staffing resources while still maintaining the core set of principles and focus that make GRACE effective.

At the program level, carefully recruiting advanced practice nurses and social workers who have geriatric experience and who can work well together as a GRACE Support Team has been vital to implementation and sustainment. Additionally, the geriatrician, pharmacist, and mental health liaison need to be highly engaged during the GRACE interdisciplinary team meeting and also available by phone as needed to answer questions from the GRACE Support Team that may arise in the course of patient care.

Barriers and Solutions

GRACE has faced some special challenges that have limited its widespread implementation. The most significant of these barriers at the health system level has been financing and reimbursement [11]. While GRACE's reduction of acute care utilization makes financial sense for capitated health systems that need to mitigate as much as possible the costs of caring for complex older patients, the GRACE model is poorly compatible with fee-for-service payment systems because much of GRACE's work, such as follow-up telephone calls and interdisciplinary team conferences, is not reimbursed under such systems.

Another reason for lower uptake of GRACE may be related to scalability concerns. Each GRACE APN/SW Support Team can care for around 80–100 complex patients which, while high-yield in terms of cost savings as long as patients are carefully and appropriately selected, will seem like a small number to health system leadership. This is especially true when compared to the "light touch," often telephone-based care management programs that can enroll high numbers of clients but may be less effective for high-risk patients with medical and psychosocial complexity. GRACE's reliance on home visits, which is one of the model's keys to success, also unfortunately limits its scalability. Home visits are inherently less efficient than clinic-based work due to the time spent driving to the patient's home, and drive time is often what limits the geographic reach of GRACE and other home visit programs. While this is true in urban areas, it is compounded even further when one considers attempting implementation in more rural settings.

Another barrier when implementing GRACE is when system leadership does not grasp its holistic focus and the benefit of having the APN and SW on the GRACE Support Team conduct home visits together. Healthcare administrators may not understand that, when a patient or family has pressing social concerns such as paying bills, finding transportation, or securing food, they struggle to make healthcare and chronic disease management a priority. By having the Team conduct the geriatric assessment together within the home, social needs can be assessed and addressed from the outset, allowing the patient and caregiver to then shift their focus to managing health concerns.

At the clinician level, an initial barrier for GRACE can be gaining primary care provider buy-in. Providers may be skeptical of the program's potential and be concerned that having to communicate about GRACE care plans with the GRACE team will be time-consuming and burdensome. This barrier can generally be overcome, however, with early investment in gaining clinician trust and by illustrating as frequently as possible the benefits to both patient and clinician of having GRACE involved. In our experience, having a unified electronic medical record that spans both inpatient and outpatient venues of a health system allows this communication to take place most efficiently and effectively and helps with primary care provider uptake of GRACE significantly.

GRACE Team Care is an evidence-based, innovative model of holistic geriatric care management that positively impacts the care of high-risk, complex older adults from the perspective of the patient, the provider, and the healthcare system. GRACE has the potential to provide better quality of geriatric and chronic disease care to medically and psychosocially complex adults and to contribute to overall cost savings in the care of this population.

References

1. Pham HH, O'Malley AS, Bach PB, et al. Primary care physicians' links to other physicians through Medicare patients: the scope of care coordination. Ann Intern Med. 2009;150:236–42.
2. National Network of Libraries of Medicine. Health Literacy. 2013. https://nnlm.gov/outreach/consumer/hlthlit.html#References. Accessed 13 Sept 2016.
3. Valcour VG, Masaki KH, Curb D, et al. The detection of dementia in the primary care setting. Arch Intern Med. 2000;160(19):2964–8.
4. Katon WJ. Epidemiology and treatment of depression in patients with chronic medical illness. Dialogues Clin Neurosci. 2011;13:7–23.
5. The American Geriatrics Society Expert Panel on the Care of Older Adults with Multimorbidity. Guiding principles for the care of older adults with multimorbidity: an approach for clinicians. JAGS. 2012;60:E1–E25.
6. ACOVE Investigators. Measuring medical care provided to vulnerable elders: the assessing care of vulnerable elders-3 (ACOVE-3) quality indicators. JAGS. 2007;55(S2):S247–487.
7. Sloss EM, Solomon DH, Shekelle PG, et al. Selecting target conditions for quality of care improvement in vulnerable older adults. JAGS. 2000;48:363–9.
8. Counsell SR, Callahan CM, Clark DO, et al. Geriatric care management for low-income seniors: a randomized controlled trial. JAMA. 2007;298(22):2623–33.
9. Schubert CC, Myers LJ, Allen K, et al. Implementing geriatric resources for assessment and care of elders team care in a Veterans Affairs Medical Center: lessons learned and effects observed. JAGS. 2016;65:1503–9.

10. Counsell SR, Callahan CM, Buttar AB, et al. Geriatric resources for assessment and care of elders (GRACE): a new model of primary care for low-income seniors. JAGS. 2006;54:1136–41.
11. Counsell SR, Callahan CM, Tu W, et al. Cost analysis of the geriatric resources for assessment and care of elders care management intervention. JAGS. 2009;57:1420–6.
12. Institute of Medicine. Crossing the quality chasm: a new health system for the 21st century. Washington, DC: National Academy Press; 2001.
13. The American Geriatrics Society Expert Panel on Person-Centered Care. Person-centered care: a definition and essential elements. JAGS. 2016;64:15–8.

Introduction to Population Health

4

James Riopelle

As I began the final draft of this chapter, I was reminded of a story that applied not only to population health but to life in general. It seems that when Christopher Columbus returned to Spain in 1492 after discovering the Americas, Queen Isabella was quite smitten. This did not go unnoticed by King Ferdinand, who was reportedly jealous. At the royal dinner celebrating Columbus' return and after several glasses of wine, the King said, "I don't think discovering the Americas was such a big deal – all you did was sail until you hit land." Columbus, remembering the courage that sailing across a believed to be flat earth took, was quite miffed. Controlling his anger, he took an egg from the royal table and asked if anyone could make the egg stand on its end. Around the table went the egg and no one could get it to balance on its end. Taking the egg from King Ferdinand, the last member of the royal party to fail, Columbus gently smashed one end to flatten the egg without breaking the entire shell. Smiling, he stood the egg on end and said, "Anything's easy when you've been shown how." I share this story because I've spent the last 25 years working on aspects of what is now called population health. I've been "shown how" so my tendency is to oversimplify the process—it's not simple or it would already be in common practice. However, it is very doable.

In reality, we are still debating the definition of population health.

Population health has been defined as "health outcomes of a group of individuals, including the distribution of such outcomes within the group" [1]. However, population health is defined differently in different settings. I will be using a more typical insurance definition, defining population health as "managing the healthcare of large groups of people, often chronically ill, to ensure that they are getting care at the right time, at the right place and at the right cost." In addition, it's impossible to discuss population health without incorporating the "triple aim"—improving the

J. Riopelle, MD
Physician Consultant Institute, Denver, CO, USA
e-mail: jfriopelle@hotmail.com

© Springer International Publishing AG 2018

M. Wasserman, J. Riopelle (eds.), *Primary Care for Older Adults*,
DOI 10.1007/978-3-319-61329-1_4

individual experience of care, improving the health of populations, and reducing the per capita costs of care for populations.

Population health also represents a transfer of insurance risk and changes the financial incentives from volume [FFS] to value. "Fee for service isn't over yet but the shift to value-based care is here and evolving rapidly. It will vary by health sector and even by geography, affecting different systems at different times. The players left standing strong will be the ones that strategically embrace innovative changes starting now. Strategic integration and deliberate organizational .transformation are essential to fully realize the benefit from the volume to value reimbursement shift and effectively manage financial and clinical risks." [2].

In my opinion, there are five critical success factors in transitioning to and maintaining a population health driven practice.

First: Physician Leadership

An essential factor for success. I cannot overstate the importance of this enough. Nonphysician business people have said things like, "It doesn't matter. We own them [or employ them], so they'll do what we tell them." One hospital ACO I worked with lost more than $5 million in their first month of operation. I joined the party late and as I was evaluating what got them where they were, an executive told me, "We couldn't generate much physician interest so we just jumped in with both feet." A virtual guarantee of failure. Organizations must understand that physicians are human and respond to incentives much like any other group. Ensuring physician leadership means taking time, making sure providers understand the upcoming processes and educating them as to the clinical, financial, and personal benefits of change for individual providers. Once this has occurred, it's important to take baby steps along the road to full risk. Perhaps start with a shared savings program, prove financial performance, gain credibility, and then move perhaps to bundled payments, again gaining experience. Try sharing upside and downside risk, each time touting improving successful involvement with these programs. Finally, the ultimate in population health management is global capitation, the end journey of successful population health practice/management. Excellent physician leadership is critical to this evolving process.

Second: Align Financial Incentives

A parallel necessity to physician leadership. It makes no sense to have the dominant component of a physician [or any provider] compensation being based on a fee-for-service production model when the organization overall wants a value-driven model. I'd hate to be the individual hospital CEO whose performance/compensation has historically been measured by heads/beds now reporting to a system CEO that just signed a value-based contract. Overnight, full beds go from a revenue center to a cost center. Careful strategic planning outlining the timeframe and necessary changes is critical to these transitional phases.

- ☐ **Bundles (bundled payments):** Instead of paying separately for hospital, physician, and other services, payments for services linked to a particular condition, reason for hospital stay, and period of time are grouped together. Providers can keep the money they save through reduced spending on some component(s) of care included in the bundle.

- ☐ **Global capitation:** An organization receives a per-person per-month payment intended to pay for all attributed individuals' care, regardless of what services they use.

- ☐ **Patient-centered medical home (PCMH):** A team-based model of care, typically led by a primary care physician who is focused on the whole person and provides continuous, coordinated, integrated, and evidence-based care. Physicians may receive additional payments (for example, care coordination and/or performance-based incentives) on top of the fee-for-service payments.

- ☐ **Shared savings:** This type of arrangement generally requires an organization to be paid using the traditional fee-for-service model, but at the end of the year, total spending is compared with a target; if the organization's spending falls below the target, it can share some of the difference as a bonus. Or, if patients have better than average quality outcomes, the provider receives a bonus for increased payment

- ☐ **Shared risk:** As a complement to shared savings, if an organization spends more than the target, it must repay some of the difference as a penalty. Or, if patients fail to have better than average quality outcomes, the provider receives a lower payment.

- ☐ **Downside risk:** Payment models in which the provider is penalized if its patients fail to have better than average quality/cost outcomes.

- ☐ **Upside risk:** Payment models in which the provider receives a bonus if its patients have better than average quality/cost outcomes.

- ☐ **CMS Bundled Payment Care Improvement (BPCI):** Initiative organizations to be paid under bundles for specific procedures/conditions. The first program is for joint replacement. After the first level of participation, participants are required to participate with gradually increasing levels of downside risk.

- ☐ **Medicare Comprehensive Joint Replacement (CJR) program:** A mandatory bundled payment model for lower extremity joint replacement services in select geographic areas.

- ☐ **Medicare Shared Savings Program (MSSP):** Initiative for organizations to develop ACOs for Medicare patients and be paid via shared savings arrangements. After the first level of the program, participants are required to participant in shared risk arrangements with gradually increasing levels of downside risk.

Fig. 4.1 Value-based payment models and CMS pilot definitions

One of healthcare systems' greatest challenges is functioning in a mixed-payment world. As noted previously, fee for service isn't just going to magically disappear, and providers must have individual/group incentives that combine overall strategic goals and a variety of payment mechanisms. The following is an "overview of value-based payment models (Fig. 4.1)."

Third: Technology

Motivated providers who are fully committed to population health must have access to cost-of-care data, care .deficiencies, and so forth available at the point of care. Most standard EMRs are woefully deficient as they grew from a fee-for-service environment. In addition, links between claim payments [not billed charges] are very complex as each provider in most systems [Kaiser being the big exception] has multiple payors and each payor guards its fee schedule as proprietary, to be kept secret at all costs. Getting BC/BS, Humana, Aetna, and UnitedHealthcare to each share its data is a herculean task, but without cost-of-care data available at the point of care, how can we expect providers to manage efficiently?

I was an HMO medical director in the 1980s when the primary care gatekeeper model had a brief flurry of popularity with payors. Although very effective at lowering costs and directing care, attributes of a good population health model, the PCP gatekeeper concept quickly fell from grace. It was cumbersome, frustrating to providers and patients alike, the technology to support it did not exist, and the financial incentives were not appropriately aligned. In many ways, population health management is the PCP gatekeeper model on steroids, adding physician leadership, proper alignment of incentives, technology, care coordination utilization review and QA, and patient satisfaction to address the issues that caused the original model to fail in the 1980s.

Fourth: Care Coordination/Utilization Review/Quality Assurance

I have combined three .historically independent functions into one of the five critical success factors because with the transfer of insurance risk from payors to providers, the integration of these functions is much more efficient across disciplines. More importantly, when these functions are carried out by providers who understand the entire clinical situation, patient satisfaction and quality are significantly improved. No longer are providers playing "Mother may I" with insurance companies. They assure responsibility for the cost and quality of care. Combining with the other four critical success factors [physician leadership, alignment of financial incentives, technology, and patient satisfaction] leads to success in a fully capitated population health-oriented delivery system.

Fifth: Patient Satisfaction

The first .challenge in identifying patient satisfaction is designing a survey that is valid and provides information for the practice. The questions should be brief and clear and include one that asks "How satisfied are you with your physician?"

Not only do patient satisfaction surveys help improve your practice, but also in the MedicareHMO world, star ratings can mean the difference between financial success and failure.

I hope any of you who choose the journey of population health management have a fun, prosperous, and successful journey.

References

1. Wikipedia—Population Health.
2. Practicing Value Based Care: What Do Doctors Need? Deloitte 2016 Survey of Physicians. Deloitte University Press.

Patient-Centered Medical Home (PCMH) and the Care of Older Adults

5

Jason F. Lee

More than 50% of older adults have multiple chronic conditions, with distinctive cumulative effects for each individual [1, 2]. As an older adult's number of chronic conditions accumulate, the risk of dying prematurely, hospitalization, functional decline, and health-care costs increases [3]. Addressing complex medical care is most effective when it is comprehensive, patient centered, and coordinated by a team of trained health-care professionals that is accessible in primary care settings where most older adults receive treatment [4].

The patient-centered medical home (PCMH) is a promising model for transforming the organization and delivery of comprehensive, cost-effective primary care. Originally introduced by the American Academy of Pediatrics (AAP) in 1967, the medical home concept initially referred to a central location for archiving patient's medical record. In 2002, the AAP expanded the medical home concept as a model of delivering primary care that is accessible, continuous, comprehensive, family centered, coordinated, compassionate, and culturally effective to every child and adolescent. The PCMH concept was adapted to patients of all ages by the American Academy of Family Physicians (AAFP) in 2004 and by the American College of Physicians (ACP) in 2006. It served as a transition away from historically episodic care toward a framework of comprehensive coordinated primary care for patients of all ages. In 2007, the AAP, AAFP, ACP, and the American Osteopathic Association developed a joint statement of principles to describe the characteristics of the PCMH and to lead changes at the physician practice level to improve outcomes in today's primary care practices [5].

Since then, the PCMH model has evolved to improve population health outcomes, enhance the patient experience, reduce per capita health-care spending, and support care team well-being through team-based coordinated care. According to

J.F. Lee, MD, MPH
UCLA Health, Los Angeles, CA 90095, USA
e-mail: JFLee@mednet.ucla.edu

© Springer International Publishing AG 2018
M. Wasserman, J. Riopelle (eds.), *Primary Care for Older Adults*,
DOI 10.1007/978-3-319-61329-1_5

the Agency for Healthcare Research and Quality (AHRQ), the PCMH encompasses five major functions and attributes: comprehensive care, patient centered, coordinated care, accessible services, and quality and safety [6]. The PCMH model of care has the potential to improve the health of older Americans, as it is uniquely aligned with the values of geriatric medicine to deliver primary care for high-cost, high-need older adults with complex health needs [7, 8]. This chapter reviews considerations for the aging population and components of PCMH highlighting that interprofessional care of older adults is oriented to the whole person, coordinated, and comprehensive, with an emphasis on patient safety and quality of care.

Comprehensive care is a vital function of the PCMH and refers to a team of health-care providers accountable for addressing the majority of a patient's physical, mental, and behavioral health-care needs, including prevention and wellness, acute care, and chronic care. The PCMH advocates for a personal physician who is informed by an interdisciplinary team, which may include consulting physicians, nurses, pharmacists, nutritionists, social workers, educators, and care coordinators, to meet the complex needs of patients with multiple comorbidities and increasing frailty and disability [9]. A core principle of geriatric medicine has been the use of interprofessional team-based care of older adults and application of comprehensive geriatric assessment to address health needs systematically and to provide age-appropriate preventive care consistent with the older adult's goals of care. Successful model of a geriatrician-led team that actively coordinates care and provides comprehensive care across disciplines has been the Department of Veterans Affairs (VA) home-based primary care (HBPC) [10]. Established in 1972, the HBPC has been expanded across VA facilities in the country to provide comprehensive, cost-effective, longitudinal primary care by an interdisciplinary team to homebound aging veterans with multiple chronic and disabling conditions [11]. The comprehensive care approach becomes more evident for older adults who experience medical and social challenges and transition through various care settings and services [12]. Geriatricians are trained to work as part of a team of health-care providers to care for older adults with complex health needs, as they are likely to experience physical and social inactivity, falls, functional decline, polypharmacy, barriers to adequate nutrition and transportation, depression and memory problems, and potential for elder abuse [13]. Geriatric medicine aligned with the PCMH model can account for these special considerations when developing comprehensive care plans for older adults.

Patient-centered care, or care that is oriented toward the whole person, is another function of the PCMH, which calls for a physician-led, team-based health-care model that focuses on building partnerships with patients and families through an understanding of and respect for culture, needs, preferences, and values. The PCMH model actively supports older adults in learning to manage and organize their own care at the level they choose, as an individual's daily life may involve various caregivers, access to independent or assisted living, management of multiple chronic conditions, and the need for advance care planning prior to functional decline [14]. Caring for older adults requires clinicians who are sensitive to whole-person care across a lifespan taking account of advance care planning for serious illness and end-of-life care and social determinants of health. Recognizing that patients and families are core members of the care team, the PCMH model focused on older adults can ensure that they are fully informed partners in establishing their own care plans [15].

Coordinated care entails the integration, management, and organization of patient care and services across various health-care systems including specialty care, hospitals, home health care, long-term care, and community services, with an emphasis on efficient and safe transitions of care. The team-based approach to care in geriatric medicine is central in assisting older adults to navigate the continuum and complexity of the health-care system to prevent them from falling through gaps in care [16]. Similarly, the PCMH model promotes care coordination to improve communication between organizations and specialists, leverages health information exchange, and facilitates follow-up with primary care providers that may reduce avoidable readmissions and improve health outcomes especially for those with complex care needs [17]. Physicians can lead teams caring for older adults to identify high-need, high-cost patients and develop individualized, coordinated plans of care that integrate medical and social issues. Based on demonstrations of various PCMH models, care coordination enables teams to address problems comprehensively and deliver age-appropriate preventive care [18]. Founded in 1978, the Programs of All-Inclusive Care for the Elderly (PACE) emerged as a successful managed-care program that coordinated comprehensive medical care and long-term services and support to frail, nursing home eligible patients to live independently in the community and with a high quality of life. Based on a recent retrospective study, PACE enrollees experienced lower rates of hospitalization, readmission, and potentially avoidable hospitalization than similar populations [19]. Older adults with multimorbidity benefit from care coordination and multidisciplinary team-based care as their health-care needs may become complex to be addressed effectively by independent primary care providers.

The PCMH framework delivers accessible services with reduced wait times for urgent care needs, enhanced and flexible office hours, and 24/7 telephone or electronic access to primary care physicians (PCPs), and alternative methods of communication through health information technology. Increasing support to PCPs with enhanced access can reduce emergency room visits and unmet health-care needs [20]. Providing accessible services is essential for caring for older adults who may lack personalized care and needs in the home and lack social support or advocacy assistance, and office visits may place a burden on patients and caregivers. The PCMH model can provide support and guidance to older adults with self-management of multiple chronic conditions and caregiver support. Extended visits in the office setting can accommodate community-dwelling older adults with physical and mental limitations.

The PCMH model is committed to continuous quality improvement and patient safety strategies through clinical decision support tools, information technology, evidence-based care, shared decision-making, performance measurement, and population health management. Measuring medical care for older patients is complex and has to account for multimorbidity, geriatric syndromes, and social issues that contribute to variations in care preferences and planning. The Assessing Care of Vulnerable Elders (ACOVE) indicators aim to evaluate the range of health-care problems experienced by vulnerable older adults in the community who are at increased risk of functional decline [21]. States and commercial payers have piloted various forms of payment alignment to support primary care, and the PCMH generally demonstrated better quality of care, patient experiences, care coordination, and access [22]. For instance, the Geriatric Resources for Assessment and Care of Elders (GRACE) model of primary care for low-income seniors and their PCPs has been demonstrated to improve the quality of geriatric care and optimize health and functional status of older adults. The GRACE support team meets with the patient in the home to conduct an initial comprehensive geriatric assessment and then meets with the larger GRACE interdisciplinary team to develop a comprehensive, patient-centered care plan in collaboration with the patient's PCP that is consistent with the patient's goals and preferences of care. The effectiveness of the GRACE intervention has shown decreased use of the emergency department and hospitalization rates of high-risk older patients and has prevented long-term nursing home placement [23]. As such, the PCMH presents an ideal opportunity to use quality indicators and metrics toward primary care of older adults.

The PCMH has been an effective model for addressing the diverse medical and complex care needs and transforming how primary care is organized and delivered in a sustainable manner for our health-care system and stakeholders. A new paper released by The John A. Hartford Foundation PCMH Change AGEnts Network offers recommendations on how PCPs can improve health outcomes for older adults through geriatric PCMHs and succeed in the emerging value-based payment health-care environment [24]. As discussed in the concept paper, PCPs can begin to transform their existing practices and workforce to address the particular concerns of older adults. PCMH steps to serve older adults include the use of the Medicare Annual Wellness Visit to create a patient-centered care plan. As PCPs cannot address all of the needs of older adults alone, they can collaborate with community organizations, such as Area Agencies on Aging, which provide services and support to older adults and their families and caregivers to become better self-managers of their care. Moreover, advance care planning conversations can help identify and update goals of care according to patient's wishes over time. As such, PCPs can facilitate better transitions of care by leading and monitoring relationships with specialists, local hospitals, and long-term care settings. Lastly, PCPs can provide training and education of all staff to deliver geriatric-competent care. A PCMH enhanced for older adults can enable PCPs to provide better care for the population they already serve.

Given the demographic imperative of an aging society, the PCMH enhanced for older adults is an ideal model to strengthen the care of all populations, as primary care becomes the focal point of complex care coordination. It has demonstrated improvement in patient care with respect to transitions of care, access to care, patient and caregiver education, chronic disease self-management, decreased hospitalizations and emergency room visits, and decreased health-care costs. The PCMH model can mature and expand to identify and address the growing, complex medical and psychosocial needs of older adults. Moving forward, geriatric medicine principles and experience of care models for older adults add to the growing national attention to patient-centered quality care and improve clinical outcomes pursued by primary care clinicians across the country.

References

1. Chronic Disease Prevention and Health Promotion. https://www.hhs.gov/ash/about-ash/multiple-chronic-conditions/index.html.
2. Gerteis J, Izrael D, Deitz D, LeRoy L, Ricciardi R, Miller T, Basu J. Multiple Chronic Conditions Chartbook. AHRQ Publications No. Q14-0038. Rockville, MD: Agency for Healthcare Research and Quality; April 2014.
3. CDC Chronic Disease Prevention and Health Promotion. https://www.cdc.gov/chronicdisease/about/multiple-chronic.htm.
4. American Geriatrics Society Expert Panel on the Care of Older Adults with Multimorbidity. Patient-Centered Care for Older Adults with Multiple Chronic Conditions: a stepwise approach from the American Geriatrics Society.
5. American Academy of Family Physicians, American Academy of Pediatrics, American College of Physicians, American Osteopathic Association. Joint principles of the patient-centered medical home. 2007. http://www.medicalhomeinfo.org/downloads/pdfs/JointStatement.pdf.
6. Defining the PCMH. https://www.pcmh.ahrq.gov/page/defining-pcmh.
7. Langston C, Undem T, Dorr D. Transforming primary care what Medicare beneficiaries want and need from patient-centered medical homes to improve health and lower costs. 2014. http://www.johnahartford.org/blog/view/policy-briefing-transforming-primary-care-what-medicare-beneficiarieswant.
8. Centers for Medicare and Medicaid Services. Chronic conditions among Medicare beneficiaries, chartbook. 2012th ed. Baltimore, MD; 2012.
9. Ensuring that patient-centered medical homes effectively serve patients with complex health needs. https://www.pcmh.ahrq.gov/page/ensuring-patient-centered-medical-homes-effectively-serve-patients-complex-health-needs.
10. Beales JL, et al. Veteran's affairs home based primary care. Clin Geriatr Med. 25(1):149–54.
11. Edes T, Kinosian B, Vuckovic NH, Olivia Nichols L, Mary Becker M, Hossain M. Better access, quality, and cost for clinically complex veterans with home-based primary care. J Am Geriatr Soc. 2014;62:1954–61. doi:10.1111/jgs.13030.
12. Transitions of care: the need for a more effective approach to continuing patient care. https://www.jointcommission.org/assets/1/18/Hot_Topics_Transitions_of_Care.pdf.
13. What is a geriatrician? American Geriatrics Society and Association of Directors of geriatric academic programs end-of-training entrustable professional activities for geriatric medicine. http://onlinelibrary.wiley.com/doi/10.1111/jgs.12825/full.
14. Lipson D, Rich E, Libersky J, Parchman M. Ensuring that patient-centered medical homes effectively serve patients with complex health needs. (Prepared by Mathematica Policy Research under Contract No. HHSA290200900019I TO 2.) AHRQ Publication No. 11. Rockville, MD: Agency for Healthcare Research and Quality; October 2011.
15. Peikes D, Genevro J, Scholle SH, Torda P. The patient-centered medical home: strategies to put patients at the Center of Primary Care. AHRQ Publication No. 11-0029. Rockville, MD: Agency for Healthcare Research and Quality; February 2011.
16. Partnership for Health in Aging Workgroup on Interdisciplinary Team Training in Geriatrics. Position statement on interdisciplinary team training in geriatrics: an essential component of quality health care for older adults.

17. Rich E, Lipson D, Libersky J, Parchman M. Coordinating care for adults with complex care needs in the patient-centered medical home: challenges and solutions. White Paper (Prepared by Mathematica Policy Research under Contract No. HHSA290200900019I/HHSA29032005T). AHRQ Publication No. 12-0010-EF. Rockville, MD: Agency for Healthcare Research and Quality; January 2012.
18. Patient-Centered Primary Care Collaborative. The outcomes of implementing patient-centered medical home interventions: a review of the evidence on quality, access and costs from recent prospective evaluation studies, August 2009.
19. Segelman M, et al. Hospitalizations in the program of all-inclusive care for the elderly. J Am Geriatr Soc. 2014;62:320–4.
20. Benefits of implementing the primary care medical home: a review of cost & quality results, 2012. https://www.pcpcc.org/guide/benefits-implementing-primary-care-medical-home.
21. Assessing Care of Vulnerable Elders (ACOVE). http://www.rand.org/health/projects/acove.html.
22. The Patient-Centered Medical Home's Impact on Cost and Quality: Annual Review of Evidence, 2014–2015. https://www.pcpcc.org/resource/patient-centered-medical-homes-impact-cost-and-quality-2014-2015.
23. Counsell SR, Callahan CM, Buttar AB, Clark DO, Frank KI. Geriatric resources for assessment and care of elders (GRACE): a new model of primary care for low-income seniors. J Am Geriatr Soc. 2006;54:1136–41. doi:10.1111/j.1532-5415.2006.00791.x.
24. Patient-centered medical homes and the care of older adults: how comprehensive care coordination, community connections, and person-directed care can make a difference. http://www.johnahartford.org/newsroom/view/patient-centered-medical-homes-and-the-care-of-older-adults-new-paper-provi.

A Geriatrician's Guide to Accountable Care Implementation: Thickets and Pathways

6

Terry E. Hill

Introduction

Your Fabulous Job Offer

Imagine getting a call from the ruler of Erewhemos, a small country ruled by a benevolent monarch who has become concerned about her nation's healthcare. One of her parents has recently died, and the other has become increasingly frail, so she has gained considerable first-hand experience with aging, death, and her healthcare delivery system. The system was developed by accretion over time so that it now has multiple layers of professions, programs, and products, each with its own rules and incentives. On good authority the queen has heard of your experience, passion, and wisdom. She asks you to come to Erewhemos and develop a sensible healthcare delivery system. You will have free rein over the reorganization and full control of the healthcare budget, which was thought to be generous until strained recently by increasing costs related to drugs, technology, and an aging population. Healthcare costs have already begun to cut into other essential services such as education and the transportation infrastructure.

You may or may not find the move to Erewhemos attractive, but my assumptions in this chapter are that you are capable of taking in a big picture view, just as this monarch must do, and that you would very much like to have a sensible healthcare delivery system. Specifically, I assume that you are interested in advocating for a full array of effective services for older adults and that you are situated as a clinician, manager, or other stakeholder at some level within a US healthcare delivery system. I will also assume that your delivery system—that is, your organization and its partnerships—is responsible for the clinical and financial outcomes for a defined population,

T.E. Hill, MD
Hill Physicians Medical Group, 2409 Camino Ramon,
San Ramon, CA 94583, USA
e-mail: terry.hill@hpmg.com

© Springer International Publishing AG 2018

M. Wasserman, J. Riopelle (eds.), *Primary Care for Older Adults*,
DOI 10.1007/978-3-319-61329-1_6

35

whether defined by enrollment, as in managed care, or attribution, as has been used in various government and private sector models. We can leave aside the challenge of further defining an accountable care organization (ACO), a term that has encompassed multiple organizational arrangements and financial imperatives under commercial and government contracts [1]; rather, in this chapter we attend to the generic challenge of taking responsibility for the health outcomes, patient experience, and total cost of care for one or more contractually defined populations. The new focus on value in the healthcare marketplace offers unprecedented overlap between the transactional logic of operating margins and the mission-driven logic of healing relationships. As advocates for older adults, we should take advantage of this overlap wherever we can.

The chapter will proceed through several domains, beginning with an extensive discussion of hospital admissions and readmissions. The costs of these are foremost in the minds of your system's decision-makers, and you can harness the Willie Sutton principle to get their attention. We then turn to new developments in post-acute and long-term care and new models for high-need populations. Next, after a review of key strategies regarding data support for your initiatives, we will address several thorny challenges, including care planning, workforce, and disparities. We conclude with new perspectives on safety, ethics, and accountability across communities. My goal is to help you with ideas, argument, and implementation. I will touch on a host of interventions and models of care that have empirical support in the published literature, but a persistent concern throughout will be the critical processes of implementation, evaluation, and adaptation. Successful new models emerge in delivery systems that are blessed with propitious leadership, data systems, culture, and luck. The degree of planning and adaptation required of other systems to replicate these models will vary, but in many cases it approaches that of *de nouveau* innovation.

Throughout this discussion I will refer to the performance of your healthcare delivery system. I recognize, however, that you may not work in a fully integrated system, and the accountable care contract(s) most pertinent to you may be held by a system component other than yours, e.g., a hospital or medical group. So what do I mean by the healthcare delivery system? I mean the full array of organizations and services that comprise a patient's healthcare experience. All delivery systems in the USA, even the most integrated, coordinate care with independent organizations, e.g., nursing facilities, home health agencies, hospices, and vendors for durable medical equipment. From the patient's point of view, all these components constitute a system that serves—more or less well—their healthcare needs. A patient-centered accountable care framework nudges us toward a similar perspective in which we feel—or at least should feel—collectively responsible for quality, cost, and the patient's experience.

You may also be interested in accountable health communities, in which multiple healthcare delivery systems collaborate with public health, education, and business to improve well-being and manage costs for the entire population. The potential synergies from these collaborations may well be worth the resource investments required, as we will address later in the chapter, but for now I will focus on an organization's accountability for its own specific population, e.g., in managed care and/or a Next Generation ACO.

Unlike the extraordinary powers you would enjoy in Erewhemos, in your current position, you work within a multitude of constraints. Nevertheless, the momentum of accountable care offers each of us an opportunity to contemplate fundamental system changes that could enable a reasonable match of remediable needs and available resources. Your advocacy is most likely to succeed if you can think along two parallel paths at once. I have begun with the Erewhemos fable to encourage blue-sky thinking. Too often our imaginations are shackled by current realities, and we miss equally real opportunities for innovation. The idealized path is simply about the fundamentals of matching patients and services; it calls for lucid delineation of your population's healthcare needs and the most effective and efficient deployment of resources to meet those needs. While on this idealized path, it would be unwise to lose sight of the real-life path that is brambled by all those pesky constraints, laws and regulations, obvious power dynamics, not-so-obvious backstories and their emotional legacies, and the complex calculus of who wins and who loses in the marketplace. As you try to make your way toward optimal care, it would be prudent to watch your flank. Many people inside and outside of your organization do not share your commitment. Their decisions and activities may hinder or thwart your efforts. What appears to be waste, from an idealized point of view, is seen as livelihood from the view of entrenched personal and organizational interests.

The Age-Neutral Option for Geriatric Programming

The use of age as a marker of need may obscure more than it illuminates. The men and women over 70 years of age who can run the Boston marathon in 4 h probably don't need your system's specialized geriatric services. Conversely, significant numbers of younger adults have problems common to aging, so it may or may not be appropriate to develop programs targeting only older adults. Continence programs, for instance, are appropriate for a range of ages; urinary incontinence is common in young women, afflicts at least half of middle-aged women, and becomes the norm in elderly women [2].

New program development is rarely done on a blank slate, of course. Even if you took that all-powerful job in Erewhemos, you would still want to build on the strengths of your existing programs, champions, and workforce. Decisions about geriatric-specific versus age-neutral programming are likely to turn on the dominant messaging and imperatives within your delivery system. A system eager to celebrate its care for older adults may favor elder-specific terminology, whereas geriatric programming in other systems may fare better if bolstered by younger alliances. Your homebound population, for example, may include a large minority of younger patients, so age-neutral programming and terminology may be appropriate, e.g., "Independence at Home."

Geriatrics has long stressed function over age with regard to organ systems and individuals. Similarly, one can list the requisites of geriatric care without reference to age, as demonstrated in Christine Cassel's argument that the principles of geriatrics should be applied throughout the broader delivery system. "Geriatric medicine asks for care based on (1) continuous healing relationships; (2) customized services devoted to individual patient needs, which also allow the patient to exercise control over care; (3) access to information that is accurate and timely and shared with patients and families; (4) interdisciplinary teams and coordination of services across different settings; (5) anticipation of needs to avoid complications and exacerbations of chronic illnesses; and (6) cooperation, communication, and collaboration among specialists working toward patient-centered goals" [3]. A healthcare delivery system organized with the requisite competencies for high-quality and efficient care of older adults can deploy those same competencies to manage complex younger populations well.

One can advocate for these principles and competencies in generic rather than geriatric fashion without sacrifice to your older patients because older patients are overrepresented among those with chronic conditions and impairments needing coordinated, interdisciplinary care. More pointedly, from the perspective of your organization's decision-makers, older patients are overrepresented in high-cost categories. Several influential foundations have argued that "high-need, high-cost" patients, defined as those with at least three chronic diseases and one functional impairment, should be our healthcare priority [4]. While only 5% of all adults fall into this category, 65% of these high-need, high-cost patients are 65 or older [5]. This distribution is why the enlightened monarch of Erewhemos has realized her need for geriatric expertise; at some point your current delivery system will come to the same realization.

On the other hand, most older patients—75% who are 75 and older, 91% who are 65–74—are neither high-need nor high-cost. Even for elders far less athletic than the marathoners above, and even for some with several chronic diseases, interdisciplinary teams and an elaborate care plan may be unnecessary and wasteful. In the transitional zone between healthy and complex, however, it is important to build in self-management supports and regular screening opportunities. The annual wellness visits promoted under Medicare, for example, offer a bundle of screening processes that improve downstream health status if tied to effective follow-up. Medication review processes, if overseen by pharmacists who are attuned to aging and multimorbidity, can also serve as intervention triggers, as can electronic registries that reveal gaps in care.

Idealized Visions and Today's Nitty-Gritty

The literature is replete with helpful frameworks that you could take to Erewhemos or use to assess your own system's readiness for accountable care [6]. In an addendum to their 2012 *Health Affairs* paper, Elliot Fisher and colleagues adopt the metaphor of journey toward accountable care. They lay out a logic model that highlights the importance of a propitious environmental and economic context, as well as the requisite governance, relationships, infrastructure elements, and implementation activities [7]. The image of journey is apt; it's also worth noting that an organization's journey is often far from linear. Early CMS ACOs often failed outright, and some commercial ACOs with initial successes have subsequently struggled with diminishing financial returns and eroding leadership commitment. Attention to the conceptual frameworks in light of these challenges may avert future grief.

Idealized models specific to older populations with complex needs are also available. Particularly thoughtful is a report from The SCAN Foundation that specifies the delivery system activities critical for enabling individuals to live as independently as possible in accordance with their values and preferences. Figure 6.1 summarizes a high-quality system's essential attributes, beginning with identification of an individual's needs and goals, which then must be addressed in a rolling fashion across multiple domains: primary/acute care, community and social supports, long-term

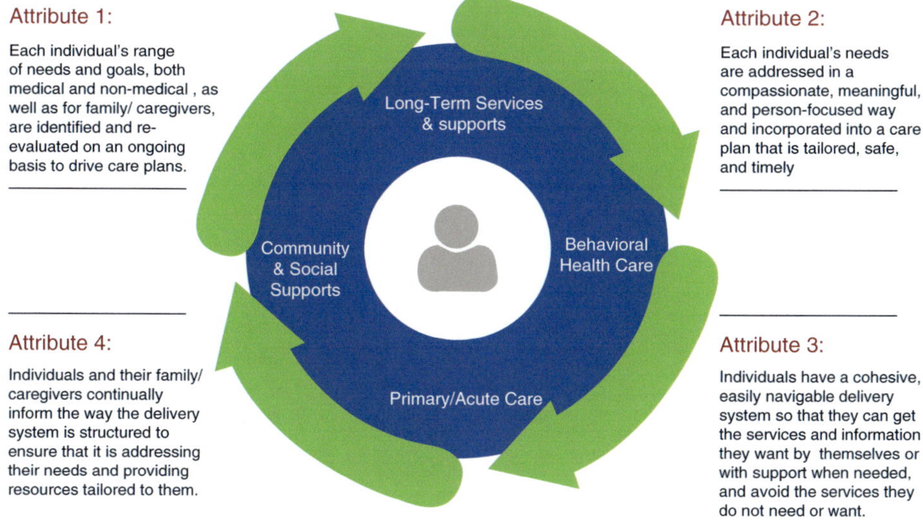

Fig. 6.1 Essential attributes of a high-quality system for adults with complex care needs (Reprinted with permission, The SCAN Foundation)

services and supports, and behavioral healthcare [8]. Notably, although ACOs have recognized the importance of behavioral health for older adults [9], progress toward improving behavioral health services has as yet been disappointing [10].

You may have opportunities within your delivery system to argue that this idealized model should be the standard of care. I agree that it should be, but you are not likely to get much traction unless you can also point to a return on investment (ROI). Fortunately, The SCAN Foundation has produced a collateral document that outlines the steps needed to make a compelling business case for person-centered care; the document includes a logic model, sample calculations, and suggestions for demonstrating an exceptionally high ROI [11]. Your argument for resources to support optimal care will turn largely on cost avoidance, which will matter to decision-makers in your organization to the extent that the delivery system as a whole has moved from fee-for-service to value. You can also quantify the financial benefits of improved patient experience. It is important as well to point out the multivalent effects of a single intervention. A robust readmission reduction program, for example, will also reduce admissions, as discussed in detail below. Interventions that are situated just before or after high-cost episodes, i.e., that are designed to prevent admissions or readmissions, tend to have the greatest near-term ROI.

The clarity of one's idealized vision can be overwhelmed when contemplating the array of needs, services, competencies, and interventions within one's actual delivery system, as illustrated in Table 6.1. Not shown here are other equally critical infrastructure elements such as information technology, data management, utilization management, contracting, and the human resource practices that are conducive to high-performance work systems [12]. In assessing your current system (or that of Erewhemos), you could ask the following questions about each of the services and other elements in Table 6.1: Does it exist? What's the range of quality? What's the

Table 6.1 Service array and competencies for geriatric population management

Illustrative needs	Services and programs	Sites and site-specific services	Modalities	Organizational competencies	Interventions
– Multimorbidity – Specific diseases, e.g., CHF, COPD, ESRD – Geriatric conditions, e.g., falls, incontinence – Dementia – Depression, anxiety – Pain – Frailty – Elder abuse	– Geriatric assessment – Geriatric comanagement – Advance care planning – Palliative care – Case management, care coordination – Care transitions – Medication management – Expertise in geriatric pharmacotherapy – Behavioral health – Social services assistance – Transportation – Durable medical equipment – Caregiver training – Interpreter services – Navigator services – Infusion services	– Primary care office – Specialist office – Urgent care – Emergency department – Acute care hospital – Acute rehabilitation – Skilled nursing facility – Home health agency – Assisted living, board, and care – Home- and community-based services – Home-based medical care – Home-based palliative care – Hospice – Dialysis – Home hemodialysis	– Face-to-face interactions – Group visits – Telehealth – Telephone visits – e-Visits – e-Consults – Video case conferences – Web-based education	– Predictive modeling – Condition-specific analyses – Multimorbidity analyses – Clinical performance measurement – Financial performance measurement – Site-specific evaluation – Program-specific evaluation – Quality improvement – Process mapping – Change management – Implementation science – Patient safety expertise – Knowledge of relevant clinical and organizational literatures	– Shared decision-making – Motivational interviewing – Patient/family experience surveys – Work process redesign – Practice coaching – Interdisciplinary team training – Clinical huddles, rapid rounds – Escalation processes – Performance feedback – Performance incentives – Provider education – Leadership development

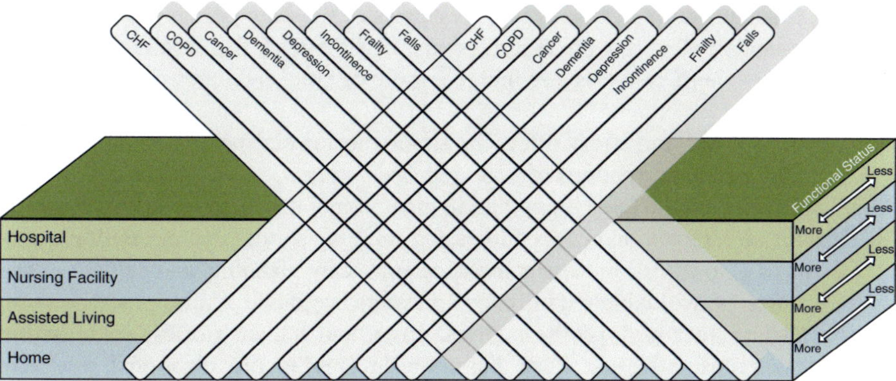

Fig. 6.2 Schematic suggesting the overlay of multimorbidity, sites of care, and functional variation in geriatric population management. For example, a patient with a primary diagnosis of CHF and concomitant COPD and depression may migrate from home to hospital, then to nursing facility or home, with or without significant functional impairment

utilization? What's the cost? Answers to the first two questions must most often come from knowledgeable insiders. Data systems can generate answers to the last two. Service utilization will always show variation across providers; the Goldilocks optimum is usually nonobvious, requiring deeper investigation.

What isn't obvious from Table 6.1 is the interplay among elements, beginning with multimorbidity itself. Your older patients are likely to have multiple conditions under the care of multiple clinicians across multiple sites. Figure 6.2 illustrates a simplified permutation of conditions and sites of care for complex patients. The schematic only hints at the intricacies of multimorbid reality, however. Medicare patients can be tiered by clinical complexity. The top tier comprising one-third of Medicare patients has over two million distinct combinations of diseases, and this third is responsible for about 80% of Medicare fee-for-service expenditures [13]. Your understanding of this complexity will protect you from the illusion that a single new program is the answer to geriatric population management. The good news is that you have multiple starting points for improvement. If you already have a spectacular team focused on congestive heart failure, for instance, you might consider supporting the extension of their work into another site of care, enhancing their behavioral health competencies, or making it easy for them to screen for geriatric conditions.

Transitions in Care as the Optical Science of Healthcare Delivery Systems

You may or may not have been paying attention to readmission reduction efforts in your current delivery system, but I will challenge you with this audacious assertion: *The delivery system that eliminates avoidable readmissions will have crossed the quality chasm.*

Don't worry, your current delivery system isn't the only one that is a long way from eliminating all avoidable readmissions. If we unpack the extravagance of my quality chasm claim, however, we find five more discrete and defensible assertions:

1. A focus on care transitions offers the single most revealing line of sight into the strengths and imperfections of your delivery system.
2. Older adults are the largest population most vulnerable to those imperfections.
3. Readmission reduction entails addressing multiple services across multiple sites of care, e.g., medication management, advance care planning, and palliative care.
4. Prevention of avoidable readmissions prevents avoidable admissions.
5. Because of their high-profile metrics, costs, and human stories, readmissions offer the most effective focal point for leveraging organizational resources toward optimal population management in geriatrics.

The power of human stories is part of why this lever works. Clinicians and associated staff draw deep satisfaction from their work when it is effective and prevents suffering. There is abundant preventable suffering among older patients and their families; readmissions in particular often represent full-scale family crises. Clinicians are disturbed when patients and families suffer needlessly; conversely, they feel their work is worthwhile when a thoughtful "plan A" is successful, or when a prearranged "plan B backup" is needed and actually works, or when they can improvise a solution for a patient in trouble. Opportunities for staff satisfaction are plentiful and excitement builds quickly when teams are making progress; this virtuous cycle yields yet more creativity.

Human stories rather than utilization and cost statistics are the most powerful drivers of frontline efforts. Readmission reviews and the stories derived from them provide the emotional hook for daily work and improvement. Clinicians are not the only ones who care, of course. Chief financial officers perk up and become more creative when good numbers are accompanied by good stories, and they too may appreciate the opportunity to reflect upon their own family experiences. Conversely, C-suites can undermine frontline compassion, intrinsic motivation, and commitment by focusing exclusively on business imperatives.

Readmission reviews will create a sense of urgency and offer lines of sight into your system—and yield promising interventions—to the extent that clinicians across disciplines, departments, and sites of care (1) are given a sustained opportunity to think together about the interplay of multilevel causes across multiple populations, (2) are informed by rich and timely data, and (3) are supported by energetic project managers. Avoidable admissions and readmissions represent a meaningful pain that calls out for healing at the individual and system level. Please note, however, that clinicians in full-time patient care cannot be expected to access data, develop reports, and drive performance improvement without the support of staff dedicated to these functions. For delivery systems on the journey away from heads-in-beds reimbursement, the cost savings and associated organizational learnings will justify the investments made toward readmission reduction.

There is now wide acknowledgement that hospitals' readmission lens has been too narrowly focused on specific diseases. The benefits of readmission reduction programs will accrue only if the programs are granted broad scope and leadership support. Restricting attention to a few diagnoses limits both scope and benefits. A 20% reduction in heart failure readmissions, for instance, might drop the overall Medicare readmission rate only from 16.0% to 15.8% [14]. Readmission programs have also been hampered by our tendency to produce reports and research as if patients have single diagnoses. Without an appreciation of multimorbidity, we cannot begin to offer person-centered care. Our data systems continue to attribute admissions and readmissions to "sepsis" with no indication of the underlying diagnoses that might be amenable to intervention. There is little acknowledgement of diagnostic overlaps, e.g., the well-demonstrated overlap of heart failure, chronic obstructive lung disease, and pneumonia [15] or the ways in which common geriatric conditions such as cognitive impairment interact with organ-specific diseases such as heart failure [16]. Delivery systems have not routinely asked clinicians with geriatric expertise to help lead their readmission reduction efforts, but they should. If not asked, clinicians with geriatric expertise should insert themselves into these efforts.

One System's Journey

Reports from two Kaiser Permanente regions offer a revealing perspective into the way readmission reduction efforts evolve over time. I will review this work in some detail, not so much because the interventions are unique, but primarily because the sequence offers a good example of a system on a journey toward accountable care. In 2008 Kaiser Permanente Northwest identified care transitions as a "pivotal opportunity" [17]. Informed by the published literature, its own research, dozens of plan-do-study-act cycles, and review sessions that brought together diverse stakeholders, the redesign team implemented an intervention bundle with the following elements:

- Risk stratification into low-, medium-, and high-risk categories
- A post-discharge "hotline" phone number for patients
- Standardized same-day discharge summaries and instructions
- Office follow-up appointments timed according to risk score
- Telephonic nurse transition management for high-risk patients
- Medication reconciliation

Readmissions decreased and patient experience scores improved for the Kaiser Permanente Northwest medical centers. In 2012 Kaiser Permanente Southern California adapted this bundle and added two major elements: a process for triggering inpatient palliative care consultations for high-risk patients and a complex case conference program to shed light on the interplay of medical conditions and social issues for high-risk patients with multiple admissions [18]. The case conferences in particular led to significant changes in the established heart failure transitions program, which evolved toward a person-centered model in which the care team aspires to recognize the patients' experience of their health problems within their particular life context [19]. Not only can this model be applied to other complex diseases but also "the knowledge we gain from successfully reducing heart failure readmission may be applied to upstream efforts to reduce index admissions."

Meanwhile, the transition program back at Kaiser Permanente Northwest has continued to evolve [17]. Readmission reviews there led to interventions addressing end-of-life issues, wound infections, and constipation, all of which contribute to readmissions. Reviews of oncology readmissions led to an expansion of the infusion clinic hours. The program involved robust participation of transition pharmacists. Invaluable lessons for patient-centeredness have come from a patient with systems improvement expertise who continues to participate in program development as an active member of the project team. Program extensions have reached to other sites of care, e.g., skilled nursing facilities and emergency departments, and have integrated the patients' care navigators and community resources. It is worth noting that even with demonstrated success on multiple performance measures, sustaining adequate attention and resources has been a challenge.

In this brief summary of the Kaiser Permanente transitions programs, I have highlighted the processes of development, adaptation, and evolution, glossing over multiple operational decisions made over multiple years. I commend these papers to those of you who want to learn more. My point here, however, is that even with the enviable resources and data systems of Kaiser Permanente, informed by rigorous reviews of the published literature and its own internal research, the program teams still had to feel their way. This is what successful journeys are like. There is an ever-present administrative temptation to bet on quick, simple, off-the-shelf solutions to complex issues. Those bets routinely result in lost money and time. A better bet is to supply advocates with access to expertise and resources and hold them to achievable program goals.

Readmissions as Marker and Leverage

But why am I going on at such length about hospital readmissions programs? The answer is purely pragmatic. If you travel to Erewhemos, you may have other options, but in the US context, for 2017 and beyond, this is likely to be your single best lever for getting resources for non-hospital programs serving elders. Even in Erewhemos, where you might be able to avoid the mental strictures imposed by 30-day windows and current bundled payment programs, readmissions will offer a fruitful starting place for your assessment.

Because admission rates skew to older ages, you can be assured that an age-neutral readmission lens entails ample geriatric focus. The Massachusetts adult all-payer database reveals that for fiscal year 2013, 57% of all 30-day readmissions occurred among adults aged 65 and over, with readmission rates of 15.1%, 16.5%, and 17.0% among adults aged 65–74, 75–84, and 85 and over, respectively [20].

In a system responsible for the total cost of care, readmission rates are one marker of overall delivery system cost-effectiveness. If decision-makers in your delivery system have emerged from their dependence on heads-in-beds reimbursement, they should take notice. Readmission rates correlate with community admission rates [21]. The apparent reason is that programs such as those using interdisciplinary team-based care for complex patients decrease both admissions and readmissions. The ROI calculation for readmission reduction, therefore, should not be limited to counting readmissions per se. Furthermore, the 30-day measure itself reflects only the initial portion of readmission vulnerability, so here again our lens has been too narrow. For both complex younger patients and for older patients, readmission rates remain high far beyond the initial 30 days [22, 23].

Readmission Reviews and the (Re)Admission Wheel of Fortune

Robust readmission reduction efforts, therefore, will reach far beyond the hospital, both downstream toward late readmissions and upstream toward index admissions, as illustrated by the evolution at Kaiser Permanente described above. Readmission reviews will point to fragmentation and vulnerabilities throughout your delivery system. Figure 6.3 begins to illustrate this process via a (Re)Admission Wheel of

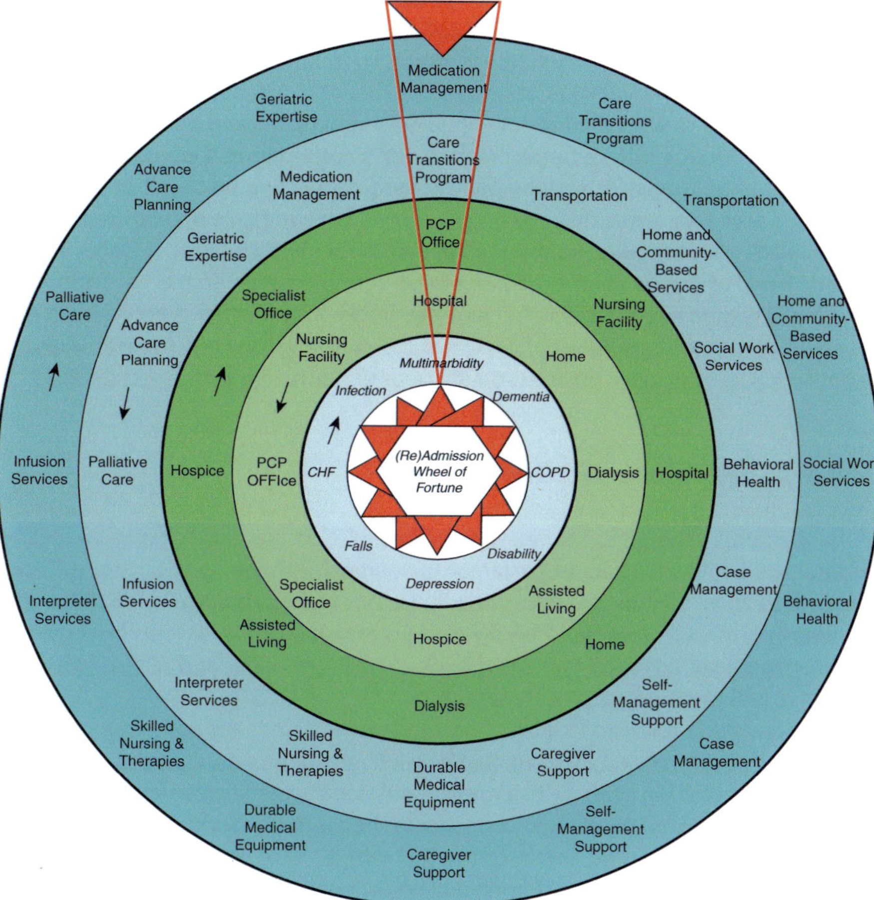

Fig. 6.3 The (Re)Admission Wheel of Fortune. Each segment of the wheel spins independently, before coming to rest within a new configuration of conditions, sites of care, and services that contribute to the occurrence or avoidance of an admission. The sites of care (in *green*) and services (in *blue*) are duplicated so as to allow for interactions between two different sites of care and between two different services. The example shown implies a medication mishap between hospital and home, not prevented by the care transition program. Not shown are patient-related biopsychosocial determinants of health

Fortune. Imagine that each segment of the wheel spins independently before coming to rest in a new configuration of sites of care and services. From the patient's perspective, the wheels can turn fast and furious during episodes of illness. From the system perspective, each readmission review is a spin of the wheel that will point to disconnects across siloed sites of care and inadequacies of the cross-cutting services. Spinning the wheel several times helps people understand the multifactorial nature of these admissions, which are resistant to magic bullet solutions.

I do not mean to imply that the majority of readmissions are preventable or even that preventability can be reliably measured; preventability lies in the eye of the beholder and depends upon the width of the beholder's lens. That said, the point of reviews is to identify factors that can be addressed. Readmissions can be roughly scored on a scale of very easy to very difficult to prevent, and they can be classified as due to clinician, system, and/or patient factors [24]. It is also useful to think through the upstream factors that contribute to the relevant clinician and patient behaviors [25]. Inadequate discharge planning, for example, might be tracked back to clinician workloads and time pressures or to lack of collaboration across nurse-physician silos. Patient no-shows at scheduled follow-up visits might be tracked back to the patient's reluctance to admit a lack of family support and transportation. Getting physicians to use standardized forms for reviews can promote "reflective practice" in which they review the care they gave; this practice alone can have impacts upon their behaviors [26]. A team with adequate representation across the delivery system, using a wide-enough lens, will soon land on most of the configurations of the (Re)Admission Wheel of Fortune and gain insights into the safety hazards that your patients must negotiate. As one editorial noted, "the real value in paying attention to readmissions is that it forces us to explore the interstitial spaces of our health delivery system" [27].

Primary Care Access and Quality

If the elements of the (Re)Admission Wheel of Fortune were drawn to scale of importance, some would loom far larger than others. Primary care access and quality certainly have an outsized effect on admissions and readmissions [28, 29]. Other functions permeate—or should permeate—across all sites of care, such as medication management, advance care planning and palliative care, and self-management support. I will mention each of these in turn.

Primary care is relevant to admissions and readmissions for many reasons, but it is prompt post-discharge follow-up that has become the standard core component of readmission reduction efforts. The operational details vary from system to system. For high-risk patients, the Kaiser Permanente Southern California bundle described above included telephonic nurse follow-up within 72 h and primary care visits within 7 days [18]. The Kaiser Permanente Northwest bundle for high-risk patients included telephonic follow-up within 48 h and office visits within 5 days; in addition, hospitalist oversight was extended to 48 h after discharge [17]. As with so many system interventions, however, the impacts are variable and clearly context dependent; there is no single best practice that will guarantee positive results. In the

Lack of Timely and Effective Post-Acute PCP visits

Hospital/transition staff behaviors

1. Hospital/transition staff do not set appointment prior to discharge
2. Hospital/transition staff do not investigate caregivers' availability, need for transportation, etc
3. Information flow from hospital is inadequate

Contributing factors
- Lack of supportive processes, time, motivation, recognition, skills, technology

Patient and caregiver behaviors

1. Patient doesn't call for appointment
2. Patient has appointment but doesn't keep it

Contributing factors
- Patient lacks transportation
- Patient lacks caregiver assistance
- Patient doesn't feel well enough to keep appointment
- Patient forgets appointment date
- Patient dosesn't want to incur co-pay
- Appointment is made for inopportune time
- Patient believes home health services preclude need for appointment
- Patient believes appointment not necessary
- Patient lacks meaningful relationship with PCP
- Patient doesn't want to bother PCP

PCP and PCP office staff behaviors

1. PCP doesn't allow hospital staff to set appointment prior to dischatge
2. PCP office offers only appointments with excessive delay or at times that are difficult for caregivers
3. PCP office doesn't take initiative to set appointment either prior to of after discharge

Contributing factors
- PCP office unaware of recent adimission and need for appointment
- PCP believes transitional care management services (TCM) or home health is adequate
- PCP office workflows are not conducive to fitting in post-acute appointments
- PCPs frustrated by inadequate information exchange from hospital and/or by high rate of appointments not kept
- PCPs and office staff do not have the bandwidth or skill sets to do process redesign
- PCPs not recognized or rewarded for making the extra effort

4. Patient appointment is timely but inadequate
- Patient seen by NP or covering MD who doesn't know patient
- Patient seen by PCP but "squeezed in" without adequate time for medication reconciliation, etc

Other

1. Need for ED visit (+/-admission) precedes PCP appointment
- May be avoidable vs unavoidable, e.g., condition change, medication mishap, DME misap, etc
2. Lack of alternatives to PCP follow-up when patients are particularly complex, e.g, transition clinic with interdisciplinary team
3. Patient has intervening SNF stay
- All factors above may apply to PCP follow-up after SNF discharge

Fig. 6.4 Behaviors that contribute to ineffective primary care visits following hospital discharge

Kaiser Permanente system, 7-day follow-up reduced readmissions of patients with congestive heart failure compared with follow-up that occurred later [30]. The timing of follow-up of medical patients at the Mayo Clinic, on the other hand, had no significant impact on readmission rates [31]. A study of Medicare claims found that the combination of early home health nursing and early office follow-up reduced readmissions of heart failure patients, but one without the other did not [32]. Regardless of this variation in research findings, the prima facie value of primary care follow-up is strong enough that you will get little pushback from stakeholders in making prompt follow-up a priority.

As yet unexplored in this literature is variation in the quality of post-acute visits that do occur. A hasty visit that occurs without a discharge summary or adequate medication review is likely to be of low value—and even less when it's with a clinician who does not know the patient. Figure 6.4 lists a number of behaviors that contribute to whether a primary care visit occurs following discharge from hospital or nursing facility, as well as why a visit might be low quality.

Medication Management

Medication management also has an outsized effect on admissions and readmissions. About 25% of adults age 75 and over have emergency department visits each year [33]. Among older adults with emergency department visits due to adverse drug events, 44% are hospitalized, a rate that is seven times higher than for younger patients [34]. The primary culprits are anticoagulants and antiplatelet agents, diabetic agents, and antibiotics. As of 2012, among adults age 75 and over, 43% were taking antihyperlipidemics, 38% were taking beta-blockers, 26% were taking diuretics, 20% were taking anticoagulants or antiplatelet agents, and 15% were taking diabetic agents [33]. The portion of older adults on five or more medications is now well over a third and rising year over year [35].

Interventions to prevent adverse drug events have become a standard component of readmission reduction efforts; as is the case with post-acute follow-up visits, they too take variable forms with variable results. One care transition program employed pharmacists to make post-hospital home visits for high-risk patients and phone calls for somewhat lower-risk patients, reducing readmissions and saving $2 for every $1 spent [36]. In another program, pharmacists reviewed medications prior to nursing facility discharge, visited patients at home after discharge, and sent notes to the primary care physicians [37]. There was a significant decrease in emergency department visits and a strong trend toward decreased hospital readmissions. This program has since moved the pharmacist upstream to do reviews in the hospital prior to nursing facility admission.

The art and science of medication management—and deprescribing in particular—have always been geriatric core competencies. We have a long way to go, however, in knowing how best to deploy geriatric and pharmacological expertise and staff in our ever-changing environment of organizational arrangements, payment streams, electronic records, and telehealth possibilities. A novel collaboration across hospitals and community pharmacies in Hawaii offered face-to-face medication management services with pharmacists for 12 months to patients identified as high risk at hospital discharge. The medication-related hospitalization rate during that year was 36% lower for the intervention group than for controls, and the ROI was 2.6 to 1 [38].

We obviously need to go further upstream and prevent medication misadventures before patients land in the hospital; our challenge is that the volume of patients who might benefit from intervention is large. Consistent with studies in other populations, a study of older veterans found that half had at least one prescribing problem; the strongest risk factor for each type of problem was the number of medications taken [39]. How can we deploy cost-effective interventions for all patients who can benefit? One key will be using lower-cost staff. Since pharmacy technicians can perform many of the routine tasks of pharmacists, there is increasing recognition that we need to integrate them into our pharmacy and interprofessional teams, with appropriate pharmacist oversight [40, 41].

Advance Care Planning and Palliative Care

When appealing to decision-makers for resources, you can legitimately claim that advance care planning is the secret sauce of cost control. Advance care planning needs to be incorporated into every service and site of care on the (Re)Admission Wheel of Fortune. It starts—or should start—with primary care, and it should extend far upstream into young and healthy populations. Simply having more care from primary care physicians increases the likelihood that patients will be able to die at home with home health or hospice care rather than in the hospital [42]. One advance care planning program reduced costs in the last 6 months of life by $14,000 per patient [43]. Fortunately, completion of formal advance directives is not a pre-requisite of benefit. Patients who report having any end-of-life conversations with physicians have been associated with having lower costs and higher quality of care at end of life [44]. The evaluation of tools and training to assist patients and providers with advance care planning is now an area of intense activity [45, 46]; excellent free resource compilations are available [47]. The enormous gap between ideal and reality suggests that this is a high-payoff opportunity for delivery systems. In a 2016 poll, 99% of physicians report that it is important to have these conversations, but less than a third had had training to do so. One in four reported that their electronic health record had no place for an advance care plan; of the rest, only 54% reported that they could access the plan's contents [48].

Evidence for cost savings from palliative care is even more robust than the evidence regarding advance care planning. One integrated delivery system deploying palliative care in home and clinic found net savings per patient per month of $4258 for cancer patients, $4017 for chronic obstructive lung disease, $3447 for congestive heart failure, and $2690 for dementia [49]. Unsurprisingly, palliative care emerged as a leading strategy among hospitals enrolled in the State Action on Avoidable Rehospitalization (STAAR) initiative [50]. In a nursing home study, consultations by palliative care nurse practitioners reduced hospital admissions at end of life; the most dramatic reductions occurred with consultations done 61–180 days before death [51]. Brian Cassel and coauthors have summarized the business case for inpatient and community-based palliative care [52]. Although the ROI is more obvious in delivery systems that are responsible for the total cost of care, there is ample evidence that inpatient palliative care programs yield financial benefits in fee-for-service models as well as a variety of risk-share models.

Readmission reviews will reveal an abundance of missed opportunities to address end-of-life decision-making, as well as opportunities to improve the impacts of the advance care planning and palliative care that do occur. In your delivery system, do advance care planning notes and documents from ambulatory care show up in the emergency department and hospital? Do inpatient palliative care consultations get to—and get read by—primary care physicians? Do inpatient palliative care consultations get read by nursing facility or home health staff? The ROIs noted above should readily motivate decision-makers to allocate resources for new program development and for repairs to gaps in these communication processes. For front-line clinicians, engagement with end-of-life patient stories—both suffering incurred and suffering averted—will be critical in motivating them to develop new skills and behaviors.

Self-Management Support

Self-management support has increasingly been recognized as critical to readmission reduction efforts, whereas earlier research and practice focused almost exclusively on structural elements such as post-discharge follow-up.

The Hospital Medicine Reengineering Network (HOMERuN) study reported that readmitted patients largely understood their discharge plan and were satisfied with the discharge process but had difficulties carrying out the plan [53]. The authors infer that more patient education is not likely to be the answer; rather, they suggest anticipatory guidance for resolving challenges, plus meaningful post-acute support at home for high-risk patients. When the HOMERuN hospitalists and primary care physicians were separately asked about the reasons for readmission of patients whom they themselves treated, they agreed on very little except the importance of patients' ability to self-manage [54]. The remedies they suggested were improving the self-management plan, engaging home and community supports, and providing resources for managing post-discharge care and symptoms. Interviews of seriously ill veterans also found that lack of caregiver support and lack of motivation to provide self-care were prominent contributors to readmissions [55].

A meta-analysis of randomized readmission reduction trials found that comprehensive bundles of support were effective [56]. These involved "a consistent and complex strategy that emphasized the assessment and addressing of factors related to patient context and capacity for self-care (including the impact of comorbidities, functional status, caregiver capabilities, socioeconomic factors, potential for self-management, and patient and caregiver goals for care)." A simple question worth asking consistently is "Can you really do what I'm asking you to do?" [57].

I have belabored these research findings because they provide objective evidence for the arguments long made by advocates for patient-centered care. After their experience in implementing the readmission bundle described above, the Kaiser Permanente Southern California clinicians concluded, "The key to reducing readmissions and avoidable hospital days may be as easy as doing the right thing for our patients" [18].

A related theme of "authentic healing relationships" emerged as a key to self-management support from interviews with patients of the successful Camden care management initiative. These relationships were characterized as being secure (accepting, attentive), genuine, and continuous (extending over multiple visits). The quality of care is often a function of the quality of relationships—both relationships between patient and clinician and relationships between clinicians. Behaviors that contribute to authentic healing relationships can be learned by team members and extended to family and friends who provide informal caregiving. The Kaiser Permanente Northern California "Caring Science" initiative offers one example of how an organization can systematically encourage such behaviors [58].

Caveats and Cautions for Your (Re)Admission Efforts

Readmissions of surgical patients involve different dynamics from readmissions of medical patients, so these readmission reviews should proceed with enhanced expertise and considerable caution. Surgical readmissions are difficult to predict at time of discharge, and most of the predictors are preoperative patient-level factors such as age, comorbidities, and functional status [59]. Because readmissions are spread out relatively evenly from time of discharge to 30 days beyond the surgery itself, early follow-up may not reduce readmissions [60]. Readmissions and surgical complications offer complementary lines of sight into the quality of care. The wide variation among surgeons in surgical site infections, the most common reason for readmission, suggests one opportunity for improvement [61]. There may also be also significant opportunities to prevent admissions following ambulatory surgery. These admissions are strongly associated with older age [62]. It may not be realistic to expect an older patient to manage medications and her wound dressings within hours of a surgical procedure.

Not all admissions and readmissions can or should be prevented. Careful manual reviews in an integrated system found that nearly half of 30-day readmissions were preventable [63], but a meta-analysis of 16 other studies found that estimates vary widely, centering around 23% [64]. The HOMERuN project found that 27% of medical admissions were potentially preventable and recommended focusing attention on many of the factors discussed above, including patient self-management, advance care planning, and medication safety [65]. The most common preventability factor, however, was the decision by emergency physicians to admit a patient who may not have needed an inpatient stay. That finding points to the need for additional care coordination and/or hospitalist resources at the point of decision in the emergency department. With rare exceptions [66], continuity of care from ambulatory sites to emergency departments has become a distant memory of aging physicians, and only a handful of readmission projects have even considered mitigating this loss by enhancing communication channels from ambulatory providers to the emergency department [67].

My final caution regarding readmission work is that you may or may not find that this is a top priority for hospital decision-makers. A careful survey of leaders at nearly 1000 hospitals conducted in 2013–2014 found that financial penalties from the federal Hospital Readmission Reduction program did have a significant impact on their behavior [68]. As a priority, however, readmission reduction efforts fell far behind initiatives on patient safety, patient experience, infections, and meaningful use of information technology. Among the morally dubious behavior changes contemplated for addressing readmissions, 27% said it was "more than moderately likely" that hospitals would increase their use of observation status, and 15% said it was "more than moderately likely" that hospitals would increasingly avoid high-risk patients. Only a minority was participating in ACO, shared savings, or bundled payment programs. It may be several years before hospitals' economic imperatives tip from fee-for-service to value.

The good news is that many hospitals have already embraced value as part of their mission, often in advance of a tidal shift away from fee-for-service incentives. The importance of this quality commitment is illustrated in a fine-grained study of readmission practices and results in the STARR project [69]. The researchers found no differences between high-performing and low-performing hospitals in terms of the actual practices deployed, such as those in the bundles described above. What they did find in the high-performing hospitals were spirited interdisciplinary collaboration, meaningful bonds with staff in post-acute settings, and enthusiasm for trial-and-error learning, often including repeated plan-do-study-act cycles. Finally, in high-performing hospitals, staff reported "that readmissions needed to be reduced primarily because they were bad for the patients, rather than to avoid Medicare fines for the hospital." These findings point to the presence of transformational leadership at the executive level and meaningful support for innovation of work processes on the clinical front lines. In addition, they point to supportive relationships and rich communication among clinicians. Particularly for the complex conditions and situations of older patients, the best course of action is often uncertain. Standard protocols and procedures are helpful but not sufficient, and patients will be best served if the clinicians have permission to improvise [70].

Post-Acute and Long-Term Strategies

Chaos and Costs

Advocates for older adults are all too aware of fragmentation in primary and specialty care, post-acute and long-term care, palliative care, and community-based services, all of which come with a dizzying array of funding sources and eligibility requirements, all of which have been plagued by perverse incentives and Balkanized by regulations. Patients and families have borne the most serious consequences, of course, but clinicians too have long suffered in their purgatorial silos. If you're lucky, the country of Erewhemos will be far less complicated.

In healthcare as in other industries, teams that coordinate with each other across different sites achieve better outcomes when their communication is frequent, timely, accurate, and problem-solving rather than finger-pointing; when the teams have mutual respect and knowledge of each other's work; and when they share common goals [71]. Unfortunately, respect and good communication, common knowledge, and common goals have often not been part of our daily experience as we struggle to care for elders with complex conditions. Each new spin of the (Re) Admission Wheel of Fortune comes to rest in a new configuration of frustration and missed opportunities. The good news is that these problems are now being recognized and addressed; we have evidence that the movement toward value and accountable care offers hope of improving our communication channels and coordination [72].

Because hospital stays incur the greatest proportion of total healthcare costs, I have suggested that advocates for older adults first look there for organizational leverage with delivery system decision-makers. The ROI from decreasing admissions and readmissions will more than cover the costs of efficient clinical interventions. Decision-makers are probably far less aware of the extraordinary costs and savings opportunities in post-acute care, which offers you another point of leverage for sensible clinical interventions. Over half of fee-for-service Medicare patients discharged from the hospital now receive formal post-acute services [73]. Those services are costly. Episodes of acute care can be divided into a 3-day preadmission segment, the inpatient segment, and a 30-day post-discharge segment. In fiscal year 2015, the proportional costs of these segments in fee-for-service Medicare were 3%, 53%, and 44%, respectively. Variation in episode costs across hospitals was largely due to variation in post-acute spending [74]. The costs of skilled nursing facilities in that 30-day period exceeded the costs of readmissions. The waste and potential savings in the post-acute period are so great that many delivery systems participating in bundled payments and shared savings ACOs are focusing almost exclusively on post-acute costs, particularly nursing facility costs, without attending to other high-opportunity areas such as medication management or palliative care. Systems with more forethought are beginning to make diverse investments across the entire post-acute and long-term care domain, which has long been starved for resources, training, and technology.

In a happy coincidence of clinical and financial interests, delivery systems have begun paving the path from hospital to home, bypassing nursing facilities whenever possible. Historically, the use of facility versus home-based services has been remarkably haphazard, subject to local custom, rather than evidence based and patient centered [75]. Participants in the Centers for Medicare and Medicaid Services (CMS) bundled payment initiatives have come to believe that "recovery from orthopedic surgery is better achieved in the beneficiary's home" [76]. One hospital, prompted in part by disruption from superstorm Sandy, decreased discharges to inpatient post-acute facilities by 49% for cardiac valve surgery and by 34% for major joint replacement—with no increases in readmission rates [77]. CMS and the Medicare Payment Advisory Commission (MedPAC) have noticed "considerable overlap in where beneficiaries are treated for similar [post-acute] needs" and are planning to implement a unified post-acute care payment system [78]. The considerable financial stakes have triggered intense interest in decision support to help clarify which patients should go where when leaving the hospital. Electronic decision-support tools developed by CMS and the private sector are promising, but they are still largely in early evaluation phase [79, 80].

Home Health Agencies

The increasing use of home health services as an alternative to nursing facilities has prompted interest in overcoming the factors that have perpetuated their suboptimal benefit. Home care nurses have been particularly frustrated by their communication with physicians—or lack thereof [81]. They feel unsupported by primary care physicians and challenged by the need to coordinate with the specialists who might be involved in the care of complex older patients. Primary care physicians themselves are often left out of the loop, given the prominent involvement of specialists and hospitalists. The need for role definition and workflow redesign is urgent [82].

Even within the current regulatory and reimbursement framework, there is ample evidence of potential for improvement and innovation. One initiative targeting all post-acute providers in 14 communities achieved significant decreases in all-cause 30-day readmissions *and* all-cause admissions in those communities, compared with controls, through the use of interventions such as transition bundles, medication reconciliation, and patient activation [83]. There is now recognition of the value in "front-loading" visit frequency and intensity during episodes of care [84], as well as the value of training home health nurses in motivational interviewing [85]. One project compared nurses' implementation of a comprehensive depression management program to usual depression management and reduced 30-day admissions by more than one-third for the intervention group [86].

Use of pharmacists in nursing facilities has been largely perfunctory and suboptimal, but they have been virtually absent in standard home care. This absence is likely to be remedied in a value-based world. One study found that integrating pharmacists into the home care team reduced admissions and emergency department visits by 40% [87]. Physicians accepted over half of the pharmacists' recommendations for medication changes.

While not a panacea for fragmentation and interdisciplinary woes, it is nevertheless true that technology promises to transform home care services. Telehealth monitoring has been effective in reducing admissions of patients with heart failure and chronic obstructive pulmonary disease, at least in demonstration projects [88, 89]. Even a simple electronic prompt for nurses and aides to report changes in condition has potential to decrease admissions [90].

Nursing Facility to Hospital (Re)Admissions

Nursing facilities have long been known as a reservoir for complex patients who make unfortunate trips to the hospital. In one study, experts rated 67% of these admissions as potentially avoidable [91]. In a more recent study, nursing facility staff rated 23% of admissions as potentially avoidable with earlier and better management of condition changes and earlier advance care planning [92]. The reasons for avoidable admissions can be clustered into nursing factors, physician factors, facility/resource factors, patient/family factors, and health system factors [93]. A movement to implement the Interventions to Reduce Acute Care Transfers (INTERACT) program may be able to reduce the national burden of unnecessary suffering and costs [94, 95]. As is so often the case, however, the attitudes, skills, and performance of clinicians make a difference. Facilities with high-admission rates tend to be associated with decision-making that has been described as "algorithmic," while low-admission facilities support individualized decision-making with meaningful clinician-family engagement during difficult decision-making [96].

More recently, attention has focused on readmissions from nursing facilities, their underlying causes, and their potential remedies. Historically, communication from hospitals to nursing facilities has been inadequate, and often abysmal [97]. Electronic access to the inpatient record is helpful but far from sufficient for downstream providers. Nurse-to-nurse and physician-to-physician communication is critical to safe care of high-risk patients. Research on early readmissions also points to the need for front-loading medical attention; getting specialist consultation as needed, either in person or via telemedicine; and focusing on goals of care [98].

Staff in hospitals and nursing facilities feel different pressures and have different perspectives on what is important and possible. When nursing facility staff performed structured root-cause analyses of unplanned 30-day readmissions using the INTERACT tool, they judged 13% to be avoidable, citing familiar reasons. Hospital-based physicians reviewing the same cases with the HOMERuN tool judged 30% to be avoidable [99]. The remarkable finding from this study was that the hospital physicians reported that the primary reason for half of the avoidable readmissions was either a missed diagnosis or inadequate treatment during the hospitalization. Standard care transition bundles will not eliminate diagnostic and treatment errors any more than they will eliminate surgical complications. Making the correct diagnosis can be challenging even in the hospital setting [100]. The challenges of diagnosis and treatment are even greater in the nursing facility setting; they necessitate expertise and resources proportionate to patient acuity if we expect to reduce avoidable transfers.

Partnerships Between Hospitals and Post-Acute Providers

The value of cross-setting readmission reviews with staff from different settings should be obvious. A prerequisite of such reviews—and real-time problem-solving, which is yet more valuable—is informal or formal partnership between the hospital and post-acute providers. Channeling patients to a limited number of home health agencies and nursing facilities through the use of either narrow-network contracts or suasion is an obvious first step toward effective partnership. An analysis of national Medicare data found that hospitals referring to fewer nursing facilities postsurgery had fewer readmissions [101]. Increasing the volume of referrals to a nursing facility by 10% resulted in a 4% decrease in readmissions. Lumbar spine surgery, coronary artery bypass, and hip fracture repair were particularly sensitive to this effect.

Common criteria used by hospitals in choosing nursing facility partners include clinical quality and satisfaction scores, readmission and length of stay performance, physician presence, time required for admission decisions, weekend admission potential, and niche competencies such as management of wounds, behavioral challenges, and palliative care [102, 103]. Criteria used in choosing home health partners are similar. Establishing highly functional relationships across the acute and post-acute divide takes time and a commitment to work through difficult clinical and contractual issues. Participants in the CMS bundled payment initiative have found this work to be fruitful [76]. Once the clinicians and managers begin to master the mental models of partnership across siloes, new creativity becomes possible. Hospitals with difficult-to-place patients, for instance, may find it worthwhile to pay for a nursing facility sitter or for a hotel stay following nursing facility discharge.

At the extreme, hospital-nursing facility partnerships can transform independent nursing facilities into the equivalent of medical-surgical units, as described in a report from the University of Michigan [104]. In this example, the ability to manage patients with postoperative solid organ transplants and left ventricular assist devices came with extra resource requirements, of course, including intensive presence of university physicians and nurse practitioners, an integrated health record, and adequate time for discussions about goals of care.

Newly Noticed Challenges and Opportunities

Until recently there has been very little recognition of adverse events following discharge from nursing facilities to home. One study of older patients discharging from nursing facilities found that 22% had emergency department visits or hospital admissions within 30 days, increasing to 38% within 90 days [105]. Another study found that 30% had hospital admissions within 30 days [106]. Among patients with end-stage renal disease, 43% had emergency department visits or hospital admissions within 30 days [107].

These volumes should not be surprising, given that there has been very little use of checklists or care transition bundles used for these discharges, and the usual deficit of information from hospital to primary care physician increases exponentially as nursing facility and home health are added to the equation. In 2016, professional organizations jointly published a minimal set of recommendations for nursing facility discharges, including appropriate communication and appointment-making with the primary care physician [108]. Pressure from both CMS and the commercial market is already leading to more robust interventions. Visits with a pharmacist in the nursing facility and then in the home, as mentioned above, can reduce hospital usage [37]. The transitional care clinic model, already popular following hospital discharge, has successfully been extended to nursing facility discharges [109].

The presence of a million people in US residential care facilities has also come to the attention of healthcare delivery systems. Hospitalization rates per year are 23.2% for long-stay nursing home residents and 23.9% for matched individuals in residential care facilities [110]. The opportunity for cost savings has prompted some systems to ensure a regular primary care presence in residential care. In one study, a dedicated primary care team dramatically reduced hospital and emergency department usage compared with control [111]. Additional interventions such as those discussed above in post-acute care are obviously appropriate. A federally funded trial to adapt the INTERACT program for assisted living is underway [112].

Home- and Community-Based Services to the Rescue

The most sustained and grievous oversight of healthcare delivery systems has been their neglect of home- and community-based services (HCBS). The Aging Network, coordinated by Area Agencies on Aging, provides services such as meals on wheels, transportation, home modifications, assistive technologies, and housing support. These and other services have operated as if in a foreign land, with shoestring funding and with scant research attention to clinical and financial outcomes. Even ACOs rarely have any meaningful collaboration with organizations delivering these services [113].

New requirements for hospital community needs assessments [114] and increasing recognition of social determinants of health are beginning to remedy this oversight. Some ACOs are partnering with schools and faith-based organizations to address population-based needs with hope of improving the ACO performance [115]. A survey of 32 ACOs in 2013–2014 found that half had formal processes for addressing patients' nonmedical needs [116]. Partners included public health agencies, churches, community centers, food banks, and fitness centers. Two of the ACOs placed HCBS representatives on the ACO governing board. Coming from the other direction, organizations with HCBS expertise have partnered with delivery systems under both fee-for-service and capitated contracts [117].

For the delivery systems, these contracts are no longer in the realm of charity funding but are executed with expectations of return. The administrative and measurement infrastructure for understanding those returns and ensuring accountability, however, is still lacking. The National Quality Forum has created a framework for measuring HCBS processes and outcomes in a broad array of domains that encompass well-being, independence, social connectedness, caregiver support, and service effectiveness [118].

Primary Care for High-Need Elders

At some point your needs assessment—and savings opportunities—will point beyond the programs and sites of care that we've discussed so far. It is abundantly clear that there are groups of patients living at home whose needs overwhelm the capabilities of traditional primary care practices. Indeed, for some their needs will overwhelm even high-performance patient-centered medical homes enhanced by electronic decision support, case management, and one or more HCBS organizations. The challenge for your organization is identifying those patients and matching them with resources that will yield benefit.

As of 2017 there are hundreds of organizations trying to figure out how to meet this challenge. About two dozen more-or-less distinct models have emerged in the literature with names that are likely familiar, e.g., PACE (Programs of All-Inclusive Care for the Elderly), GRACE (Geriatric Resources for Assessment and Care of Elders), Guided Care, and CareMore. Readily available overviews describe the target populations and program characteristics [119, 120], and the Commonwealth Fund has sponsored multiple detailed case studies that you may find useful, so I will not dwell here long.

PACE, the oldest US model serving frail elders, has set the gold standard for interdisciplinary team-based care for four decades. The newest program to receive federal blessing is Independence at Home. Its predecessor was the Home-Based Primary Care program of the US Department of Veterans Affairs, which offered ongoing team-based primary care in the home to high-risk, high-need patients who were not necessarily home bound. Based on the success of this program, the Congress passed legislation sponsoring a demonstration project [121]. The program targets patients with multiple chronic conditions and functional limitations who have had hospital and post-acute care within the last year. In the MedStar Washington Hospital Center House Call Program, physicians made same-day urgent home visits as needed and followed patients into the hospital; costs over 2 years were 17% lower than controls, with 9% fewer hospital admissions and 27% fewer nursing facility days [122]. In year 1 the national demonstration saved an average of $3070 per patient, and in year 2 it saved $1010 per patient [123]. Quality scores have been high. The US Senate Committee on Finance Bipartisan Chronic Care Working Group enthusiastically recommended extension of the demonstration [124].

Whether replicating a standard model or developing a new approach for high-need, high-cost patients, it would help to know the core principles that are critical for success. For PACE, these include medication management, advance care planning and palliative care, prompt response to clinical red flags, patient and caregiver support, and care coordination [125]. A survey of 45 diverse programs highlighted the following key processes: targeting high-need, high-cost patients likely to benefit from the program; adapting to the local environment and evolving over time; providing the structure and time to support rich, generally face-to-face interactions and relationships among clinicians and with patients; assembling the right staff personalities and skill sets; encouraging disseminated leadership; reducing physician workload; providing timely, actionable data to the care team; and attending to care transitions [126]. Your success is likely to turn on whether your program can embody these principles, whether or not you are developing programs within prescribed regulatory constraints.

Overlapping Populations with Complex and Serious Illness

Many of the high-need, high-cost patients we have been discussing are living out the last chapters of their lives, but many are not. It is important to understand the degree of overlap across your chronic and terminal populations, since this overlap will have clinical and financial implications. The 2-year mortality of Medicare homebound patients is 40%; for semi-homebound patients it is 21% [127]. Fully half of Medicare patients are homebound in the last year of their lives, making it difficult if not impossible to get adequate care in primary care offices. Mortality in the MedStar

House Call Program was 40% over 2 years. We have ample evidence of cost savings from programs designed both as home-based primary care [128] and as home-based palliative care [49].

Just as these patient populations overlap, there is also significant overlap of geriatric and palliative care principles. The commonalities include interprofessional teams focused on patients' individual goals of care and biopsychosocial needs, as well as robust caregiver support [129]. As an advocate for the care of older adults in your delivery system, this overlap of needs and principles is more a blessing than a problem. Your decision to pursue new program development using a geriatric versus palliative care model—or both—will likely turn on the clinical resources that you already have in place, your alliances, and your potential new sources of support. Palliative care programs, of course, include younger populations; 29% of Medicare hospice users are under 65 [73]. As discussed above, program nomenclature can be age specific or neutral.

Home-based programs for high-need, high-cost patients need staff with both geriatric and palliative care competencies in order to achieve program quality and efficiency standards [130]. Assembling staff with this breadth of skill sets is a nontrivial challenge. Hospice professionals, for instance, may not be comfortable with advance care planning for chronically ill but nonterminal patients. Teams are likely to benefit from extra training and tools to address symptoms such as breathlessness, which is common across these populations and which is a key driver of hospital utilization [131, 132].

Data as *Sine Qua Non* of Survival and Accountability

Your success in advocating for the full array of geriatric services and for improvement of those services will depend upon your ability to demonstrate clinical need and financial value based on data from your information systems. Advocates need good patient stories and good data in order to catalyze change in their delivery systems. Healthcare delivery systems are increasingly strained for resources, and services for older adults are typically resource intensive, so even the most successful programs are subject to budgetary review and potential reduction.

Budgetary battles are complicated by the ever-present reality that different components of your delivery system variably contribute to and reap the benefits of resource-intensive programs. A provider's program investment may reduce the total cost of care and yield an impressive ROI, but all too often the benefits accrue to health plan or payer. For example, even when a medical group's programs for high-need, high-cost patients are effective, the group may bear considerable costs without adequate benefit from shared savings. A related dynamic occurs when hospitals invest in improving care transitions; the total cost of care may fall, but even in many ACOs, the hospitals themselves lose topline admission revenue that far exceeds their readmission penalties. These disconnects and contradictions are obvious when the ACO is based upon multi-organizational collaborations, but they are also present and troublesome across the intraorganizational divisions and departments of integrated delivery systems such as Kaiser.

The challenge for eldercare advocates is demonstrating value to executive decision-makers of the delivery system as a whole. This value may take the form of straightforward financial ROI, but it can also take the form of clinical performance scores that can yield increased market share because of public reporting [11]. Demonstrating value is easier when one has access to good data and analytics; your ability to develop and sustain geriatric programs may depend upon your ability to obtain and present credible data on clinical and financial performance. If you do not have informatics or business intelligence staff dedicated to your programs, then you would be advised to make good friends in those departments.

Your clinical priorities should be informed by the available data from your own delivery system, by the literature, and by your knowledge of other systems. Keeping an open mind, i.e., avoiding premature closure regarding the nature of your challenges, will be easier if you ask open-ended questions such as *What's going on?* Strategic thinking, like Shewhart quality plan-do-study-act (PDSA) improvement efforts, should be cyclical, so follow-up questions include *Is there a need for intervention?*, *How will we know if an intervention works?*, *Did the intervention work?*, and then back to *What's going on?*

These questions can be directed to any component of the triple aim (health status, cost, experience). Answering the questions depends upon your ability to access data for specific patient populations (clinical condition, age category), delivery system components (site of care, discipline, program), and business groups (Medicare Advantage, fee-for-service ACO), at any level of granularity (system, region, practice, physician). The process of asking questions and gathering data itself requires time and resources; your knowledge of the literature and other systems will increase the likelihood of high-payoff queries. Analyses will often replicate what can be found in the published literature, but decision-makers are much more likely to be swayed when confronted with patient experiences and costs from their own system. Additional issues concerning measurement are addressed in the appendix to this chapter.

Targeting Patients for High-Touch Interventions

The good news is that we have made significant headway in understanding how to match services to high-need, high-cost patients who can benefit from those services. The first lesson learned was that many high-cost patients do not remain high-need or high-cost from year to year, so targeting a group that recently incurred high costs will not necessarily generate savings or clinical benefit. A series of CMS care management demonstration projects floundered because they could not generate sufficient savings to overcome this regression-to-the-mean phenomenon [133].

Studies of "super-utilizers" reflect the same phenomenon. Patients with a run of emergency department visits and admissions are likely to settle down without specialized care management intervention. A Denver Health study found that over half of the super-utilizers were no longer super-utilizers after 7 months and 72% were no longer super-utilizers after 12 months [134]. A study of Medicare fee-for-service patients found that 1% were super-utilizers, responsible for 11% of costs, but this was a heterogeneous group resistant to standardized intervention [135]. Clustering patients into smaller, more clinically coherent categories was more promising. The challenge in financial terms is to identify low-cost patients who will soon become high-cost and who are amenable to your interventions. If you have limited high-touch, high-cost resources, you would be advised not to spend them in whack-a-mole fashion based solely on retrospective cost experience.

The second lesson is that many high-touch interventions generate savings only from the highest-risk tier of patients. The MedStar Washington Hospital Center House Calls Program discussed above achieved savings only in the highest frailty category [122]. A similar pattern emerged from the Department of Veterans Affairs Home-Based Primary Care program [128]. The Washington University Medicare Coordinated Care Demonstration achieved its entire overall savings from the highest acuity patients. In this program, care managers used high-touch processes, including face-to-face meetings, in order to form trusting relationships with high-risk patients; lower risk patients were served by less-expensive care manager assistants [136].

A useful survey of 17 industry-leading delivery systems found that these systems were using a variety of approaches to identify high-risk patients who could benefit from care management [137]. Claims-based predictive models can be purchased off-the-shelf or derived from one's own data using split derivation and validation samples. The LACE index is a non-claims tool derived from clinical data (length of stay, acuity, comorbidity, emergency department utilization) that predicts readmission [138]. One organization cited in the survey segmented high-risk patients by diagnoses well known to be high cost, such as chronic kidney disease, but also focused on patients with nonspecific symptom diagnoses such as syncope and abdominal pain, since those patients are likely to return for more care.

Most organizations allow for clinician referral to care management of patients who are not automatically identified. Some use a formal process of presenting an algorithmically generated list to physicians who then identify patients most amenable to intervention. With modest instructions, physicians can distinguish high-risk patients who are likely versus unlikely to benefit from care management [139]. Physicians take into account patient factors such as literacy, home environment, insight, coping skills, and financial resources [140]. Physicians can also identify highly activated patients who may not need assistance because they are already managing their chronic conditions well.

Organizations that enlist clinicians into the process of developing predictive models may be able to automate some of the clinicians' insights and thereby exclude patients who are unlikely to benefit from care management [141]. Denver Health has described its iterative process of incorporating clinical feedback into model development so as to enable actionable risk stratification at the point of care [142]. The risk stratification process can be enhanced to indicate not merely who is likely to benefit from intervention, but also which intervention is most likely to help.

An unfortunate current reality is that functional assessment is notable for its absence in most electronic health records. Functional status outperforms demographics and clinical conditions in predicting hospital readmission from rehabilitation settings [127, 143]. The combination of functional status and clinical conditions effectively predicts likelihood of hospitalization, costs, and mortality among older adults [144]. In particular, this combination identifies seriously ill older adults, while there is still time to intervene rather than just prior to end of life. Kaiser Permanente used proxy measures, such as the use of a hospital bed at home, to enrich its Senior Segmentation Algorithm. This algorithm yielded four groups: robust seniors, those with one or more chronic conditions, those with advanced illness and end-organ failure, and those with advanced frailty or at end of life. Mortality in this last group was 50% in 2 years [145]. Recent receipt of assistive devices can also serve as a proxy for function.

More Caveats, Cautions, and Hope

Many medical and engineering challenges, such as determining the optimal dose of antibiotic or launching a satellite, are complicated but solvable. "Wicked problems," on the other hand, are those that "defy efforts to delineate their boundaries and to identify their causes," so their "would-be solutions are confounded by a still further set of dilemmas posed by the growing pluralism of the contemporary publics, whose valuations… are judged against an array of different and contradicting scales" [146]. There are plentiful wicked problems regarding healthcare services and performance accountability, but I will touch on only several that are most pertinent in this context: the challenges of care planning, competencies and workforce, and disparities.

The Challenges of Care Planning and Care Plans

The foundation of Joanne Lynn's vision for the reorganization of frail eldercare is the care plan, and her manual for reform [147] elaborates on many of the elements shown in Fig. 6.5. Similarly, The SCAN Foundation's essential attributes for eldercare systems begin with identification of a patient's needs and goals, which must be operationalized within a "cohesive, easily navigable delivery system" that is responsive to patient, family, and caregiver input [8].

The foundation of care planning is good patient assessment. With a modicum of process redesign, geriatric assessment tools can be deployed in primary care offices [149, 150]. CMS reimbursement for annual wellness visits has been a boon to eldercare advocates in many systems, although meaningful adoption of this intervention is not yet widespread [151]. As is obvious from Fig. 6.5, however, care planning is inherently complex, requiring iterative attention to the intricate interplay of multiple factors, including the patient's situation, values, preferences, and goals. Care planning for an older adult with multiple chronic conditions and an evolving social situation can be challenging even for a high-functioning interdisciplinary team and is far beyond what an isolated primary care physician can do. In particular, as per

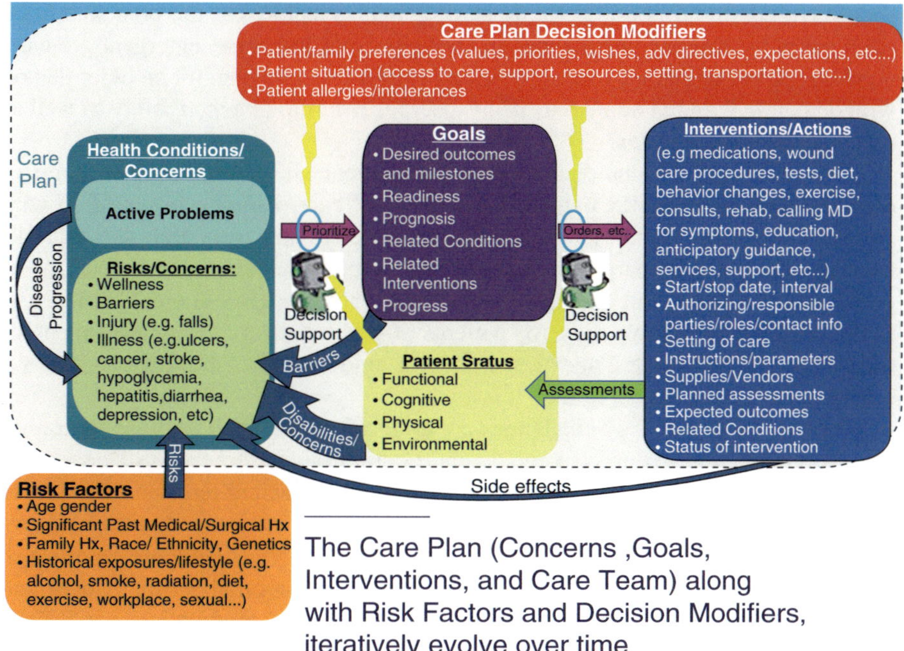

Fig. 6.5 How a meaningful care plan emerges and evolves [148]

Dr. Lynn's understatement, "It turns out that articulation of preferences and goals is an underdeveloped art form."

In the setting of PACE or a geriatric home care program, an interdisciplinary team can get to know patients well enough and have enough time to develop a finely tuned plan and adapt it as needed. A POLST form or a hospital discharge plan, while important, is obviously only a piece of the picture. To be fair to the clinicians struggling to integrate all these separate pieces, however, we should acknowledge that care planning has been fraught with challenges, the most obvious of which are terminology, time, and technology.

One analysis addressed the terminology challenge by deriving a typology of care plans and care planning based on such factors as whether the perspective taken is that of patient or provider, whether the focus is on goals or behaviors, and whether the plan involves one or many disciplines [152]. The appropriate type of plan will vary by condition and setting. An asthma care plan will include instructions for specific medication adjustments based on peak flows. A diabetes care plan may focus on goals related to self-efficacy. In nursing facilities or assisted living, a care plan may need to include a pocket card for unlicensed aides with instructions regarding how to manage a particular resident's difficult behaviors on the evening shift. An awareness of diversity within the care plan typology can help prevent us from believing that care plans can be all things to all people. Muriel Gillick has advised that care plans should focus on foreseeable problems: "Specifying exactly what should happen in all possible circumstances is impossible, but the plan should be sufficiently precise to guide the patient, caregiver, visiting nurse, emergency department physician, or primary care physician" [153]. The care plan for an older person with dementia living at home may need specifics regarding kitchen safety as well as a POLST for emergencies.

Time poses an obvious challenge to development of comprehensive, iterative care planning for complex patients. One study of care planning for children with chronic conditions found that creation of an effective care plan took 4–6 h [154]. Getting an interdisciplinary team to sit around a table (whether real or virtual), compare notes and ideas, and document a comprehensive plan is a clinical luxury. It is likely to be cost-effective only for patients at highest risk of incurring expensive care. Fortunately, as noted above, we do have evidence of cost-effectiveness for a number of high-touch programs.

Many of the technology challenges are all too familiar, such as those stemming from fragmentation in our systems. A report commissioned by the US Department of Health and Human Services found that providers in long-term and post-acute care "have important information that is generally not exchanged, such as functional and cognitive status, potential risks (e.g., fall history), elder abuse reports, use of services such as DME and homemakers, and information about the patient and family/caregivers that may be relevant to care" [155]. A comprehensive RAND report, however, found that the technical challenges of care planning go deeper than fragmentation alone [156]. Confusion regarding the definition of a care plan, as just discussed, gets reflected in information technology. Developers are also hampered by the lack of definition for a "team member." Who exactly is on the care team, and how does the team composition change over time? And what are the rules regarding who can change a care plan? Developers at proprietary software companies have had to make a multitude of decisions in the absence of clinical standards, so providers should take appropriate cautions in their purchasing decisions.

Finally, clinicians should be cautious about how much to rely on care plan decisions made in advance of current circumstances. In addition, while protocols, guidelines, and best practices are valuable, clinicians should remember that evidence-based medicine for older adults rests on a very thin base. Uncertainty abounds, so evidence should be combined with expertise based on experience. In particular, team members often bring invaluable expertise in the form of tacit knowledge and intuition [157]. And as discussed in the context of readmission reduction efforts, they will benefit from encouragement to improvise solutions as needed, navigating uncertainty with all the creativity they can muster [70]. The care planning process should be shaped so as to support competent and caring decisions made in the context of trusting relationships.

Prospects for Adequate Competencies and Workforce

The shortage of clinicians with specialized training in the care of older adults is well known and needs little elaboration here. The three recommendations made by the Institute of Medicine are pertinent at the delivery system level as well [158]. First, delivery systems must aggressively recruit clinicians with geriatric competencies in order to increase supply within the system. Second, in light of the shortage, it is imperative that systems invest in training and tools to enhance the skills and performance of the current workforce. And third, systems should redesign the models of care for older adults, as discussed above, particularly in ways that engage patients and caregivers as active partners in the care process.

Delivery systems interested in improving performance for high-need, high-cost populations will need to craft strategies for enhanced training of their nurses, physicians, pharmacists, and other clinicians managing these patients. Fortunately, considerable progress has been made in defining the core competencies needed within the disciplines serving older adults. Competency sets that have been formally approved by national organizations are gathered on the website of the American Geriatrics Society [159]. The American Academy of Home Care Medicine has also defined the requisite competencies of home care clinicians [160]. Competency gaps in your own delivery system will show up in reviews of avoidable readmissions and other adverse outcomes. Evidence from a comprehensive Veterans Affairs training program suggests that these gaps can be closed, with the added benefit of increasing job satisfaction among participating physicians, nurse practitioners, physician assistants, pharmacists, psychologists, and social workers [161]. Less-intensive office-based education for community physicians is a viable alternative strategy for closing the gaps related to geriatric syndromes, especially if educators can form collaborative alliances with key staff in the physician offices [162]. Excellent web-based educational resources are also available [163].

The movement toward accountable care, with its incentives for cost-effective population management, may propel reform of antiquated scope-of-practice restrictions and thus optimize the use of high-cost clinicians [164]. It may also prompt reform of regulations and payment models that contribute to rote, task-dominated mindsets of clinicians treating older adults. To take just one example, nursing facilities have traditionally engaged pharmacists to perform only the minimal work required by CMS regulation. Pharmacists have been virtually absent in the work of home health agencies, which are not required to offer their services, although that may change with increasing evidence of their effectiveness in reducing ED visits and hospitalizations [87]. Delivery systems should be aware, however, that an effort to develop new models of team-based care and redesign work roles will almost certainly provoke resistance among the professions, reducing the potential for savings [165]. One is advised to proceed with caution to avoid triggering unnecessary professional turf wars.

There is no controversy regarding the need for delivery systems to improve the performance and prospects of the nonprofessional workforce currently serving older adults. Nursing assistants are a core part of workflows that have made the INTERACT program successful in reducing transfers from nursing facility to hospital, as discussed above [95]. Even a brief training for nursing assistants can yield reductions in pressure ulcer development [166]. Although the demand for unlicensed direct care workers in long-term care facilities and home settings is growing, their wages have been stagnant, recruitment is often challenging, and the high turnover is costly to organizations. Exemplary programs have begun to respond by developing enhanced training and job lattices for these workers [167].

The most exciting recent workforce development is the integration of new lay health worker roles into care teams. Lay care guides can improve quality measures in primary care offices by leveraging their face-to-face relationships with both patients and physicians [168]. Lay health workers can be trained to identify household safety hazards of vulnerable elders [169]. Lay health workers can also successfully conduct advance care planning conversations in the home. Community health workers in Indiana University Center for Aging Research's Aging Brain Care (ABC) Program were able to increase documentation of advance care planning by an order of magnitude [170]. In the process they reduced hospitalizations and ED visits of older patients with dementia and other chronic conditions. Based upon these results, the Indiana University healthcare delivery system has agreed to fund community health worker positions. Tools are now available to assist systems in recruiting staff with appropriate skills for these positions, including the ability to express caring and empathy [171]. Only a few of our geriatric and palliative care models of care have optimized the use of lay health workers within their team-based workflows. Doing so holds the promise of significant improvements in costs and efficiency.

Disparities, *Quo Vadis*?

It is yet unclear whether the movement toward accountable care will decrease healthcare disparities. ACOs can improve the quality of care, but physicians practicing in zip code areas with high concentrations of poverty, disability, black race, and low educational levels are less likely to participate in ACOs [172]. If this pattern persists, disadvantaged populations could be differentially left behind. This dynamic may well be accelerated in post-acute care. We know that Medicare and Medicaid dual-eligible patients are more likely to be discharged from hospitals to nursing facilities with lower nurse staffing, longer lengths of stay, and lower rates of discharge back to the community [173]. Obese patients are also more likely to be sent to lower-quality nursing facilities [174]. Finally, nurse and nursing assistant staffing is lower in nursing facilities with higher concentrations of minority residents [175]. In light of that background, what will be the consequences of the tighter hospital-nursing facility partnerships that we discussed earlier as one of the imperatives of accountable care? Hospitals are choosing to partner with higher-quality facilities, channeling high-reimbursement patients away from lower-quality to higher-quality facilities, and in some cases directly investing resources in those higher-quality facilities. Resource-poor organizations caring for minority patients are likely to become yet more resource-poor.

On a brighter note, the community health workers just discussed are typically more culturally aligned with the patients they serve than are the physicians and other professionals. Indeed, this alignment is part of what makes them effective. As delivery systems achieve more integration, these community health workers can serve as boundary spanners across healthcare and social service organizations [176]. Health status disparities among older populations are persistent and in some respects worsening [177], but interventions outside the healthcare system itself can address social determinants of health and thus reduce disparities [178]. Some delivery systems are well into a journey that goes beyond the formal healthcare borders and into the community. Kaiser Permanente began producing equitable care reports in 2009, invested in geographically enriched sociodemographic data systems, and launched its Equitable Care Health Outcomes (ECHO) Program with leadership at all levels of the organization [179]. One of its projects systematically and proactively identifies the unmet social needs of high-risk patients and connects them to community services [180].

Steering Clear of Implementation Failure in Healthcare

Organizations trying to replicate interventions that proved successful elsewhere sometimes fail. Indeed, we often fail, even though the interventions may be "evidence based." In some cases, the original evidence derived from settings of unmitigated fragmentation, so there was plenty of low-hanging fruit to be had via any reasonably executed improvement effort. You may not have an abundance of low-hanging fruit in your setting. In some cases, we lack adequate knowledge of the requisite execution strategy, rather like having only the ingredient list of a plum pudding recipe. In some cases, the failure is due to unstated or unknown differences in culture or context. An organization's ability to innovate often depends upon informal, tacit relational contracts between administrators, clinicians, and lower managerial staff. These relational contracts, in turn, depend upon credibility, trust, and clarity of roles and tasks [181]. Finally, we often under-resource the development phase, which tends to be under-described in the original reports. Just-do-it approaches can work, but only in good weather with favorable winds. Starting out with an inexperienced crew, uninformed management, and meager analytics will likely yield suboptimal adaptation and eventual disappointment. Rather than encouraging blind optimism, leaders should ask early on, "If this fails, what will have been the most likely causes?" The answers from all those involved may be surprising, and at least some of the risk factors may be remediable.

Thoughtful reports about replication failures are worthy of close attention. For example, in the years 2002–2010, the care management program of Health Quality Partners significantly reduced hospitalizations and costs for its high-risk Medicare patients. In this program, 60% of the contacts between patients and nurse care managers were face to face, occurring in patient homes, physician offices, and inpatient settings, and guided by individualized care plans, with particular attention to care transitions. The replication phase in the years 2010–2014 failed to reduce hospitalizations and costs compared to controls, however, probably because the usual care for this control group had improved over time, making it difficult to show improvement with the intervention [182].

In a Canadian intervention that used now-standard care transition processes, the dedicated transition nurses in the hospital handed off to rapid response nurses who made home visits, reconciled medications, devised care plans, provided self-management support, and referred patients to chronic disease clinics. The intervention failed to yield reductions in facility utilization, however, in part due to lack of role clarity, communication, and trust between the inpatient and outpatient nurses, in part due to lack of attention to advance care planning and appropriate pathways for the frailest patients [183]. The researchers noted that appropriate investment in relational coordination [184], feedback loops, and pathway adaptations could potentially address these deficiencies.

We could save ourselves considerable grief by attending to richly detailed descriptions of program implementation and evolution. One example is found in the Kaiser Permanente readmission papers discussed above, which offer ample particulars and insights. Yet more detailed is the evolution story of the practice-based Care Management Program at Massachusetts General Hospital, which moved from its original CMS demonstration phase to an ACO model with a disciplined focus on patient targeting and assessment, physician engagement, behavioral health, and advance care planning [185].

To assist organizations with program replication, the Centers for Disease Control and Prevention has developed a framework that highlights the critical preconditions and the pre-implementation, implementation, and maintenance factors for success. A version of this framework proved helpful in adapting a Veterans Affairs care transitions program to a non-VA setting, with significant reductions in the cost of care [186].

As discussed in relation to the STARR readmission initiative, however, an unpropitious culture and half-hearted leadership can sink replication of the best of best practices. The scholarship on learning organizations is particularly pertinent to ACOs, which need spirited collaboration within and across organizations in order to change deeply ingrained work practices. The demand for performance should be balanced with explicit support for a learning perspective and tolerance for a learning curve [187]. In the STARR experience, the hospitals that succeeded were those that supported trial-and-error learning of teams implementing new readmission reduction processes [69]. The inherent uncertainty of improvement efforts in complex environments calls for leadership generously enriched with humility and for ongoing give-and-take among participants. New programs merit "peripartum monitoring" with the best quantitative and qualitative data one can muster, but established programs need routine evaluation as well. Washington University has offered a good example of lessons learned after their care coordination program failed to reduce hospitalizations or cost; a subsequent wholesale redesign with more face-to-face contacts reduced hospitalizations by 12% and monthly Medicare costs by $217 per patient [136]. The pertinent advice from *To Err Is Human* is "It's more helpful to think like a farmer than an engineer or architect in designing a health care system" [188].

Unchartered Territories

As healthcare boundaries expand outward beyond hospital and clinic into the community, encompassing socioeconomic determinants of health, the landscape of several medical disciplines becomes less familiar. New challenges arise, for instance with regard to patient safety, and we more frequently bump into ethical questions without obvious answers. But we also meet people beyond the traditional healthcare sector who share our commitment to community well-being. Partnering with these stakeholders may make it possible for us to get closer to our newly perceived goals.

Navigating to Safety

When healthcare professionals venture beyond inpatient and clinic walls into the community, they must negotiate for their very presence with patients and caregivers. Here the rules of the game dictate expectations for performance reliability and patient safety that are different from those found in hospitals. Hospitals have been seen as the most challenging settings of care, requiring the finest skill sets and commanding the greatest prestige and rewards, but many of the care processes there are truly evidence based and bolstered by an array of team and management supports, whereas a clinician in the home is often very much on her own. Even in hospitals, there is increasing recognition that patient safety depends on staff attributes such as emotional commitment and respectful interactions [189]. In the home setting, achieving desired outcomes is supremely dependent upon clinicians' interpersonal and technical skills, exquisite attention to early signals of trouble, and tolerance of uncertainty. Evidence-based protocols apply to blood transfusions but not necessarily to decisions such as when and whether to insist on modification of fall risks in the home environment.

Charles Vincent and René Amalberti have pointed out that "as more types of harm have come to be regarded as preventable, the perimeter of patient safety has expanded" [190]. We once viewed hospital admissions caused by an adverse drug reaction or fall at home as regrettable, but not within our particular sphere of influence. Now, because we are part of a system with population health accountability, we are being held responsible for these unfortunate events, and our clinical teams are struggling to improve patient safety in the home.

Meanwhile patients and caregivers are also experiencing dramatic new realities. Elderly patients with multiple chronic conditions find themselves at home within hours of ambulatory surgery, with or without caregivers, faced with the challenges of wound dressings and postoperative medications. Following through on care plans is often harder than we or patients or caregivers want to admit. Vincent and Amalberti go on to say, "Family and other unpaid caregivers often make promises out of love and a sense of responsibility to keep the client at home, without being aware that this may be beyond their capacity." A large study of patients who refused post-acute care services found that their 30-day and 60-day readmission rates were twice as high as the group accepting services even though the refusing group was younger, healthier, and better educated [191]. As discussed earlier, one of our new challenges is developing effective ways to improve patients' self-management support; we also need to improve our ability to get patients to accept our help, which in turn depends upon our success in establishing trusting relationships. Thoughtfully integrating patients into governance and redesign teams can dramatically enhance providers' appreciation of patient needs and improve intervention effectiveness [192].

Unfortunately, our initiatives to improve patient safety in the home come with a price tag that unsettles decision-makers. An expensive new medication or operative technology is usually approved as soon as we have evidence of superior outcomes—or even prior to such evidence—regardless of the cost; our high-touch interventions in the home, however, face a much steeper budgetary climb even after they have been found to be clinically and financially effective. Advocates for older adults should be quick to point out this discrepancy, but we should also acknowledge that our organizations are staring cost calamity in the face. Other industries have put the tradeoff between cost and safety out on the table and developed guidelines for how much risk is tolerable [193]. In ambulatory care and home settings, we need to get better at articulating the spectrum of risk consequences (from small to catastrophic), matrixing with the frequency of occurrence (from rare to frequent), and then calculating the cost of risk mitigation. Meanwhile we should be sensitive to the burden of responsibility being felt by patients, caregivers, and our clinical teams as they attempt to prevent mishaps and disasters.

Ethics and Value

What's new in accountable care is our explicit commitment to value, generally conceived as healthcare quality divided by cost, and to the triple aim concept, which aspires to integrate patient experience, quality outcomes, and efficiency. To date we have been less explicit about the moral questions and contradictions inherent in this bundle of aspirations.

As human beings we swim in a sea of moral values; indeed, we cannot imagine otherwise. In healthcare we have developed ways of thinking and behaving that enable us to swim past most of the ethical dilemmas that emerge around us every day, when principles such as autonomy, beneficence, and justice come into tension. As we increasingly move care for high-risk, high-cost patients into the home, a number of ethical issues become accentuated anew. Self-management support, for example, raises questions about the impact of patient autonomy on our ability to do good (beneficence) and the availability of high-touch programs (justice). Routines for managing such issues are far less established in community settings than in the hospital, and clinicians working in community settings have far less support for even raising such questions.

Our new focus on analytical prediction models for identifying high-risk patients also raises new questions. The overlap between clinical benefit and cost-effectiveness is not perfect; that is, some interventions would yield meaningful benefit for patients but not yield financial savings. Even where the clinical and financial incentives overlap, someone must still decide where to set the cut point for the targeted population. Should we target patients who are likely to receive only modest benefit if the financial impact is only breakeven? Our advanced analytics do not magically resolve this question, which is hardly an esoteric concern to clinicians on the front lines [194].

Accountable care raises yet more practical questions. With rising costs and a growing sense of austerity, we are under increasing pressure to perform early and ongoing assessments of our new clinical programs. Even our long-established programs and practices merit examination. Perhaps the core question to ask is *Does this healthcare activity (or program, service) add value?* One can ask whether an activity adds value from several perspectives, however. For example:

- Does it benefit the patient in a meaningful way?
- Does it benefit my delivery system as a whole? My component of the delivery system?
- Is the benefit worth the cost? Does it involve other burdens or risk?
- Would other patients benefit more?

These questions should be encouraged at every level of the delivery system. Just as hospitals that encourage trial-and-error learning are more likely to be high performing, I suspect that delivery systems capable of engaging such questions will also be more likely to succeed in the new world of accountable care. A companion question is *whether there might be an altogether different process or provider that could more efficiently achieve the goal of this activity.* It would be naïve, however, to expect entrenched clinicians and managers to engage with enthusiasm in creative destruction of their own care practices or livelihoods. Transformation in healthcare is indeed hard, so systems need to invest in change management; mitigation measures may be appropriate.

Institutional Logics, both Aligned and at Odds

Elizabeth Goodrick and Trish Reay have pointed out that the triple aim—defined as improving patient experience (including quality and satisfaction), improving the health of populations, and reducing costs—maps roughly onto the "logic" of profession, government (the state), and market, that is, the individual and organizational guide to thought and behavior for each of these entities [195]. Professionals are charged with quality and patient experience, the government with overall population health, and the market with cost-effectiveness. The mapping is obviously not exact. Market forces, for instance, are indeed associated with costs and incentives for reducing cost, but patient experience also drives market share. Similarly, government is concerned with both population health and costs.

In spite of these imperfect mappings, research using the institutional logics model can elucidate the contradictory challenges of ACOs. A leading concern is whether physicians will embrace or reject the need to reduce costs and what organizations can do to achieve a modicum of harmony. An extended longitudinal study in Alberta, Canada, followed the medical profession's response to the provincial government's 1994 initiation of businesslike healthcare. Physicians tenaciously insisted on their control of medical decisions and quality, resulting in an "uneasy truce" between the logic of businesslike healthcare and the logic of medical professionalism. Over time, however, both parties settled into an acceptance of pragmatic coexistence in which the two logics were held in creative tension. Goodrick and Reay suggest that delivery systems should advance via thoughtful and pragmatic introduction of new practices that are respectful of professional, government, and market logics.

This trio of logics can also map to professional association, government agency, and trade association. Many of us in healthcare have some connection to all three and perhaps even to multiple professional and trade associations and government agencies. These entities operate at one level up from the delivery system itself, and each of these tends to embody a single dominant logic in fierce unfettered fashion. Advocates for the common good of care for older adults may find themselves disheartened by the sometimes short-sighted self-interest on display in policy disputes. It can be helpful to remember that each of these entities espouses support for an ideal of high-quality healthcare for all, to remind them of that stated mission, and to rejoice when they collaborate creatively for a common purpose.

Toward a Community Vision for Accountable Care

My focus throughout this guide has been on organizing for improvements in care for high-need, high-cost older patients within healthcare delivery systems. In all but the most rural of areas, however, each healthcare delivery system shares an ecosystem with other healthcare delivery systems; this ecosystem is itself embedded in a broader community of organizations (business, government, education) that have an impact upon population health status. Community-based intersectoral initiatives across healthcare delivery systems are now an area of intense interest, both because they promise to help us achieve the triple aim and because achieving the triple aim may be impossible without community collaboration. Alert advocates for older patients may be able to hitch a valuable ride on such initiatives—or perhaps even initiate one yourself.

If you are extremely fortunate, you live in a community with a history of community-wide healthcare organizing. In San Diego, for example, the Right Care Initiative prompted delivery system leaders in 2010 to begin joint efforts toward reduction of heart attacks and strokes, and they began pooling patient-level data in 2012 [196]. The commitment to community well-being prevailed over narrow competitive interests, and the data helped create momentum for clinical practice change within and across the participating organizations. Early results suggest that San Diego has far surpassed the rest of California in reducing heart attacks.

Advance care planning has been a frequent focus of community-wide organizing efforts since the success of the effort in La Crosse County, Wisconsin [197]. In Oregon and elsewhere, limitations specified within electronic POLST registries have led to markedly less hospitalization at end of life [198]. Creation of POLST registries requires operational and political collaboration across delivery systems. It is not an accident that the counties chosen for ePOLST pilots in California were San Diego, with the history just noted, and Contra Costa, where the local medical association has long supported cross-system collaboration for improved end-of-life care [199].

What delivery system leaders have not fully appreciated, in spite of extraordinary costs, is how much they are dependent upon a shared ecosystem for post-acute and long-term care services and supports, as illustrated in Fig. 6.6. This entire ecosystem has been hampered by low expectations, regulatory mindsets, and a lack of workforce incentives; the result has been a kind of persistent ebb tide lowering all

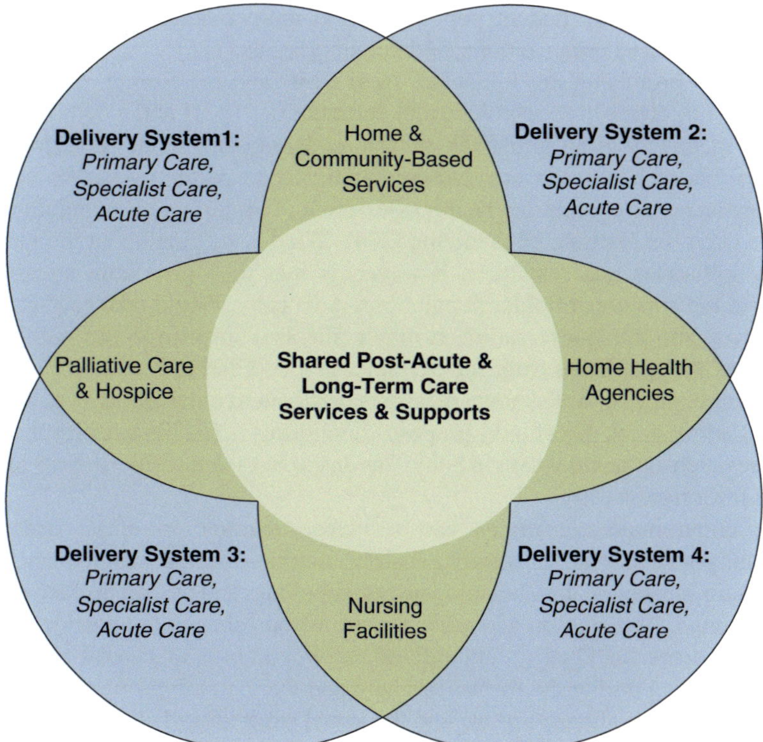

Fig. 6.6 The post-acute and long-term care ecosystem. Some delivery systems have their own post-acute programs, but none are entirely self-contained

boats. Some delivery systems have their own post-acute programs, e.g., home health and hospice agencies or home-based medical care. Even the most integrated systems, however, require services beyond their organization; most systems acquire post-acute services via arm's-length contracting [200]. Standards for staffing, training, and performance tend to be uniformly low and shared by all delivery systems within the community.

As noted earlier, some delivery systems are developing specific post-acute partnerships, but as yet there has been little collaboration across delivery systems with regard to the post-acute and long-term care ecosystem. The same is true for community-based interventions in general. A 2015–2016 survey of hospital-based ACOs revealed a disconnect between the espoused mission, vision, and values of ACOs on the one hand and activities directed toward improving the overall health of the community on the other; meaningful collaboration even with their own community benefit departments was rare [113]. Promising exceptions were noted, however. A few ACOs have stepped up efforts to organize community resources for patients with mental illness and substance use issues. Another study of private-sector ACOs found that all were involved in at least some initiatives beyond caring for their own specific patient population; the more mature were engaged with schools, faith-based organizations, and neighborhoods [115].

Yet more promising are initiatives from CMS and the Robert Wood Johnson Foundation to create accountable health communities [201] and a culture of health [202], respectively. Both initiatives go beyond the medical model to address social determinants of health via creative community-wide partnerships. We now have new approaches to community health assessment [114, 203], plus population health metrics from the Institute of Medicine [204]. What is striking about the new community initiatives and resources, however, is that they give little attention—or none—to the concerns of older populations. Advocates should take heed and insert themselves into this conversation. It may come as a surprise to our public health colleagues that palliative care, for example, is a population health issue [205]. In addition to deploying well-known measures pertinent to older adults, e.g., avoidable hospital admissions, we should propose monitoring population health using new measures such as "healthy days at home," as discussed at length in the 2015 MedPAC Report to Congress [206].

The commitment, creativity, and resilience required to create and sustain community-wide partnerships across societal sectors—or even within the healthcare sector—are substantial, but the rationale is compelling, and we can take advantage of past learnings. Research on an earlier Robert Wood Johnson Foundation initiative, Aligning Forces for Quality, highlighted the importance of careful collaborative decision-making during the formative phase and the increasing importance of dedicated leadership as alliances move into the actual work toward common goals [207].

An empirical study of an HIV collaboration in Washington, DC, highlighted the well-known need for leadership and collaborative decision-making, but it also described how mistrust and competition can undermine relationship building among the organizations [208]. Studies from other industries stress that there must be an economic logic supporting organizations' commitments, and issues such as membership and power dynamics must be carefully negotiated [209]. Collaborating because "it's the right thing to do" is not good enough to motivate this level of individual and organizational investment. Advocates for older adults should seek sweet spots common to all participants, such as support for community-based services or a POLST registry. The increasing maturity of our knowledge in this area is suggested by the publication of an action guide from the National Quality Forum [210].

Conclusion

This survey of the prospects and challenges for accountable care has covered considerable ground, sprinkled generously with empirical studies that don't yet provide definitive guidance. But early in your journey, a modicum of common sense will yield ample dividends. You can start anywhere, though you would be wise to begin by pushing against open doors. For example, adopt and evolve care transition bundles. Deploy pharmacists liberally throughout your care transition programs. Match your high-touch, high-cost teams to high-need, high-cost patients who can benefit. Promote advance care planning and palliative care. Pursue partnerships with post-acute providers and home- and community-based services. Train and empower non-licensed lay workers so as to optimize the use of scarce professionals. Train your current professionals in geriatric principles and practices.

We have also touched on number of thorny issues resistant to easy, off-the-shelf solutions. The complexity of the issues will come as no surprise to clinicians and managers experienced in the care of older adults and other high-need, high-cost populations. Understandably, delivery system decision-makers have little appetite for exploring such dense thickets. Rather than exhaustively search for optimal solutions, they "satisfice," often choosing the first reasonable-sounding solution at hand [211]. As a result, the healthcare industry is beset by "fads, fashions, and bandwagons" [212].

I hope that my discussions of these issues will help you clarify your own perspectives and facilitate your explanations to others in your delivery system and beyond. I have referenced a great many resources that you may find useful. Throughout I have also highlighted the processes of program development and replication, implementation, evaluation, and adaptation. Achieving optimal performance requires relentless creativity chastened by experience, now generally known as organizational learning. The alternatives are complacency or foolishness, neither of which will get us to the triple aim. The prospects for significant improvements in the healthcare of these populations have never been greater, but progress is by no means assured.

An economist once noted in reference to Latin America that "development depends not so much on finding optimal combinations for given resources and factors of production as on calling forth and enlisting for development purposes resources and abilities that are hidden, scattered or badly utilized" [213]. For better or worse, no one is trying to impose a master plan for achieving the triple aim for older adults. No one has a formula for the precise combination of resources and processes that we need. What we can agree on is that we have resources and abilities that are hidden, scattered, and badly utilized. When it comes to the aging demographic, we are all living in the developing world. We have just landed in Erewhemos with a charge to make the healthcare delivery system better. We've never been here before, and we have no map and no preset GPS course around hazards and siren songs. As advocates for older adults and their healthcare workforce, then, we must stay alert to opportunities, fend off threats, and find our way around impasses toward a more promising future.

Appendix on Measurement: Necessary, Potent, and Imperfect

If your delivery system has begun taking risk for a defined population, then your information systems presumably include a data warehouse supplied by claims, (facility, professional, laboratory, radiology, pharmacy), authorizations, and patient experience data. You may be missing some of these elements; you may also have additional elements, e.g., clinical data from electronic health records and care coordination systems. At a minimum, your business intelligence capacities will yield the performance measures shown in Table 6.2. While you may be most interested in data related to older and/or high-need, high-cost populations, these need to be understood in the context of the delivery system performance as a whole, since that is the perspective the system's decision-makers must take.

Monitoring these basic measures will reveal variation across time and across providers (physicians, acute and post-acute settings) and thus serve as a starting point for your questions. Your business intelligence capacities should assist your search for answers by allowing you to drill down to the individual provider, e.g., clinic or hospital, and to trend performance over time. Additionally, you will need to filter measures by line of business and product and to segment if possible by risk tier, diagnoses, and service lines. While it is important to identify, understand, and address negative outlier performance, it may be more valuable to identify, understand, and replicate superior performance.

In addition to these claims data, most ACOs have access to measures of patient experience. Note that utilization may be more illuminating than cost when there are significant differences in unit costs and/or missing data on costs. When possible, you should take advantage of authorization data, which have shorter lag times than claims.

Table 6.2 Typical claims-based performance measures for various providers

Delivery system	Primary care	Hospital	Nursing facility	Home health
– Facility utilization (admissions/1000, length of stay, days/1000, ED visits/1000) – Readmission (3, 7, 30, 90 days) – Leakage to non-contracted or non-preferred providers – Pharmacy usage	– Clinical quality measures – Facility utilization – Readmission (3, 7, 30, 90 days)	– Average length of stay – Readmission (3, 7, 30, 90 days) – Percentage of patients seen in ED and admitted – Use of post-acute facilities and home health – Clinical quality measures	– Average length of stay – Hospital utilization: ED and (re) admission, both directly from SNF and after discharge home – Discharge destinations	– Hospital utilization: ED, (re) admission

Measurement in Older and High-Risk Populations

- Claims-based quality measures include the Medicare Stars specified by CMS, e.g., screening for colon cancer and renal insufficiency and management of diabetes and osteoporosis.
- Of particular interest for management of older populations are:
  - Annual wellness visits
  - Primary care claims for care coordination and care transitions
  - Lag times from hospital discharge to outpatient follow-up and nursing facility discharge to outpatient follow-up
- Claims will enable at least bare-bones monitoring of specialized programs, e.g., the patient enrollment, visits, and facility utilization of a home-based medical care program. There is interest in development of standardized quality metrics for such programs, but these as yet do not exist [214].
- Claims will enable identification of "hidden" high-risk populations such as patients in domiciliary settings (assisted living, board-and-care homes) or custodial nursing facilities or on dialysis.
- To monitor the channeling of patients to preferred post-acute home health agencies and nursing facilities, I suggest using the Herfindahl-Hirschman Index, which is the standard formula for market concentration. Your goal is to concentrate patients as much as possible with preferred providers.

You may find useful variation in monitoring claims for advance care planning, although those claim numbers are not a measure of the quality of advance care planning conversations. Similarly, you are likely to find variation in the volumes of inpatient and outpatient palliative care consultations. If you access dates of death from state or federal agencies and match those data with your claims, you will be able to create robust end-of-life quality and utilization measures reflecting the use of primary care, specialty care, emergency department, hospital, and chemotherapy in the patient's final weeks and months.

Risk Adjustment and Socioeconomic Determinants of Health

Risk adjustment is critical for comparing performance across providers, but it continues to be challenging. The Hierarchical Condition Category (HCC) model employed by CMS does not adequately account for the resource use of complex older patients [215]. There is now intense interest in using socioeconomic determinants of health as adjustments in risk estimates, quality measures, and payment, but methodologies are not yet in widespread use [216].

Socioeconomic factors also have potential clinical utility in patient management and program development, particularly for high-need, high-cost populations. The SCAN Foundation report discussed earlier outlined four essential attributes of delivery systems caring for adults with complex care needs. The National Quality Forum has since reported on data and measurement systems that are being used to support progress toward the four essential attributes [217]. One of the promising examples described is the Protocol for Responding to and Assessing Patients' Assets, Risks, and Experiences (PRAPARE). This 22-question tool captures biopsychosocial determinants of health, including race and ethnicity, housing status, neighborhood, social integration, and social support. It is freely available for incorporation into electronic health records.

Characteristics of Good Measures

The simplest way to evaluate a given measure is to ask, *How accurately does this measure reflect meaningful variation in a process or outcome?* Criteria for measure selection typically used by CMS, the National Quality Forum, and the Institute of Medicine [218] include the following:

- Impact: importance for health status and/or cost, i.e., does the measure really matter?
- Improvability: existence of gap between current practice and best practice, as well as evidence that the gap can be closed (whether the measure is actionable).
- Feasibility, including data availability and the burden of data collection.
- Scientific soundness and methodological rigor of the measure, including validity (credibility, or how well the measure captures the process or outcome it is intended to assess) and reliability (consistency, or whether the measure produces similar results under consistent conditions).
- Understandability of the measure, e.g., obvious specifications versus "black box."
- Timeliness: the turn-around time and frequency of measurement (e.g., monthly versus annually).

Measurement criteria become more stringent along a continuum from low stakes, e.g., quality improvement feedback, to high stakes, e.g., payment for performance.

- For rapid-cycle quality improvement purposes, low-rigor measures and nonrandom small samples can suffice for adequate insight, as long as the stakes as perceived by providers are low.
- Imprecise or "noisy" but directionally accurate data may suffice when an organization is giving performance feedback to a provider but not sharing the data more widely.
- Clinicians within a setting, practice, or specialty may also appreciate getting variation data regarding a process when the "correct number" or Goldilocks optimum is unknown. Such data can trigger a useful conversation within the group members about why they vary in their decision-making.
- Sharing data openly throughout a specialty can have significant positive impact among physicians, who are typically quite competitive, but doing so also increases the demand for rigor. Sharing data on specialists with primary care physicians can influence referrals, increasing the stakes even higher. Paying incentives for performance multiplies the demand for rigor.

Measurement Challenges

Increasing recognition of the burdens of measurement has led to calls for reduction and harmonization of measure sets. In addition, CMS has recently emphasized the unintended consequences of performance feedback and incentives, including worsening quality in unmeasured areas ("teaching to the test"), providing overtreatment or unnecessary care, gaming of the data, avoiding high-risk or challenging patients, and worsening disparities in care [219].

Many clinical domains lack meaningful measures that can be derived from existing data sources. Before giving up on a domain, delivery systems should consider the use of manual sampling strategies. Guidance for efficient and reliable sampling is readily available [220]. It remains true that some important domains defy direct measurement. We have no measures addressing the act of diagnosis, for example, yet that act is central to the practice of medicine [100]. We often find ourselves looking for substitute measures that may be distant from the area of interest, rather like the story of the drunk looking under a streetlight for the keys that he dropped in a distant dark alley. That said, good estimates of key processes are invaluable in quality improvement and program development, and we now have excellent guides for improving the quality of our estimates [221].

Attribution of responsibility is often a nontrivial task. Responsibility for an outcome such as readmission, for example, is shared across settings. Additionally, although appropriate attribution of patient to primary care provider is largely straightforward in managed care, it is less precise in CMS ACOs and in managed care populations with high turnover. An obvious question, most pertinent in the pay-for-performance context, is whether the provider has a meaningful amount of control over what is being measured.

The unit of analysis often dictates what measures may be available. The unit of interest may be a county population, a health plan's enrollees, a medical group's enrollees, a practice, or a provider. As the analysis becomes more fine-grained, e.g., down to the physician level, small denominators may render a measure unusable because of unreliability (more noise than signal) [222]. The most common approach to the small denominator problem is to exclude providers below a certain cutoff, e.g., 30 patients in the denominator [223]. Bayesian reliability adjustment (smoothing) is sometimes used—and would arguably be fairer to all—but is less intuitive.

Measures that are not robust enough for public reporting or pay for performance may nevertheless be invaluable for the other uses noted above. Also, whereas "noise" may overwhelm "signal" in a one-time use of a measure with small denominators, the signal-to-noise ratio improves with repeat use over time.

Finally, you should not be surprised or overly dismayed to find that you sometimes have difficulty getting reliable data from your information systems. You are not alone. No one has a single electronic health record that unifies all sites of care, and critical data may reside in any of dozens of other applications. Your delivery system encompasses multiple separate organizations contracted to care for your patients. Data flows across these applications and organizations are immensely challenging [224], and few organizations of any kind have invested adequate resources in data management [225]. Decision-makers may remedy this deficit as pressures to manage performance—and the need for measurement insights—continue to increase [156].

References

1. Fulton BD, Pegany V, Keolanui B, Scheffler RM. Growth of accountable care organizations in California: number, characteristics, and state regulation. J Health Polit Policy Law. 2015;40(4):669–88.
2. Qaseem A, Dallas P, Forciea MA, Starkey M, Denberg TD, Shekelle P. Nonsurgical management of urinary incontinence in women: a clinical practice guideline from the American College of Physicians. Ann Intern Med. 2014;161(6):429–40.
3. Cassel C. Medicare matters: what geriatric medicine can teach American health care. Berkeley: University of California Press; 2005.
4. Blumenthal D, Chernof B, Fulmer T, Lumpkin J, Selberg J. Caring for high-need, high-cost patients – an urgent priority. N Engl J Med. 2016;375(10):909–11.
5. Hayes SL, Salzberg CA, McCarthy D, et al. High-need, high-cost patients: who are they and how do they use health care? A population-based comparison of demographics, health care use, and expenditures. Issue Brief (Commonw Fund). 2016;26:1–14.
6. Evans J, Grudniewicz A, Baker GR, Wodchis W. Organizational context and capabilities for integrating care: a framework for improvement. Int J Integr Care. 2016;16(3):15.
7. Fisher ES, Shortell SM, Kreindler SA, Van Citters AD, Larson BK. A framework for evaluating the formation, implementation, and performance of accountable care organizations. Health Aff (Millwood). 2012;31(11):2368–78.
8. The SCAN Foundation. What matters most: essential attributes of a high-quality system of care for adults with complex needs (full report). 2016. http://www.thescanfoundation.org/what-matters-most-essential-attributes-high-quality-system-care-adults-complex-needs-full-report.
9. Fullerton CA, Henke RM, Crable E, Hohlbauch A, Cummings N. The impact of Medicare ACOs on improving integration and coordination of physical and behavioral health care. Health Aff (Millwood). 2016;35(7):1257–65.
10. Busch AB, Huskamp HA, McWilliams JM. Early efforts by Medicare accountable care organizations have limited effect on mental illness care and management. Health Aff (Millwood). 2016;35(7):1247–56.
11. Tabbush V, Kogan AC, Mosqueda L, Kominski GF. Person-centered care: the business case. SCAN Foundation. 2016. http://www.thescanfoundation.org/person-centered-care-business-case-full-report.
12. Gittell JH. High performance healthcare: using the power of relationships to achieve quality, efficiency and resilience. New York: McGraw Hill Professional; 2009.
13. Sorace J, Wong HH, Worrall C, Kelman J, Saneinejad S, MaCurdy T. The complexity of disease combinations in the Medicare population. Popul Health Manag. 2011;14(4):161–6.
14. Boutwell AE, Noga PM, Defossez SM. State of the state: reducing readmissions in Massachusetts. Burlington: Massachusetts Hospital Association; 2016. www.mhalink.org.
15. Dharmarajan K, Strait KM, Tinetti ME, et al. Treatment for multiple acute cardiopulmonary conditions in older adults hospitalized with pneumonia, chronic obstructive pulmonary disease, or heart failure. J Am Geriatr Soc. 2016;64(8):1574–82.
16. Agarwal KS, Kazim R, Xu J, Borson S, Taffet GE. Unrecognized cognitive impairment and its effect on heart failure readmissions of elderly adults. J Am Geriatr Soc. 2016;64(11):2296–301.
17. Rice YB, Barnes CA, Rastogi R, Hillstrom TJ, Steinkeler CN. Tackling 30-day, all-cause readmissions with a patient-centered transitional care bundle. Popul Health Manag. 2016;19(1):56–62.
18. Tuso P, Huynh DN, Garofalo L, et al. The readmission reduction program of Kaiser Permanente Southern California-knowledge transfer and performance improvement. Perm J. 2013;17(3):58–63.
19. Tuso P, Watson HL, Garofalo-Wright L, et al. Complex case conferences associated with reduced hospital admissions for high-risk patients with multiple comorbidities. Perm J. 2014;18(1):38–42.

20. Center for Health Information and Analysis. Hospital-wide adult all-payer readmissions in Massachusetts: 2011–2013. 2015. http://www.chiamass.gov/assets/docs/r/pubs/15/CHIA-Readmissions-Report-June-2015.pdf.
21. Epstein AM, Jha AK, Orav EJ. The relationship between hospital admission rates and rehospitalizations. N Engl J Med. 2011;365(24):2287–95.
22. Jackson CT, Trygstad TK, DeWalt DA, DuBard CA. Transitional care cut hospital readmissions for North Carolina Medicaid patients with complex chronic conditions. Health Aff (Millwood). 2013;32(8):1407–15.
23. Dharmarajan K, Hsieh A, Dreyer RP, Welsh J, Qin L, Krumholz HM. Relationship between age and trajectories of rehospitalization risk in older adults. J Am Geriatr Soc. 2017;65(2):421–26.
24. Patel KK, Vakharia N, Pile J, Howell EH, Rothberg MB. Preventable admissions on a general medicine service: prevalence, causes and comparison with AHRQ prevention quality indicators-a cross-sectional analysis. J Gen Intern Med. 2016;31(6):597–601.
25. Hesselink G, Zegers M, Vernooij-Dassen M, et al. Improving patient discharge and reducing hospital readmissions by using intervention mapping. BMC Health Serv Res. 2014;14:389.
26. Kashiwagi DT, Burton MC, Hakim FA, et al. Reflective practice: a tool for readmission reduction. Am J Med Qual. 2016;31(3):265–71.
27. Atkins D, Kansagara D. Reducing readmissions—destination or journey? JAMA Intern Med. 2016;176(4):493–5.
28. Nyweide DJ, Anthony DL, Bynum JP, et al. Continuity of care and the risk of preventable hospitalization in older adults. JAMA Intern Med. 2013;173(20):1879–85.
29. Gruneir A, Bronskill SE, Maxwell CJ, et al. The association between multimorbidity and hospitalization is modified by individual demographics and physician continuity of care: a retrospective cohort study. BMC Health Serv Res. 2016;16:154.
30. Lee KK, Yang J, Hernandez AF, Steimle AE, Go AS. Post-discharge follow-up characteristics associated with 30-day readmission after heart failure hospitalization. Med Care. 2016;54(4):365–72.
31. Kashiwagi DT, Burton MC, Kirkland LL, Cha S, Varkey P. Do timely outpatient follow-up visits decrease hospital readmission rates? Am J Med Qual. 2012;27(1):11–5.
32. Murtaugh CM, Deb P, Zhu C, et al. Reducing readmissions among heart failure patients discharged to home health care: effectiveness of early and intensive nursing services and early physician follow-up. Health Serv Res. 2016. [Epub ahead of print].
33. National Center for Health Statistics. Health, United States, 2015: with special feature on racial and ethnic health disparities. 2016. https://www.cdc.gov/nchs/data/hus/hus15.pdf.
34. Shehab N, Lovegrove MC, Geller AI, Rose KO, Weidle NJ, Budnitz DS. US Emergency Department visits for outpatient adverse drug events, 2013–2014. JAMA. 2016;316(20):2115–25.
35. Qato DM, Wilder J, Schumm LP, Gillet V, Alexander GC. Changes in prescription and over-the-counter medication and dietary supplement use among older adults in the United States, 2005 vs 2011. JAMA Intern Med. 2016;176(4):473–82.
36. Polinski JM, Moore JM, Kyrychenko P, et al. An insurer's care transition program emphasizes medication reconciliation, reduces readmissions and costs. Health Aff (Millwood). 2016;35(7):1222–9.
37. Reidt SL, Holtan HS, Larson TA, et al. Interprofessional collaboration to improve discharge from skilled nursing facility to home: preliminary data on postdischarge hospitalizations and emergency department visits. J Am Geriatr Soc. 2016;64(9):1895–9.
38. Pellegrin KL, Krenk L, Oakes SJ, et al. Reductions in medication-related hospitalizations in older adults with medication management by hospital and community pharmacists: a quasi-experimental study. J Am Geriatr Soc. 2017;65(1):212–9.
39. Steinman MA, Miao Y, Boscardin WJ, Komaiko KD, Schwartz JB. Prescribing quality in older veterans: a multifocal approach. J Gen Intern Med. 2014;29(10):1379–86.
40. Najafzadeh M, Schnipper JL, Shrank WH, Kymes S, Brennan TA, Choudhry NK. Economic value of pharmacist-led medication reconciliation for reducing medication errors after hospital discharge. Am J Manag Care. 2016;22(10):654–61.

41. Pevnick JM, Shane R, Schnipper JL. The problem with medication reconciliation. BMJ Qual Saf. 2016;25(9):726–30.
42. Kim SL, Tarn DM. Effect of primary care involvement on end-of-life care outcomes: a systematic review. J Am Geriatr Soc. 2016;64(10):1968–74.
43. Colaberdino V, Marshall C, DuBose P, Daitz M. Economic impact of an advanced illness consultation program within a Medicare advantage plan population. J Palliat Med. 2016;19(6):622–5.
44. Zhang B, Wright AA, Huskamp HA, et al. Health care costs in the last week of life: associations with end-of-life conversations. Arch Intern Med. 2009;169(5):480–8.
45. Austin CA, Mohottige D, Sudore RL, Smith AK, Hanson LC. Tools to promote shared decision making in serious illness: a systematic review. JAMA Intern Med. 2015;175(7):1213–21.
46. Reidy J, Halvorson J, Makowski S, et al. Health system advance care planning culture change for high-risk patients: the promise and challenges of engaging providers, patients, and families in systematic advance care planning. J Palliat Med. 2017;20(4):388–94.
47. Coalition for Compassionate Care of California. Advance care planning tools & resources. http://coalitionccc.org/tools-resources/advance-care-planning-resources.
48. Fulmer T. Talking with patients about end-of-life care: new poll reveals how physicians really feel. 2016. http://www.johnahartford.org/blog/view/talking-with-patients-about-end-of-life-care-new-poll-reveals-how-physician.
49. Cassel JB, Kerr KM, McClish DK, et al. Effect of a home-based palliative care program on healthcare use and costs. J Am Geriatr Soc. 2016;64(11):2288–95.
50. Cherlin EJ, Brewster AL, Curry LA, Canavan ME, Hurzeler R, Bradley EH. Interventions for reducing hospital readmission rates: the role of hospice and palliative care. Am J Hosp Palliat Care. 2016. [Epub ahead of print].
51. Miller SC, Dahal R, Lima JC, et al. Palliative care consultations in nursing homes and end-of-life hospitalizations. J Pain Symptom Manag. 2016;52(6):878–83.
52. Cassel JB, Kerr KM, Kalman NS, Smith TJ. The business case for palliative care: translating research into program development in the U.S. J Pain Symptom Manag. 2015;50(6):741–9.
53. Greysen SR, Hoi-Cheung D, Garcia V, et al. "Missing pieces"—functional, social, and environmental barriers to recovery for vulnerable older adults transitioning from hospital to home. J Am Geriatr Soc. 2014;62(8):1556–61.
54. Herzig SJ, Schnipper JL, Doctoroff L, et al. Physician perspectives on factors contributing to readmissions and potential prevention strategies: a multicenter survey. J Gen Intern Med. 2016;31(11):1287–93.
55. Enguidanos S, Coulourides Kogan AM, Schreibeis-Baum H, Lendon J, Lorenz K. "Because I was sick": seriously ill veterans' perspectives on reason for 30-day readmissions. J Am Geriatr Soc. 2015;63(3):537–42.
56. Leppin AL, Gionfriddo MR, Kessler M, et al. Preventing 30-day hospital readmissions: a systematic review and meta-analysis of randomized trials. JAMA Intern Med. 2014;174(7):1095–107.
57. Mair FS, May CR. Thinking about the burden of treatment. BMJ. 2014;349:g6680.
58. Foss Durant A, McDermott S, Kinney G, Triner T. Caring science: transforming the ethic of caring-healing practice, environment, and culture within an integrated care delivery system. Perm J. 2015;19(4):e136–42.
59. Morris MS, Graham LA, Richman JS, et al. Postoperative 30-day readmission: time to focus on what happens outside the hospital. Ann Surg. 2016;264(4):621–31.
60. Merkow RP, Ju MH, Chung JW, et al. Underlying reasons associated with hospital readmission following surgery in the United States. JAMA. 2015;313(5):483–95.
61. Leape LL. Hospital readmissions following surgery: turning complications into "treasures". JAMA. 2015;313(5):467–8.
62. De Oliveira GS Jr, Holl JL, Lindquist LA, Hackett NJ, Kim JY, RJ MC. Older adults and unanticipated hospital admission within 30 days of ambulatory surgery: an analysis of 53,667 ambulatory surgical procedures. J Am Geriatr Soc. 2015;63(8):1679–85.

63. Jackson AH, Fireman E, Feigenbaum P, Neuwirth E, Kipnis P, Bellows J. Manual and automated methods for identifying potentially preventable readmissions: a comparison in a large healthcare system. BMC Med Inform Decis Mak. 2014;14:28.
64. van Walraven C, Jennings A, Forster AJ. A meta-analysis of hospital 30-day avoidable readmission rates. J Eval Clin Pract. 2012;18(6):1211–8.
65. Auerbach AD, Kripalani S, Vasilevskis EE, et al. Preventability and causes of readmissions in a national cohort of general medicine patients. JAMA Intern Med. 2016;176(4):484–93.
66. Meltzer DO, Ruhnke GW. Redesigning care for patients at increased hospitalization risk: the comprehensive care physician model. Health Aff (Millwood). 2014;33(5):770–7.
67. Luu NP, Pitts S, Petty B, et al. Provider-to-provider communication during transitions of care from outpatient to acute care: a systematic review. J Gen Intern Med. 2016;31(4):417–25.
68. Joynt KE, Figueroa JE, Oray J, Jha AK. Opinions on the hospital readmission reduction program: results of a national survey of hospital leaders. Am J Manag Care. 2016;22(8): e287–94.
69. Brewster AL, Cherlin EJ, Ndumele CD, et al. What works in readmissions reduction: how hospitals improve performance. Med Care. 2016;54(6):600–7.
70. McKenna K, Leykum LK, McDaniel RR Jr. The role of improvising in patient care. Health Care Manag Rev. 2013;38(1):1–8.
71. Gittell JH, Fairfield KM, Bierbaum B, et al. Impact of relational coordination on quality of care, postoperative pain and functioning, and length of stay: a nine-hospital study of surgical patients. Med Care. 2000;38(8):807–19.
72. Rundall TG, Wu FM, Lewis VA, Schoenherr KE, Shortell SM. Contributions of relational coordination to care management in accountable care organizations: views of managerial and clinical leaders. Health Care Manag Rev. 2016;41(2):88–100.
73. Medicare Payment Advisory Commission. A data book: health care spending and the Medicare program. 2016. http://www.medpac.gov/docs/default-source/data-book/june-2016-data-book-health-care-spending-and-the-medicare-program.pdf?sfvrsn=0.
74. Das A, Norton EC, Miller DC, Chen LM. Association of postdischarge spending and performance on new episode-based spending measure. JAMA Intern Med. 2016;176(1):117–9.
75. Sacks GD, Lawson EH, Dawes AJ, et al. Variation in hospital use of postacute care after surgery and the association with care quality. Med Care. 2016;54(2):172–9.
76. Lewin Group. CMS bundled payments for care improvement initiative models 2–4. 2016. https://innovation.cms.gov/Files/reports/bpci-models2-4-yr2evalrpt.pdf.
77. Jubelt LE, Goldfeld KS, Chung WY, Blecker SB, Horwitz LI. Changes in discharge location and readmission rates under Medicare bundled payment. JAMA Intern Med. 2016;176(1):115–7.
78. Crosson FJ. Letter from MedPAC to CMS regarding file code CMS-1648-P. 2016. http://www.medpac.gov/docs/default-source/comment-letters/20160824_cy17_hha_pps_nprm_medpac_comment_rev_rev_sec.pdf?sfvrsn=0.
79. American Hospital Association. Private sector discharge tools. 2015. http://www.aha.org/content/15/15dischargetools.pdf.
80. Bowles KH, Chittams J, Heil E, et al. Successful electronic implementation of discharge referral decision support has a positive impact on 30- and 60-day readmissions. Res Nurs Health. 2015;38(2):102–14.
81. Press MJ, Gerber LM, Peng TR, et al. Postdischarge communication between home health nurses and physicians: measurement, quality, and outcomes. J Am Geriatr Soc. 2015;63(7):1299–305.
82. Shih AF, Buurman BM, Tynan-McKiernan K, Tinetti ME, Jenq G. Views of primary care physicians and home care nurses on the causes of readmission of older adults. J Am Geriatr Soc. 2015;63(10):2193–6.
83. Brock J, Mitchell J, Irby K, et al. Association between quality improvement for care transitions in communities and rehospitalizations among Medicare beneficiaries. JAMA. 2013;309(4):381–91.

84. O'Connor M, Bowles KH, Feldman PH, et al. Frontloading and intensity of skilled home health visits: a state of the science. Home Health Care Serv Q. 2014;33(3):159–75.

85. Hennessey B, Suter P. The community-based transitions model: one agency's experience. Home Healthc Nurse. 2011;29(4):218–30; quiz 231-212

86. Bruce ML, Lohman MC, Greenberg RL, Bao Y, Raue PJ. Integrating depression care management into Medicare home health reduces risk of 30- and 60-day hospitalization: the depression care for patients at home cluster-randomized trial. J Am Geriatr Soc. 2016;64(11):2196–203.

87. Reidt SL, Larson TA, Hadsall RS, Uden DL, Blade MA, Branstad R. Integrating a pharmacist into a home healthcare agency care model: impact on hospitalizations and emergency visits. Home Healthc Nurse. 2014;32(3):146–52.

88. O'Connor M, Asdornwised U, Dempsey ML, et al. Using telehealth to reduce all-cause 30-day hospital readmissions among heart failure patients receiving skilled home health services. Appl Clin Inform. 2016;7(2):238–47.

89. Baker LC, Macaulay DS, Sorg RA, Diener MD, Johnson SJ, Birnbaum HG. Effects of care management and telehealth: a longitudinal analysis using Medicare data. J Am Geriatr Soc. 2013;61(9):1560–7.

90. Dean KM, Hatfield LA, Jena AB, et al. Preliminary data on a care coordination program for home care recipients. J Am Geriatr Soc. 2016;64(9):1900–3.

91. Ouslander JG, Lamb G, Perloe M, et al. Potentially avoidable hospitalizations of nursing home residents: frequency, causes, and costs: [see editorial comments by Drs. Jean F. Wyman and William R. Hazzard, pp 760–761]. J Am Geriatr Soc. 2010;58(4):627–35.

92. Ouslander JG, Naharci I, Engstrom G, et al. Root cause analyses of transfers of skilled nursing facility patients to acute hospitals: lessons learned for reducing unnecessary hospitalizations. J Am Med Dir Assoc. 2016;17(3):256–62.

93. Trahan LM, Spiers JA, Cummings GG. Decisions to transfer nursing home residents to emergency departments: a scoping review of contributing factors and staff perspectives. J Am Med Dir Assoc. 2016;17(11):994–1005.

94. Ouslander JG, Lamb G, Tappen R, et al. Interventions to reduce hospitalizations from nursing homes: evaluation of the INTERACT II collaborative quality improvement project. J Am Geriatr Soc. 2011;59(4):745–53.

95. Tena-Nelson R, Santos K, Weingast E, Amrhein S, Ouslander J, Boockvar K. Reducing potentially preventable hospital transfers: results from a thirty nursing home collaborative. J Am Med Dir Assoc. 2012;13(7):651–6.

96. Cohen AB, Knobf MT, Fried TR. Avoiding hospitalizations from nursing homes for potentially burdensome care: results of a qualitative study. JAMA Intern Med. 2017;177(1):137–39.

97. King BJ, Gilmore-Bykovskyi AL, Roiland RA, Polnaszek BE, Bowers BJ, Kind AJ. The consequences of poor communication during transitions from hospital to skilled nursing facility: a qualitative study. J Am Geriatr Soc. 2013;61(7):1095–102.

98. Ouslander JG, Naharci I, Engstrom G, et al. Hospital transfers of skilled nursing facility (SNF) patients within 48 hours and 30 days after SNF admission. J Am Med Dir Assoc. 2016;17(9):839–45.

99. Vasilevskis EE, Ouslander JG, Mixon AS, et al. Potentially avoidable readmissions of patients discharged to post-acute care: perspectives of hospital and skilled nursing facility staff. J Am Geriatr Soc. 2017;65(2):269–76.

100. National Academies of Sciences Engineering and Medicine. Improving diagnosis in health care. Washington: The National Academies Press; 2015.

101. Schoenfeld AJ, Zhang X, Grabowski DC, Mor V, Weissman JS, Rahman M. Hospital-skilled nursing facility referral linkage reduces readmission rates among Medicare patients receiving major surgery. Surgery. 2016;159(5):1461–8.

102. Maly MB, Lawrence S, Jordan MK, et al. Prioritizing partners across the continuum. J Am Med Dir Assoc. 2012;13(9):811–6.

103. Lage DE, Rusinak D, Carr D, Grabowski DC, Ackerly DC. Creating a network of high-quality skilled nursing facilities: preliminary data on the postacute care quality improvement experiences of an accountable care organization. J Am Geriatr Soc. 2015;63(4):804–8.

104. Joshi DK, Bluhm RA, Malani PN, Fetyko S, Denton T, Blaum CS. The successful development of a subacute care service associated with a large academic health system. J Am Med Dir Assoc. 2012;13(6):564–7.
105. Toles M, Anderson RA, Massing M, et al. Restarting the cycle: incidence and predictors of first acute care use after nursing home discharge. J Am Geriatr Soc. 2014;62(1):79–85.
106. Donovan JL, Kanaan AO, Gurwitz JH, et al. A pilot health information technology-based effort to increase the quality of transitions from skilled nursing facility to home: compelling evidence of high rate of adverse outcomes. J Am Med Dir Assoc. 2016;17(4):312–7.
107. Hall RK, Toles M, Massing M, et al. Utilization of acute care among patients with ESRD discharged home from skilled nursing facilities. Clin J Am Soc Nephrol. 2015;10(3): 428–34.
108. Lindquist LA, Miller RK, Saltsman WS, et al. SGIM-AMDA-AGS consensus best practice recommendations for transitioning patients' healthcare from skilled nursing facilities to the community. J Gen Intern Med. 2017;32(2):199–203.
109. Park HK, Branch LG, Bulat T, Vyas BB, Roever CP. Influence of a transitional care clinic on subsequent 30-day hospitalizations and emergency department visits in individuals discharged from a skilled nursing facility. J Am Geriatr Soc. 2013;61(1):137–42.
110. Grabowski DC, Caudry DJ, Dean KM, Stevenson DG. Integrated payment and delivery models offer opportunities and challenges for residential care facilities. Health Aff (Millwood). 2015;34(10):1650–6.
111. Bynum JP, Andrews A, Sharp S, McCollough D, Wennberg JE. Fewer hospitalizations result when primary care is highly integrated into a continuing care retirement community. Health Aff (Millwood). 2011;30(5):975–84.
112. Wagner L. Focus on integrated care fosters transformation in assisted living. Provider. 2012;38(8):22–4, 27–30, 33 passim
113. Premier Research Institute. Performance evaluation: what is working in accountable care organizations? 2016. https://www.premierinc.com/wp-content/uploads/2016/10/What-Is-Working-In-ACOs-Report-10.16.pdf.
114. King CJ, Roach JL. Community health needs assessments: a framework for America's hospitals. Popul Health Manag. 2016;19(2):78–80.
115. Hefner JL, Hilligoss B, Sieck C, et al. Meaningful engagement of ACOs with communities: the new population health management. Med Care. 2016;54(11):970–6.
116. Fraze T, Lewis VA, Rodriguez HP, Fisher ES. Housing, transportation, and food: how ACOs seek to improve population health by addressing nonmedical needs of patients. Health Aff (Millwood). 2016;35(11):2109–15.
117. Solomon J, Peterson L. Preparing California's community-based organizations to partner with the health care sector by building business acumen: case studies from the first cohort of linkage lab grantees. The SCAN Foundation. 2015. http://www.thescanfoundation.org/sites/default/files/linkage_lab_case_studies_final_august_2015.pdf.
118. National Quality Forum. Quality in home and community-based services to support community living: addressing gaps in performance measurement 2016. file:///C:/Users/teh02010/Downloads/hcbs_final_report.pdf.
119. Davis K, Buttorff C, Leff B, et al. Innovative care models for high-cost Medicare beneficiaries: delivery system and payment reform to accelerate adoption. Am J Manag Care. 2015;21(5):e349–56.
120. Hong CS, Siegel AL, Ferris TG. Caring for high-need, high-cost patients: what makes for a successful care management program? New York: The Commonwealth Fund; 2014. http://www.commonwealthfund.org/~/media/files/publications/issue-brief/2014/aug/1764_hong_caring_for_high_need_high_cost_patients_ccm_ib.pdf
121. Edes T, Burris JF. Home-based primary care: a VA innovation coming soon. Phys Leadersh J. 2014;1(1):38–40. 42
122. De Jonge KE, Jamshed N, Gilden D, Kubisiak J, Bruce SR, Taler G. Effects of home-based primary care on Medicare costs in high-risk elders. J Am Geriatr Soc. 2014;62(10): 1825–31.

123. Centers for Medicare & Medicaid Services (CMS). Independence at home demonstration performance year 2 results. 2016. https://www.cms.gov/Newsroom/MediaReleaseDatabase/Fact-sheets/2016-Fact-sheets-items/2016-08-09.html.
124. Taler G, Kinosian B, Boling P. A bipartisan approach to better care and smarter spending for elderly adults with advanced chronic illness. J Am Geriatr Soc. 2016;64(8):1537–9.
125. Stefanacci RG, Reich S, Casiano A. Application of PACE principles for population health management of frail older adults. Popul Health Manag. 2015;18(5):367–72.
126. Anderson GF, Ballreich J, Bleich S, et al. Attributes common to programs that successfully treat high-need, high-cost individuals. Am J Manag Care. 2015;21(11):e597–600.
127. Soones T, Federman A, Leff B, Siu AL, Ornstein K. Two-year mortality in homebound older adults: an analysis of the National Health and Aging Trends Study. J Am Geriatr Soc. 2017;65(1):123–9.
128. Edes T, Kinosian B, Vuckovic NH, Nichols LO, Becker MM, Hossain M. Better access, quality, and cost for clinically complex veterans with home-based primary care. J Am Geriatr Soc. 2014;62(10):1954–61.
129. Pacala JT. Is palliative care the "new" geriatrics? Wrong question—we're better together. J Am Geriatr Soc. 2014;62(10):1968–70.
130. Leff B, Carlson CM, Saliba D, Ritchie C. The invisible homebound: setting quality-of-care standards for home-based primary and palliative care. Health Aff (Millwood). 2015;34(1):21–9.
131. Smith AK, Currow DC, Abernethy AP, et al. Prevalence and outcomes of breathlessness in older adults: a national population study. J Am Geriatr Soc. 2016;64(10):2035–41.
132. Bone AE, Gao W, Gomes B, et al. Factors associated with transition from community settings to hospital as place of death for adults aged 75 and older: a population-based mortality follow-back survey. J Am Geriatr Soc. 2016;64(11):2210–7.
133. Urato C, McCall N, Cromwell J, Lenfestey N, Smith K, Raeder D. Evaluation of the extended Medicare Care Management for High Cost Beneficiaries (CMHCB) demonstration: Massachusetts General Hospital (MGH). 2013. Prepared for Center for Medicare and Medicaid Innovation, Centers for Medicare & Medicaid Services. Available at https://innovation.cms.gov/Files/reports/CMHCB-MassGen.pdf.
134. Johnson TL, Rinehart DJ, Durfee J, et al. For many patients who use large amounts of health care services, the need is intense yet temporary. Health Aff (Millwood). 2015;34(8):1312–9.
135. Lee NS, Whitman N, Vakharia N, Ph DG, Rothberg MB. High-cost patients: hot-spotters don't explain the half of it. J Gen Intern Med. 2017;32(1):28–34.
136. Peikes D, Peterson G, Brown RS, Graff S, Lynch JP. How changes in Washington University's Medicare coordinated care demonstration pilot ultimately achieved savings. Health Aff (Millwood). 2012;31(6):1216–26.
137. Kivlahan C, Gaus C, Webster AM, et al. High-risk-patient identification: strategies for success. 2016. https://www.aamc.org/download/470456/data/riskid.pdf.
138. van Walraven C, Dhalla IA, Bell C, et al. Derivation and validation of an index to predict early death or unplanned readmission after discharge from hospital to the community. CMAJ. 2010;182(6):551–7.
139. Vogeli C, Spirt J, Brand R, et al. Implementing a hybrid approach to select patients for care management: variations across practices. Am J Manag Care. 2016;22(5):358–65.
140. Haime V, Hong C, Mandel L, et al. Clinician considerations when selecting high-risk patients for care management. Am J Manag Care. 2015;21(10):e576–82.
141. Cohen CJ, Flaks-Manov N, Low M, Balicer RD, Shadmi E. High-risk case identification for use in comprehensive complex care management. Popul Health Manag. 2015;18(1):15–22.
142. Johnson TL, Brewer D, Estacio R, et al. Augmenting predictive modeling tools with clinical insights for care coordination program design and implementation. EGEMS (Wash DC). 2015;3(1):1181.
143. Shih SL, Zafonte R, Bates DW, et al. Functional status outperforms comorbidities as a predictor of 30-day acute care readmissions in the inpatient rehabilitation population. J Am Med Dir Assoc. 2016;17(10):921–6.

144. Kelley AS, Covinsky KE, Gorges RJ, et al. Identifying older adults with serious illness: a critical step toward improving the value of health care. Health Serv Res. 2017;52(1):113–31.
145. Zhou YY, Wong W, Li H. Improving care for older adults: a model to segment the senior population. Perm J. 2014;18(3):18–21.
146. Rittel HW, Webber MM. Dilemmas in a general theory of planning. Policy Sci. 1973;4(2):155–69.
147. Lynn J. MediCaring communities: getting what we want and need in frail old age at an affordable cost. Ann Arbor: Altarum Institute; 2016.
148. Garber L, Harvell J, Gallego E. New standards to support coordinated care planning: overview for NY Department of Health. Washington: The Office of the National Coordinator for Health Information Technology; 2014. https://www.healthit.gov/sites/default/files/nydohcareplanning_082014_.pdf
149. Quinn TJ, McArthur K, Ellis G, Stott DJ. Functional assessment in older people. BMJ. 2011;343:d4681.
150. Morley JE, Adams EV. Rapid geriatric assessment. J Am Med Dir Assoc. 2015;16(10):808–12.
151. Hu J, Jensen GA, Nerenz D, Tarraf W. Medicare's annual wellness visit in a large health care organization: who is using it? Ann Intern Med. 2015;163(7):567–8.
152. Burt J, Rick J, Blakeman T, Protheroe J, Roland M, Bower P. Care plans and care planning in long-term conditions: a conceptual model. Prim Health Care Res Dev. 2014;15(4):342–54.
153. Gillick MR. The critical role of caregivers in achieving patient-centered care. JAMA. 2013;310(6):575–6.
154. Adams S, Cohen E, Mahant S, Friedman JN, Macculloch R, Nicholas DB. Exploring the usefulness of comprehensive care plans for children with medical complexity (CMC): a qualitative study. BMC Pediatr. 2013;13:10.
155. Byrne C, Dougherty M. Long-term and post-acute care providers engaged in health information exchange: final report. Washington: U.S. Department of Health and Human Services; 2013. https://aspe.hhs.gov/report/long-term-and-post-acute-care-providers-engaged-health-information-exchange-final-report
156. Rudin RS, Gidengil CA, Predmore Z, Schneider EC, Sorace J, Hornstein R. Identifying and coordinating care for complex patients. Santa Monica: RAND Corporation; 2016. http://www.rand.org/content/dam/rand/pubs/research_reports/RR1200/RR1234/RAND_RR1234.pdf.
157. Klein DE, Woods DD, Klein G, Perry SJ. Can we trust best practices? Six cognitive challenges of evidence-based approaches. J Cogn Eng Decis Mak. 2016;10:244.
158. Institute of Medicine. Retooling for an aging America: building the health care workforce. Washington: The National Academies Press; 2008.
159. American Geriatrics Society. Existing formal geriatrics competencies and milestones. http://www.americangeriatrics.org/health_care_professionals/education/curriculum_guidelines_competencies/existing_formal_geriatrics_competencies.
160. American Academy of Home Care Medicine. American Academy of Home Care Medicine Clinical Competencies. 2016. http://c.ymcdn.com/sites/www.aahcm.org/resource/resmgr/Homepage/HomeCareMedicineComptencies_.pdf.
161. Kramer BJ, Creekmur B, Howe JL, et al. Veterans affairs geriatric scholars program: enhancing existing primary care clinician skills in caring for older veterans. J Am Geriatr Soc. 2016;64(11):2343–8.
162. Warshaw GA, Modawal A, Kues J, et al. Community physician education in geriatrics: applying the assessing care of vulnerable elders model with a multisite primary care group. J Am Geriatr Soc. 2010;58(9):1780–5.
163. Portal of Geriatrics Online Education (POGOe). https://www.pogoe.org.
164. Dower C, Moore J, Langelier M. It is time to restructure health professions scope-of-practice regulations to remove barriers to care. Health Aff (Millwood). 2013;32(11):1971–6.
165. Bohmer RM, Imison C. Lessons from England's health care workforce redesign: no quick fixes. Health Aff (Millwood). 2013;32(11):2025–31.
166. Wogamon CL. Exploring the effect of educating certified nursing assistants on pressure ulcer knowledge and incidence in a nursing home setting. Ostomy Wound Manag. 2016;62(9):42–50.

167. The Institute of Medicine and National Research Council. The future of home health care: workshop summary. Washington: The National Academies Press; 2015.

168. Adair R, Wholey DR, Christianson J, White KM, Britt H, Lee S. Improving chronic disease care by adding laypersons to the primary care team: a parallel randomized trial. Ann Intern Med. 2013;159(3):176–84.

169. Gershon RR, Dailey M, Magda LA, Riley HE, Conolly J, Silver A. Safety in the home healthcare sector: development of a new household safety checklist. J Patient Saf. 2012;8(2):51–9.

170. Litzelman DK, Inui TS, Griffin WJ, et al. Impact of community health workers on elderly patients' advance care planning and health care utilization: moving the dial. Med Care. 2017;55(4):319–26.

171. Cottingham AH, Alder C, Austrom MG, Johnson CS, Boustani MA, Litzelman DK. New workforce development in dementia care: screening for "caring": preliminary data. J Am Geriatr Soc. 2014;62(7):1364–8.

172. Yasaitis LC, Pajerowski W, Polsky D, Werner RM. Physicians' participation in ACOs is lower in places with vulnerable populations than in more affluent communities. Health Aff (Millwood). 2016;35(8):1382–90.

173. Rahman M, Gozalo P, Tyler D, Grabowski DC, Trivedi A, Mor V. Dual eligibility, selection of skilled nursing facility, and length of Medicare paid postacute stay. Med Care Res Rev. 2014;71(4):384–401.

174. Zhang N, Li Y, Rodriguez-Monguio R, Barenberg A, Temkin-Greener H, Gurwitz J. Are obese residents more likely to be admitted to nursing homes that have more deficiencies in care? J Am Geriatr Soc. 2016;64(5):1085–90.

175. Li Y, Harrington C, Mukamel DB, Cen X, Cai X, Temkin-Greener H. Nurse staffing hours at nursing homes with high concentrations of minority residents, 2001–11. Health Aff (Millwood). 2015;34(12):2129–37.

176. Martin LT, Plough A, Carman KG, Leviton L, Bogdan O, Miller CE. Strengthening integration of health services and systems. Health Aff (Millwood). 2016;35(11):1976–81.

177. Freedman VA, Spillman BC. Active life expectancy in the older US population, 1982–2011: differences between blacks and whites persisted. Health Aff (Millwood). 2016;35(8):1351–8.

178. Thornton RL, Glover CM, Cene CW, Glik DC, Henderson JA, Williams DR. Evaluating strategies for reducing health disparities by addressing the social determinants of health. Health Aff (Millwood). 2016;35(8):1416–23.

179. Bartolome RE, Chen A, Handler J, Platt ST, Gould B. Population care management and team-based approach to reduce racial disparities among African Americans/Blacks with hypertension. Perm J. 2016;20(1):53–9.

180. Shah NR, Rogers AJ, Kanter MH. Health care that targets unmet social needs. NEJM Catalyst; 2016. http://catalyst.nejm.org/health-care-that-targets-unmet-social-needs.

181. Gibbons R, Henderson R. Relational contracts and organizational capabilities. Organ Sci. 2012;23(5):1350–64.

182. Peterson GG, Zurovac J, Brown RS, et al. Testing the replicability of a successful care management program: results from a randomized trial and likely explanations for why impacts did not replicate. Health Serv Res. 2016;51(6):2115–39.

183. McNeil D, Strasser R, Lightfoot N, Pong R. A "Simple" evidence-based intervention to improve care transitions for frail patients with complex health conditions: why didn't it work as expected? Healthc Q. 2016;19(2):67–72.

184. Gittell JH, Weiss L. Coordination networks within and across organizations: a multi-level framework. J Manag Stud. 2004;41(1):127–53.

185. Kodner DL. Managing high-risk patients: the Mass General care management programme. Int J Integr Care. 2015;15:e017.

186. Kind AJ, Brenny-Fitzpatrick M, Leahy-Gross K, et al. Harnessing protocolized adaptation in dissemination: successful implementation and sustainment of the veterans affairs coordinated-transitional care program in a non-veterans affairs hospital. J Am Geriatr Soc. 2016;64(2):409–16.

187. Nembhard IM, Tucker AL. Applying organizational learning research to accountable care organizations. Med Care Res Rev. 2016;73(6):673–84.

188. Plsek P. Appendix B: redesigning health care with insights from the science of complex adaptive systems. Crossing the quality chasm: a new health system for the 21st century. Washington: The National Academies Press; 2001.
189. Vogus TJ, Iacobucci D. Creating highly reliable health care: how reliability-enhancing work practices affect patient safety in hospitals. Ind Labor Relat Rev. 2016;69:911–38.
190. Vincent C, Amalberti R. Safer healthcare: strategies for the real world. New York: SpringerOpen; 2016.
191. Topaz M, Kang Y, Holland DE, Ohta B, Rickard K, Bowles KH. Higher 30-day and 60-day readmissions among patients who refuse post acute care services. Am J Manag Care. 2015;21(6):424–33.
192. Greenhalgh T, Humphrey C, Woodard F. User involvement in health care. Oxford: Wiley; 2010.
193. Marszal EM. Tolerable risk guidelines. ISA Trans. 2001;40(4):391–9.
194. Cohen IG, Amarasingham R, Shah A, Xie B, Lo B. The legal and ethical concerns that arise from using complex predictive analytics in health care. Health Aff (Millwood). 2014;33(7):1139–47.
195. Goodrick E, Reay T. An institutional perspective on accountable care organizations. Med Care Res Rev. 2016;73(6):685–93.
196. Fremont A, Kranz AM, Phillips J, Garber C. Improving population health through an innovative collaborative: The Be There San Diego Data for Quality Group. Santa Monica: RAND Corporation; 2016. http://www.rand.org/pubs/research_reports/RR1622.html
197. Hammes BJ, Rooney BL, Gundrum JD. A comparative, retrospective, observational study of the prevalence, availability, and specificity of advance care plans in a county that implemented an advance care planning microsystem. J Am Geriatr Soc. 2010;58(7):1249–55.
198. Moss AH, Zive DM, Falkenstine EC, Fromme EK, Tolle SW. Physician orders for life-sustaining treatment medical intervention orders and in-hospital death rates: comparable patterns in two state registries. J Am Geriatr Soc. 2016;64(8):1739–41.
199. California Health Care Foundation. CHCF to fund pilot project to develop an electronic POLST registry in California. 2016. http://www.chcf.org/media/press-releases/2016/polst-eregistry.
200. Peiris D, Phipps-Taylor MC, Stachowski CA, et al. ACOs holding commercial contracts are larger and more efficient than noncommercial ACOs. Health Aff. 2016;35(10):1849–56.
201. Alley DE, Asomugha CN, Conway PH, Sanghavi DM. Accountable health communities—addressing social needs through Medicare and Medicaid. N Engl J Med. 2016;374(1):8–11.
202. Chandra A, Miller CE, Acosta JD, Weilant S, Trujillo M, Plough A. Drivers of health as a shared value: mindset, expectations, sense of community, and civic engagement. Health Aff (Millwood). 2016;35(11):1959–63.
203. Bhatia R, Corburn J. Lessons from San Francisco: health impact assessments have advanced political conditions for improving population health. Health Aff (Millwood). 2011;30(12):2410–8.
204. National Academies of Sciences Engineering and Medicine. Metrics that matter for population health action: workshop summary. Washington: The National Academies Press; 2016.
205. Casarett D, Teno J. Why population health and palliative care need each other. JAMA. 2016;316(1):27–8.
206. Medicare Payment Advisory Commission (MedPAC). Medicare and the health care delivery system. 2015. http://www.medpac.gov/docs/default-source/reports/june-2015-report-to-the-congress-medicare-and-the-health-care-delivery-system.pdf?sfvrsn=0.
207. D'Aunno T, Alexander JA, Jiang L. Creating value for participants in multistakeholder alliances: the shifting importance of leadership and collaborative decision-making over time. Health Care Manag Rev. 2017;42(2):100–11.
208. Aldoory L, Bellows D, Boekeloo BO, Randolph SM. Exploring use of relationship management theory for cross-border relationships to build capacity in HIV prevention. J Community Psychol. 2015;43(6):687–700.
209. Gulati R, Puranam P, Tushman M. Meta-organization design: rethinking design in interorganizational and community contexts. Strateg Manag J. 2012;33(6):571–86.
210. National Quality Forum. Improving population health by working with communities: action guide 3.0. 2016. http://www.qualityforum.org/Publications/2016/08/Improving_Population_Health_by_Working_with_Communities__Action_Guide_3_0.aspx.

211. Simon HA. Rational choice and the structure of the environment. Psychol Rev. 1956;63(2):129.
212. Kaissi AA, Begun JW. Fads, fashions, and bandwagons in health care strategy. Health Care Manag Rev. 2008;33(2):94–102.
213. Hirschman AO. The strategy of economic development. New Haven: Yale University Press; 1958.
214. Leff B, Weston CM, Garrigues S, Patel K, Ritchie C. Home-based primary care practices in the United States: current state and quality improvement approaches. J Am Geriatr Soc. 2015;63(5):963–9.
215. Min L, Wenger N, Walling AM, et al. When comorbidity, aging, and complexity of primary care meet: development and validation of the Geriatric CompleXity of Care Index. J Am Geriatr Soc. 2013;61(4):542–50.
216. National Academies of Sciences, Engineering, and Medicine. Accounting for social risk factors in Medicare payment: data. Washington: The National Academies Press; 2016.
217. National Quality Forum. Essential attributes of a high-quality system of care: how communities approach quality measurement. 2016. file:///C:/Users/teh02010/Downloads/scan_final_report.pdf.
218. Institute of Medicine. Toward quality measures for population health and the leading health indicators. Washington: The National Academies Press; 2012.
219. Centers for Medicare and Medicaid Services. National impact assessment of the centers for Medicare and Medicaid services (CMS) quality measures report. Baltimore: CMS; 2015.
220. Valente E. An explanation of the "8 and 30" file sampling procedure used by NCQA during accreditation survey visits. 2001. http://www.ncqa.org/portals/0/programs/8-30.pdf.
221. Hubbard DW. How to measure anything: finding the value of intangibles in business. 3rd ed. New York: Wiley; 2014.
222. Hofer TP, Hayward RA, Greenfield S, Wagner EH, Kaplan SH, Manning WG. The unreliability of individual physician "report cards" for assessing the costs and quality of care of a chronic disease. JAMA. 1999;281(22):2098–105.
223. Ryan AM, Tompkins CP. Efficiency and value in healthcare: linking cost and quality measures. National Quality Forum; 2014.
224. Fihn SD, Francis J, Clancy C, et al. Insights from advanced analytics at the Veterans Health Administration. Health Aff (Millwood). 2014;33(7):1203–11.
225. Aiken P. EXPERIENCE: succeeding at data management: BigCo attempts to leverage data. J Data Inf Qual. 2016;7(1–2):1–35.

Primary Care Clinic Model

Jeremy V. Phillips and Steven L. Phillips

Over the years, primary care and its meaning has evolved to include more than just the care that is delivered. Between the quality metrics, meaningful use, and value-based payment modifiers, clinicians are being scored on and therefore spending more time on nonclinical activities. This doesn't even begin to address the amount of nonclinical paperwork that clinicians and their staff are dealing with on a daily basis when working with an elderly population, for example, housing forms, VA forms, durable medical equipment, Medicaid applications, etc.

Our practice focuses on offering a healthcare experience that allows every individual the opportunity to age gracefully and be able to make the most of their years by maximizing their ability to engage with all that life has to offer and ensuring they have the chance to spend as much meaningful time as possible with families and friends in the comfort of their own homes and routines. While hospital stays can't always be avoided, a clinical practice that allows seniors to thrive and live to their full potential is one that provides a continuum of care and support.

Despite an ever growing awareness that health and wellness has a significant social and cultural component that stems from the daily actions of individuals, healthcare delivery systems, historically, have placed themselves at the center of the care continuum with their focus primarily being on the treatment of disease rather than facilitating healthier living. As a result, the de facto healthcare approach to seniors is often reactive rather than proactive, with endless referrals to specialists, increased prescriptions, and hospitalizations in response to issues as they present themselves. While 85% of seniors (60+) are relatively free of serious chronic conditions that account for the majority of healthcare spend and hospitalizations, the lack of social support combined with a less than 9% penetration of regular screening and

J.V. Phillips (✉) • S.L. Phillips, MD
Geriatric Specialty Care, 5250 Neil Road Suite 207, Reno, NV 89502, USA
e-mail: jeremy@gscnv.com; sphillips@gscnv.com

© Springer International Publishing AG 2018
M. Wasserman, J. Riopelle (eds.), *Primary Care for Older Adults*,
DOI 10.1007/978-3-319-61329-1_7

annual wellness visits in this population contribute to the onset of identifiable cognitive, emotional, and physical diseases that often lead to hospitalization and a deterioration of end of life potential.

To reinforce how important it is to develop an effective network of services for this population, it's important to know that 27.5% of the current population falls into the at-risk category of senior citizenship, with this number projected to grow to 30.3% within the next 5 years. Secondly, the cost of care for seniors who have more than five chronic conditions in the community accounts for 76% of the healthcare expenditure in the United States.

The following assessment represents a community profile based on compiling data from a variety of data sources, including a community health needs assessment (CHNA) for Washoe County conducted by the Washoe County Health District [1]. This study illustrated some of the most significant challenges faced by the 60+ senior community, which highlighted issues related to economic security, frailty, social isolation, caregiver support and awareness and utilization of community services.

Affordability of healthcare is a significant boundary to seniors in Washoe County. Over 41% of seniors have annual income of less than $30,000 with 9% reporting an income of less than $10,000. This directly contributes to seniors not seeking medical care or maintaining their prescribed medications with 10% of seniors reporting that they had to forego medical care and skip medications due to income constraints. The populations most likely to report that they had insufficient means to pay bills and those who scored moderate to high in regard to frailty (18% reporting inability to pay) and social isolation (19%), minorities (20%), and women (49% with incomes under $30,000 versus 31% of men) cover the cost of care.

One of the key indicators of risk for seniors is where they lie on the frailty index. The index measures an individual's levels of activity and self-sufficiency. Seniors who score as mildly, moderately, severely, or very severely frail are measured specifically to exhibit higher risk of mortality and hospitalization. Part of this risk comes from having a limited ability to perform activities of daily living (ADL) such as dressing, eating, ambulation, toileting, and hygiene and instrumental activities of daily living (IADL) such as managing finances, handling transportation, managing medications, and performing housework and basic home maintenance. According to the community profile, 28% of the population aged 60+ and 39% of those aged 80+ were categorized as mildly frail or above. This equates to nearly 23,000 seniors within the community who are at significant risk of hospitalization within the next 5 years and over 30,000 projected for the 5 years following. Additionally, 15% of those aged 60+ experienced periods of depression, with that number increasing to 42% for those with incomes of less than $10,000 per year.

Another key indicator of risk is social isolation. Social isolation and loneliness are measured by an individual's perceptions on relationships, social activity, feelings about social activity, and the robustness of their network. Seniors that exhibit these factors have less support in the performance of ADLs and IADLs and are less likely to be aware of or have access to social services that may help prevent illness, injury, and ultimately hospitalization. Twenty-five percent of seniors aged 60+ in the community are estimated to be moderately to highly socially isolated, with that figure growing to 37% of unmarried seniors, 40% for those with incomes less than $30,000, and 42% of seniors aged 80+. Fourteen percent of seniors aged 60+ no longer drive and are dependent on alternate forms of transportation.

The community profile also indicates a need for additional caregiving support in the community to assist at-risk seniors. Some caregivers report receiving less than 3 h of sleep per night as a result of meeting the physical and social demands required by seniors ranking higher on the frailty index. Nineteen percent of caregiver's report have accumulated significant debt in the process of supporting seniors, with 29% needing additional emotional, financial, or housekeeping support for seniors in their care beyond what they were capable of providing. Twenty-eight percent of caregivers indicated needing respite during the process of providing care.

These social determinants of health in seniors all play a critical role in the well-being of the community. There are numerous exceptional nonprofit and social service agencies working on different aspects of senior health and well-being.

Our practice is unique with an emphasis on the frail, elderly population providing visits in the patient's place of residence: skilled nursing facilities, group homes, long-term care, assisted living facilities, and private homes. The CHNA along with our years of providing care across Northern Nevada helped shape the principles and recommendations to help address our community and the needs of the seniors that live in it, the continuous onslaught of reporting requirements, and help transition from volume to value.

Mission

Geriatric specialty care is committed to provide high-quality, compassionate, and patient-centered healthcare for the frail and vulnerable aging population.

Vision

To be recognized as a unique and superior geriatric care practice with an emphasis on enhancing the quality of senior health and well-being in Northern Nevada.

Values

Compassionate, comprehensive, collaborative, communicative, responsive, solution seeking

Principle 1: Create a high value primary care experience.

The Centers for Medicare and Medicaid Services (CMS) views value as quality over resource utilization (cost). In order to provide high value primary care, one has a few approaches that they may take. They may increase quality and keep costs the same, they may increase quality and decrease cost, they may keep quality the same while decreasing cost, or they may increase quality and cost but at higher levels for quality and less cost. CMS has also shared with us their "quality strategy" which they say may be summed up in three words: better, smarter, and healthier (Triple AIM) [2]. Their focus on quality is the basis for a patient centric approach to care. Listed are their quality strategy goals and the framework for our practice.

- Make care safer by reducing harm caused while care's delivered:
    - Improve support for a culture of safety.
    - Reduce inappropriate and unnecessary care.
    - Prevent or minimize harm in all settings.
- Help patients and their families be involved as partners in their care.
- Promote effective communication and coordination of care.
- Promote effective prevention and treatment of chronic disease.
- Work with communities to help people live healthily.
- Make care affordable.

Recommendation 1: Familiarize, Educate, Manage, and Reevaluate

When we first started down this path of implementing the quality strategy goals that CMS has based all of their value-based payment and alternative payment models upon, we needed to first familiarize ourselves with our population. This required us to understand what we knew about our patients, but more importantly begin to figure out what we didn't know but needed to understand in order to achieve success. We started with data that was readily available to us via electronic health records (EHRs). During this exercise, we realized that EHRs are very good at capturing clinical data that has a quality measure such as continuous quality management (CQM), meaningful use (MU), and/or physician quality reporting system (PQRS) tied to it, although there was an entire subset of information that is required to fully understand your patient population needs not readily available within EHRs. This subset of data consists of biological, psychological, and social information which helps to shed light on social determinants and how they affect your population and how patients with similar conditions but different social needs require a different approach to care. Table 7.1 shows the data points that we settled on to best manage our patients from a population level.

Table 7.1 (Population health data requirements)

Data	Currently captured	Transfer ability	Actionable items
Diagnoses	EHR	HL7 or claims	Hierarchical categorical conditions (HCC), risk stratification, chronic conditions, measures, care plans
Biological, psychological, social	Modified EHR/not readily available	None, potentially HL7	Diagnosis support/validation, risk stratification, functional, clinical support, care plans
Labs/diagnostics	Lab companies/EHR	HL7	Diagnosis support/validation
Outreach	Modified EHR/not readily available	Potentially HL7	Care plan
Wearables	Individual systems	Custom APIs	Vitals, care plan
Vitals	EHR/wearables	HL7/custom APIs	Diagnosis support/validation (BMI, blood pressure, respiratory rate, heart rate, etc.)
Medications	EHR	HL7 (NDC)	Risk stratification, measures, care plans

Once we had the data that we desired and began to identify the different subsets of populations (chronic condition 0–1, 2–4, 5+, robust, pre-frail, frail, etc.) within our greater population, we set out to educate our clinicians and care team on how to best care for these different populations. Our practice has a higher volume of patients with dementia and behavioral impairments so we hired a geriatric psychiatrist to offer greater quality of care to this population. Once we had educated our clinical team on the populations that we deal with, we wanted to ensure that we were achieving success at the individual patient level, and so we set out to help the patients and their families be involved as partners in their care. We began to educate the patient, family members, and caregivers on each patients' individual clinical and social needs, although during this process, we realized that we were still missing critical information about our patients and that was their individual goals that they want to be able to achieve, consisting of their desires, wants, and needs. In order to gain access to this information, we were required to create an environment in which our patients become a part of the care team and collaborate on the care they receive based upon their individual goals. This allows us to measure our practices' success by the number of goals that are achieved; there is nothing more rewarding than seeing an individual achieve their goal that they previously thought was unattainable. We modified the data points that we were capturing to now include the ability to capture these patient's goals and measure their outcomes.

After familiarizing and educating our clinical care team and our patient care team, we needed a platform that allowed us to manage our progress, successes, and areas for improvement. This platform has allowed us to promote effective communication and coordination of care between all involved parties. Our solution was a patient centric, goal oriented, interactive care plan. This care plan over its different iterations has finally helped solve the familiarized and educate portions of our overall quality success system. These care plans focus on the patients' wants, desires, and needs. They are created collaboratively between the patients and clinicians and are evidence based and/or best practiced. Rather than the check box measures that we have all become so accustomed to, we focus on these patient centric goals. The more robust and far reaching the care team, the more opportunities present themselves to achieve the patient's goals. It is vital for the care team to interact, collaborate, and engage in new and alternative ways, to help manage the patient's goals.

The last step to the cycle that we created is to reevaluate our overall processes and to incorporate everything that we have learned to be able to offer a better experience to everyone involved. This can be anything from new educational materials to viewing data a different way.

Recommendation 2: Create a Chronic Condition Solution

As we were familiarizing ourselves with our patient population, one of the data points that we focused on was chronic conditions. The benefits to the patient and their families to have a coordinated approach to their chronic conditions were a huge motivating factor, especially after we read this. "The average Medicare patient with one chronic condition sees four physicians a year, while those with five or more chronic conditions see 14 different physicians a year [3]." Of course another factor is the resource use associated with patients who have multiple chronic conditions. In 2002, beneficiaries with five or more chronic conditions accounted for 76% of Medicare expenditures [4].

At the center of our chronic condition solution is our patient-centered care plans, which help promote effective intervention and treatment of chronic diseases. These care plans are shared with all specialists, community resources, and healthcare members in order to better manage our patients and to create a collaborative experience.

Along with the data points mentioned above, our care plans include and are created from the following sections:

- Initial/ongoing assessment—This initial assessment is reviewed on an as-needed basis with a mandatory assessment done each quarter.
  - Personal goal/wishes—These are tracked and relayed back to the support team.
  - ADL (activities of daily living).
  - IADL (instrumental activities of daily living).
  - Support team—Including, but not limited to, family members, caregivers, community resources, available contact hours, support rendered.
  - Residence—Single-story home, two-story home, group home, assisted living facility, retirement home.
  - Advanced care planning.
- Chronic conditions—Including conditions from the CMS Chronic Condition Data Warehouse (CCW) along with those conditions that last a year or more and require ongoing medical attention and/or limit activities of daily living [5, 6]. Care plans are created that incorporate the following six domains based off of the patients chronic conditions:
  - Educational
  - Functional
  - Medical
  - Psychological
  - Social
  - Environmental
- Care tracking—Includes information from clinician encounters, patient and support team outreach, and community clinical and nonclinical interactions. Some of our tracking includes:
  - Referral's—creation through completion
  - Condition specific—for example, PT/INR tracking
  - Quality measures

Principle 2: Promote patient, family, and caregiver activation/engagement.

To have the highest impact, we encourage our patients, family members, and caregivers to take an active role in the creation of the care plans and in the management of them. Chronically ill patients with higher activation levels are more likely than those with lower levels to adhere to treatment, perform regular self-monitoring at home, and obtain regular chronic care [7].

Recommendation 3: Collaborate with the patient, family, and caregiver to develop and maintain a care plan that reflects the patient's goals, needs, and preferences.

Without the buy-in of the patient, family, and/or caregiver, the care plan will not be as effective or meaningful. Active engagement and participation have been shown to improve adherence to the plan of care and overall satisfaction. We are a high outreach practice which helps us facilitate and ensure that our patients and their support team are constantly involved in the creation and maintenance of the care plans. In an average month, we review and/or update 70% of the care plans which we have created.

The personal goals/wishes section of our care plans helps our patients and their support team stay more engaged with their health and care plan. As their goals/wishes are accomplished, our staff can continue to encourage them to follow the current collaboratively created plan by reminding them of all that they have achieved so far. This also helps to motivate our staff when the going gets tough.

Principle 3: Focus on work that promotes high quality care and minimize work that does not contribute.

Primary care clinicians, irrespective of their discipline or specialty, have high administrative burden [8], excessive reporting and documentation of care [9, 10], and transactional relationships with patients. It is imperative to focus on the work that promotes high-quality care, such as direct patient care and care team collaboration, and to minimize the excessive work that does not contribute to the quality of care. By streamlining and/or removing the administrative burden along with the reporting and documentation requirements from clinicians, this will allow them to focus on the care of the individual and also allow for greater satisfaction. It is critical to start to transition from volume-based transactional care and move toward a just-in-time delivery model that focuses on the whole patient and engages with them when necessary, with the appropriate method and appropriate team member.

Recommendation 4: Allow all care team members to work at the top of their professional capacity which in turn creates a more positive and rewarding work environment.

Within healthcare an effective team is one in which all members understand, support, and work toward a shared objective of caring for and serving the needs of their patients. This requires a clear understanding of each team member's roles and responsibilities. In addition, there must be shared goals, mutual trust, and effective communication with measurable processes and outcomes [11].

One tool that allows for each team member to work at the top of their professional capacity is our patient-centered care plan which encourages them to contribute to the overall plan of care for each patient. Before we introduced our patient-centered care plans, much of our clinical staff were frustrated and felt underutilized. We had clinicians performing tasks that could be handled by nursing staff, nursing staff performing tasks that could be handled by certified medical assistants (CMA), and CMAs performing tasks that could be handled by medical records and/or office assistants. Our patient-centered care plans helped our clinical staff navigate which tasks may be best performed by which appropriate team member.

This has led to higher satisfaction along with a greater use of our resources. If a task is above their scope, the processes that have been created along with the care plans will help them reach out to the appropriate team member to help them complete the task and achieve overall success. We have discovered that fostering a clinical team environment and supporting all members create a more rewarding workplace and one in which every member has ownership, pride, and respect for the outcomes that are achieved.

The future of healthcare will rely upon every member in the system to perform at the top of their professional capacity. With a shrinking workforce, increasing patient loads, and continued expanse of administrative burden, efficiencies will need to be created and achieved.

Recommendation 5: Capture the data that is required to achieve success during that encounter and the overall plan of care.

Electronic health records in general were never created with the intent of being mobile, and while many EHRs are now cloud based, this still does not solve the workflow for an office without walls practice. This becomes very apparent with the quality measures, meaningful use, and many of the other programs that CMS has created over the years. Many of these data points that are required to be captured would be done by ancillary staff within an office-based setting, though since our clinicians do home visits without any support staff, they are the receptionist, MA, RN, as well as clinician on the day of the visit.

In order to better utilize our clinicians' time and to allow them to perform at the top of their professional capacity, we have created "focused" encounter templates that guide them to capture the pertinent information for the type of visit that is occurring that day. While not revolutionary, it helps our clinicians to be able to focus on the patient-centered care that we strive for while meeting all of the administrative documentation burdens that go along with being a clinician.

Allowing our clinicians to focus on the care task at hand has created an environment in which we are now able to watch our own utilization of services. Having specific encounter types help our clinicians focus on the high-quality care that we as an organization are striving for. It allows for the clinician to focus on the task at hand and document accordingly.

Principle 4: Enhance collaboration with specialists, hospitals, emergency departments, other healthcare professionals, and community resources to deliver timely, appropriate, and efficient care.

In order to offer true value to our patients and their families, we need to ensure that they are receiving the appropriate services to be able to achieve their goals. This requires not only just interacting and collaborating with these outside entities but also facilitating our patients' wishes throughout the entire healthcare continuum. Our practice uses two systems/solutions to support the success of this principle, the HIE, care tracking tools, and our care plans.

Recommendation 6: Have systems in place that help with the flow of data.

Our practice is in the fortunate position of being located in Nevada where there is only one state run HIE, HealtHIE Nevada. We have also been fortunate that HealtHIE NV has worked very well with us and allows us to identify our patients and notifies us when there are new documents posted to the HIE for our patients. This has allowed us to have a better view of our patients as they utilize services from the hospital, emergency medical systems (EMS), outpatient diagnostics, or emergency departments.

The care tracking tools help facilitate the flow of the information that we receive from the HIE, clinicians, and facilities. These tools are also utilized to help close gaps in care, facilitate our medical delivery system, and help with reporting results to our partners.

As previously mentioned, our patient-centered care plans are the cornerstone to our collaboration with and throughout our community. These care plans while initially created to monitor chronic conditions have evolved to help our clinical staff monitor and address coordination of care throughout the continuum. We have integrated our tracking tools to the care plans for ease of use.

Recommendation 7: Promote a just-in-time (JIT) medical delivery system.

In order to remove redundancy as well as to offer the greatest value to our patients, we strive to offer the appropriate level of service, in the appropriate setting, at the appropriate time. This includes but is not limited to interactions with the clinician, clinical staff, or nonclinical staff in a face-to-face visit or over the phone. Our care tracking helps facilitate some of this, although like with any JIT system, one needs to be able to adapt to the unknown/unexpected event and be able to deploy the appropriate resources. Our practice has been fortunate to be able to partner with the local EMS under the Community Healthcare Paramedic program, in which they are able to send their trained paramedics to handle acute cases and help avoid potential hospitalizations.

EMS used the protocols from INTERACT III with reporting through the SBAR when they were contacted by our office to do a community health assessment for one of our patients that had one of the following suspected conditions: UTI, cellulitis, worsening of CHF, or pneumonia. The paramedic would then relay their assessment to the corresponding clinician who would initiate the treatment plan, and there would be a follow-up with the patient within 24 h by either the EMS team or the clinician. This program is a wonderful service and helps our patients help achieve their goals.

Principle 5: Promote excellent clinical and patient experience outcomes that reflect patient goals and whole person care.

Directly tied to our patient-centered care plans are the patients' goals, and the education piece of our care plans along with the care tracking system helps our office track patient experience, goals, and whole person care. To ensure that our office consistently offers quality care, it is imperative to have a workforce that is also having a positive experience.

Recommendation 8: Focus on quality measures that are meaningful to this patient population.

With the advent of meaningful use (MU), the Physician Quality Reporting System (PQRS), and value-based payment modifier (VBPM), quality measures began to take center stage, along with the burdens of reporting these measures. There was very little guidance around which measures an organization or practice should report on, leading to many just reporting on the simplest measures to capture in order to fulfill this burdensome request, missing the overall intent of the programs creation which was to enhance patient care and outcomes. It is vital for organizations to choose measures that are not only appropriate for their patient population but also measures that will lead to a meaningful impact for their patients.

Next year, 2017, will be the start of a brand new Quality Payment Program (QPP) the Merit-based Incentive Payment System (MIPS). In an effort to get more dollars tied to value MIPS which is comprised of four pillars, three involving measures and one involving cost, now is the time for clinicians to focus on which of the 271 Quality Measures are pertinent for their patient population.

Principle 6: Create a collaboration between primary care, behavioral health, and community resources to address determinants of health.

This can either be done internally within the group practice or by partnering with local resources.

Recommendation 9: Integrate with behavioral health.

For many years, our practice had a working relationship with a gero-psychiatrist to help facilitate care for our population. In 2016, we hired the gero-psychiatrist in order to better serve our population, focusing on our patients that have been diagnosed with dementia, depression, and other behavioral health conditions. For us to fully integrate our new clinician into our fold, we enhanced our care plans with a focus on behavioral health, integrated measurement, and tracking tools into our EHR and informed the community of our recent addition. Having our own gero-psychiatrist has been beneficial for our clinicians, allowing them to call at any time and receive a curbside consult adds tremendous value to our patients; however, reimbursement for these activities has been lacking. There are new payment codes for 2017 that promote Behavioral Health Integration (BHI). These codes similar to CCM will help those organizations that are prepared to begin to receive compensation for work that is already being done. Though more importantly, it will allow for greater integration between behavioral health and primary care.

Recommendation 10: Educate patient, family, and caregivers on community services that are provided.

The incorporation of community services into an individual patient's care plan requires a thorough understanding of those resources that are available within the community. Effective usage of community services is dependent upon care planning that goes beyond the identification of medical needs. For example, Medicare's Second Generation Social/Health Maintenance Organization (S/HMO) Program allowed primary care teams to provide expanded care benefits for eligible patients. These expanded benefits included care coordination programs, in which multidisciplinary ambulatory care teams conducted health-risk screenings, identified at-risk patients, developed care plans, and regularly contacted at-risk patients to identify potential emergent health issues. Where appropriate, the S/HMO Program reimbursed primary care teams (via prospective PBP) to provide transportation, respite care, house cleaning, emergency response, and adult day care benefits, at a nominal cost to patients (via copays). Evaluations of the S/HMO Program identified reductions in the utilization of intensive services (e.g., emergency department visits) and increases in the utilization of less intensive services (e.g., physical therapy) for high risk-patients, while at the same time improving functional status in comparison to a control group that did not receive expanded benefits [12].

Other examples of coordination and contracting between primary care and community services include integration of social determinants screening in patient care workflows, embedding community health workers or nonclinical specialists (e.g., public interest lawyers in a medical-legal partnership model) in healthcare settings, data sharing and referral management with nonclinical community-based organizations, contracting with community health workers and other nonmedical professionals, educational and occupational support, in-home improvement/adaptation to accommodate physical disabilities, and aging and disabilities resource centers.

Recommendation 11: Conduct patient, family, and caregiver satisfaction surveys to continually improve our product line.

The active solicitation of feedback, positive or negative, cannot be overlooked in order to improve the overall service quality and intent. Over the years, these surveys have helped our practice achieve greater patient, support team, and payer's satisfaction.

Principle 7: Attempt to create partnerships with payers (ADD Stuff).

Once our delivery system was created and working effectively, we began to seek out commercial payer contracts that focus on value and not volume. Some of the contracts that we have created over the years have included HRA assistance, TCM for the costliest, skilled nursing assistance, etc.

Recommendation 12: Collaborate with payers to create meaningful measures for this population (MDX Senior Dimensions, Wellness Clinic, Complex Discharge, etc....).

With an eye toward alternative payment models and meeting the CMS Triple Aim goals for value-based care, there are several opportunities for partnering with local Medicare Advantage Plans and Medicare Shared Savings Programs (MSSP).

Collaborative payer agreement:

We entered into a Transitional Care Program agreement with a Medicare Advantage Plan to help facilitate the care for their at-risk senior population. We agreed upon the following criteria for admittance into the program, the services to be provided, and the measures we would be scored upon.

- Criteria for admission: Two or more of the following (for MAP members/patients who reside in Washoe County geographic area):
  - LOS > 7 days
  - Previous readmissions in past 3 months
  - Three or more admissions within a 12-month period
  - Five or more chronic conditions with associated dementia diagnosis
  - Member identified by MAP data mining for patients at risk for palliative needs and/or predictive readmission to the hospital
  - Members/patients that decline recommended transfer to skilled or acute rehab level of care

- Members/patients that decline home healthcare or other recommended health-related services
- Members/patients who meet current homebound criteria due to frailty or debility
- Taxing effort to leave home
- Cognitive impairments
- Deficits with ADL and IADL
- TCM services
  - Clinician visit within 72 h of discharge
  - Provide medication reconciliation with patient and/or caregiver
  - Review "red flag" signs and symptoms with patient and/or caregiver and educate when and how to report health concerns
  - Follow-up with referrals from discharge entity: home health, hospice, DME, specialists
  - Directs to community resources to assist in the burden of financial or clinical care
  - Develop comprehensive patient-centered care plan
  - Advance Care Planning discussion
  - Medication adherence and potential interactions
- Measures (results)
  - 30-day all-cause readmission rate (7.9%)
  - RAF Scores—Closing HEDIS gaps (pass)
  - Acute admission/K hospital (220/1000)
  - Average length of stay (<4.8 Days)
  - Acute bed days/K (<1000)
  - Admission/K skilled nursing facility (65/1000)
  - Average length of stay (<14 Days)
  - Bed days/K skilled nursing facility (<950)
  - Clinician visit within 48 h (100%)
  - PCP visit within 7 days upon discharge from Transitional Care Program (100%)

In order to achieve these results, we rely upon the principles and recommendations that have been discussed. This Transitional Care Program relies heavily upon our clinical staff within the office, the community relationships we have created over the years, and our care tracking system. To help create the experience that we are striving for in some cases our clinical office staff have been mobilized and gone into the field in order to help assure we continue to see the results we want. The results have helped show the value of this program to the health plan and have helped our office look to expand this offering to other health plans in the area.

References

1. https://www.renown.org/wp-content/uploads/CHNA_Final-1.pdf.
2. https://www.cms.gov/Medicare/Quality-Initiatives-Patient-Assessment-Instruments/Value-Based-Programs/CMS-Quality-Strategy.html.
3. Cogeli C, et al. Multiple chronic conditions: prevalence, health consequences, and implications for quality, care management, and costs. J Gen Intern Med. 2007;22(3 Supp):391–5.
4. Thorpe KE, Howard DH. The rise in spending among medicare beneficiaries: the role of chronic disease prevalence and changes in treatment intensity. Health Aff. 2006;25:w378–88. (published online 22 August 2006; 10.1377/hlthaff.25.w378).
5. Hwang W, Weller W, Ireys H, Anderson G. Out-of-pocket medical spending for care of chronic conditions. Health Aff. 2001;20:267–78.
6. HCUP, Chronic Condition Indicator http://www.hcup.us.ahrq.gov/toolssoftware/chronic/chronic.jsp , Accessed 12 Dec 2016.
7. Hibbard JH, Greene J. What the evidence shows about patient activation: better health outcomes and care experiences; fewer data on costs. Health Aff. 2013;32(2):207–14.
8. http://medicaleconomics.modernmedicine.com/medical-economics/news/why-primary-care-physicians-are-seeing-fewer-patients?page=full.
9. http://www.modernhealthcare.com/article/20160307/news/160309890.
10. http://www.elske-ammenwerth.de/Publikationen/z55.pdf.
11. https://www.nationalahec.org/pdfs/vsrt-team-based-care-principles-values.pdf.
12. Newcomer R, Harrington C, Kane R. Challenges and accomplishments of the second-generation social health maintenance organization. Gerontologist. 2002;42(6):843–52.

Keys to Successful Primary Care Operations

Shelly Thomas

Many healthcare consultants, practice owners, and authors have studied and analyzed the most successful practices in the United States and have published key factors of success. A publication by the Total Success Center summarized the key success factors after studying for over 25 years and found what works best. A primary care practice is a business. "Over time it became apparent that many of these consultants and authors were saying basically the same thing, just using different language." [1].

Five keys to a successful practice [2]:

1. Managing and developing people
2. Strategic focus
3. Operations
4. Physical resources—the finances
5. Customer relations

It takes more than just knowing the five factors; the entire practice must be engaged, committed, and willing to work together to achieve success.

The most valuable assets of a practice are its people and recognizing this is the start to a successful practice. Managing and developing people is a primary aspect of building and maintaining a primary care practice. It is difficult to accomplish an organization's goals unless their people are motivated and have good teamwork. Building a strong team and developing positive relationships among team members are the keys to a positive successful environment. This can be achieved by understanding and addressing the individual needs and concerns of your staff.

S. Thomas
Rocky Mountain Senior Care, Golden Colorado
A member of the American Academy of Professional Coders, New York, USA
e-mail: shellyshell315@aol.com

© Springer International Publishing AG 2018
M. Wasserman, J. Riopelle (eds.), *Primary Care for Older Adults*,
DOI 10.1007/978-3-319-61329-1_8

People at work share fundamental needs that tend to never change, regardless of generation, geography, nationality, or gender:

- We all want to be informed.
- We want our opinions to matter.
- We want to be involved in creating changes and improvements.
- We want to be acknowledged for our efforts.

Develop winning leaders within the organization and work with people who can coach good employees to become better people. "There is a difference between being a boss and a leader. One manages their employees, while the other inspires them to innovate, think creatively, and strive for perfection. Every team has a boss, but what people need is a leader. Not sure how to tell the difference between the two? Here are some key traits that differentiate bosses from leaders." [3]. It is the people that matter at the end of the day and ultimately drive the success or failure of the practice. Winning leaders can be a "boss" or a coach if their style includes awareness and responsibility. Employees respond well to these qualities.

A primary care practice must continually work on the organization's strategic focus which is always changing. It is ultimately unknown who will control the healthcare market because it is externally driven, and being able to adjust and plan for changes is an important aspect of any management team. It is important that all employees understand the goals, the mission, and the values of the organization so they too are part of where you are headed. Hiring and retaining employees who understand and are committed to carrying out the mission and values are necessary to carry out strategic plans. It is important to infuse pride among the employees through the implementation of the organization's goals, mission, and values. This takes time and requires constant interaction among the team.

You cannot have a strategic focus or direction without operations to carry out the vision. In a primary care practice, whether the title is manager, medical practice manager, physician practice manager, administrator, practice administrator, executive director, office manager, CEO, COO, director, division manager, department manager, or any combination thereof, people who manage physician practices must understand the day-to-day operations. These people perform some combination of the responsibilities listed here or manage and/or oversee people who do:

- Human resources
- Facilities and machines
- Ordering and expense management
- Legal
- Accounting
- Payroll
- Billing, claims, accounts receivable
- Marketing
- Strategic planning

- Day-to-day operations
- Insurance contracting
- Incentive plan management (HEDIS, PQRS, MACRA, etc.)
- Stay current

Operations are largely internally focused, whereas strategic focus is externally driven.

A comprehensive strategic plan includes analysis of an organization's internal strength (i.e., the operations). An internal evaluation allows you to focus on areas that will increase productivity, efficiency, quality standards, and overall performance. "Analyzing a company's current strengths and weaknesses provides a wealth of insight helpful in accomplishing internal goals and internal analyses can provide advantages for achieving external goals, as well. Analyze all components of your business when identifying internal strengths and weaknesses. Look into the education, experience and overall competence of your employees to discover competitive advantages in your workforce. Review your production systems to spot any competitive advantages or clear impediments. Review your cost structure, pricing policies and financial ratios to determine you financial strength or weakness compared with competitors." [4].

Now that you have the people, the strategic plan and the operations team ready, how are you going to pay for everything? "Failing to manage cash flow is the number 1 reason for business failure." [5]. By selecting a few key performance indicators (KPIs) to review frequently, you will be able to concentrate efforts on areas key to financial success and will be able to observe trends or spot potential issues in a timely manner. A key area to financial performance is successful medical billing. Weather you outsource this function or perform this function in-house, it is important to understand how the practice is performing.

KPIs to review and monitor:

1. Monitor claim volume, submission trends, and clean claim rates.
2. Isolate/prevent rejections by reviewing denials by payer and provider.
3. Understand where rejections/denials are occurring (coding, eligibility, not covered, patient demographics, etc.).
4. Monitor charge lag/time to payment from DOS to clearinghouse to full payment for cash flow indicators.
5. Monitor and evaluate payments by CPT code.
6. Know your contracted payment amounts.
7. Monitor/trend percentage of the allowed amount paid.
8. Monitor credentialing and timing of effective dates.

Knowing how you are performing will allow the practice to make necessary operational changes and adjustments to ensure clean claims are being sent out with the quickest turnaround leading to efficient cash flow. Communication among all leaders in the practice is necessary to bring about any type of change impacting financial success.

Customer relations may be listed as number five; however, it is actually probably the number one key to any successful practice. The definition of a "customer" is a person or entity that obtains a service or product from another person or entity in exchange for money. Customers can buy either goods or services. Healthcare is classified by the government as a service industry because it provides an intangible thing rather than an actual thing. Many practices are now focusing on "patient-centered" care, which, because they are businesses, means that they are focusing on keeping customers by providing good customer service. Understanding patient needs is more important than what you are selling. Clinical care is rarely the reason a patient is not satisfied with the practice. Typically, dissatisfaction comes from an interaction with staff, a billing error, or frustration with getting through to the office. "By keeping in touch with customers and asking the following questions often, you will do a great job at developing customer loyalty and keeping the competition away" (see Ref. [1]).

1. What do you need?
2. What problem would you like solved?
3. What deficiency would you like filled?

If the team can accomplish these keys, a successful practice and a rewarding sense of teamwork will follow. It's not always the task at hand that challenges teams in their progress, it's the relationships and the little things that happen day to day. Maintaining a team that cares about each other and the organization is the ultimate key to successful operations.

References

1. The 5 key success factors: a powerful system for total business success. E.W. "Buck" Lawrimore; 2011.
2. http://totalsuccesscenter.com/business-success/key-success-factors.
3. https://acetechontarioblog.wordpress.com/2015/08/.
4. http://smallbusiness.chron.com/internal-external-strategic-plan-development-12123.html.
5. http://totalsuccesscenter.com/business-success/key-success-factors.

Primary Care Across the Care Continuum

9

Steven Atkinson

The model of geriatric primary care has undergone some dramatic changes over the last decade. Both nursing homes and assisted living facilities (ALFs) are developing into a framework where patients live out the rest of their days comfortably. Traditionally, neither environment was ideal, but the shift in services those facilities can now provide has shaped how a primary care provider (PCP) can also practice medicine comfortably with all the amenities of resources they may have utilized in a traditional office setting. If PCPs can envision this environment as a delivery method for quality primary care, unbound by the boxed-in walls they may have been accustomed to, then management of chronic care can be done in both a cost-effective way and also one in which the practice thrives. However, there may be some who believe primary care practices cannot make it in this environment; this chapter is dedicated to transcending that barrier.

Practices can, and do, thrive in a place where the services are brought to the patient rather than the patient going to get the services [1]. Labs, X-rays, ultrasound, barium swallows, and EKGs all are delivered in ALFs and nursing homes nowadays. These services have been extended to wound care, podiatry, psychological services, dentistry, and audiology to give a few additional examples. Now specialty services, such as neurology, psychiatry, and orthopedists, are being asked to join. In some cases, the setting makes it's even easier to deliver primary care medicine since everything comes to the patient rather than the patient going out to seek the service. In keeping that focus in mind and understanding the place where modern medicine and technology have taken us, thoughts have long been emerging about the best way to deliver that care.

S. Atkinson, PA-C, MS
Twin Cities Physicians, Minneapolis, MN 55427, USA
e-mail: satkinson@twincitiesphysicians.net; steven.atkinson@health.utah.edu

© Springer International Publishing AG 2018
M. Wasserman, J. Riopelle (eds.), *Primary Care for Older Adults*,
DOI 10.1007/978-3-319-61329-1_9

Fragmented Care

Fragmentation of the current delivery system of medicine in the United States is what initially created a costly and counterproductive environment. It's not surprising that families utilize an emergency department, or even a hospital, as a "one-stop shop" for the healthcare delivery system. Those environments allow a patient to get every test and every specialist, all housed in one environment, quickly, even though the cost is outrageous. However, since the product of this environment is high-paced, the care becomes fragmented, which compromises the patients personal safety. The safety net of the holistic care a primary care provider can provide, is simply overlooked just by the nature of the environment.

Various models have been developed to try to reduce fragmentation but have had difficulty implementing them. The GRACE model, discussed later in this chapter, is an example of a recently successful approach that combines care coordination with the expertise of a clinical geriatric provider [2]. Studies clearly show that single provider interventions are rarely successful in reducing readmissions [3]. A successful transition of care model has been shown to be effective if the services extend throughout the transition of care. Furthermore, well-known philosophical geriatric models have demonstrated in the real world the ability to reduce emergency department visits as well as hospitalizations to improve overall healthcare costs. In the earlier models, GeriMed of America and Senior Care of Colorado set the tone for more care-coordinated models such as Twin Cities Physicians and Rocky Mountain Senior Care. These newly developed models have, to some degree, been able to extend services along the continuum of care.

So why haven't organizations like this spread? One reason is those models described above have not had an effective payment model to support such efforts. Our existing healthcare system doesn't take a vested interest in incentivizing care coordination when multiple specialists are involved. Fee for service—the Medicare model—is a barrier to successful implementation of these types of care coordination programs. In fact, hospitals and private payers have made attempts to provide additional programs supporting continuity of care, only to find the care is still not completely coordinated because the teams involved in the patient's care poorly communicate with one another along those different environments. Additional barriers include the absence of evidence-based treatment decisions, lack of healthcare provider teams that are accountable for that particular patient, inaccurate medication reconciliation, delay in the transfer of medical records, lack of timely follow-up, duplicative testing and services, and substandard communication with patient's families [4].

Questions then arise: can states effectively handle the booming elderly population as they move along the spectrum of care? Will states find alternatives that combat those barriers described above? Will communities expand down the roads to include skilled nursing sectors or stick with assisted living communities only? Or, even more dramatic, will assisted living communities become what most would envision as a nursing home?

Given those over 65 years of age will increase to over 98 million older persons living in America by 2060 (Fig. 9.1) and those 85 are expected to increase to 19

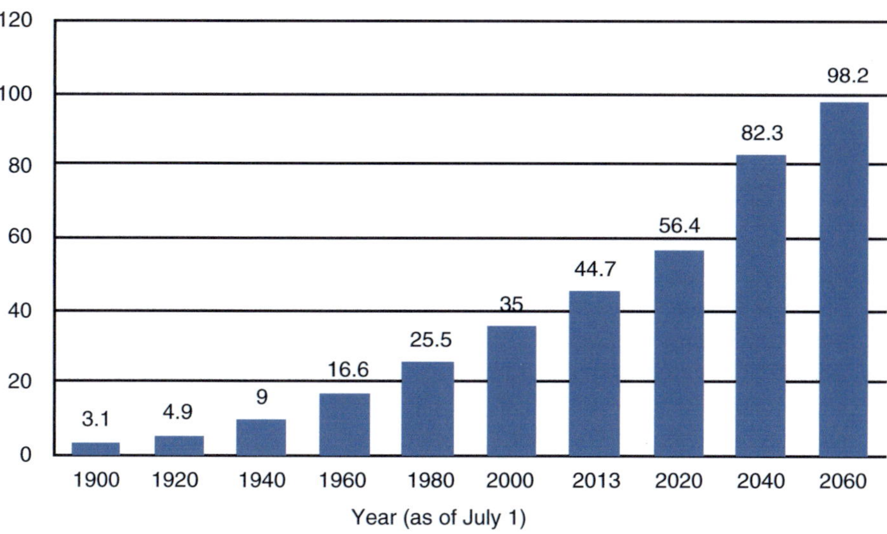

Fig. 9.1 US Department of Health and Human Services projections for adults aged 65 and older

million people by 2050 [5], there is going to be a huge shortage of providers. These are just a few of those questions that need to be answered to prepare for the influx of aging seniors to meet their needs.

One reason for concern is Medicare alone won't be able to cover healthcare needs for seniors given that influx. Those projections indicate that nearly one-fifth of the US adult population will be over 65 by approximately 2040. The traditional fee-for-service model will collapse under the weight of all those seniors.

Senior living communities that desire to stand apart have started to catch on to the idea and are now building "neighborhoods" that are servicing all types of care within that community. Newer housing developments for seniors are steering away from exclusively assisted living, independent living, or skilled nursing and instead working within a framework like that of continuing care retirement communities (CCRCs). These communities set aside space for a percentage of skilled nursing beds in relation to independent living, assisted living residences, and memory care. For the model to embrace continuity, at the helm, there is a physician with a handful of physician assistants and nurse practitioners delivering all of the hands-on care, alongside a designated care coordinator—oftentimes a social worker—who is coordinating the services those patients may need, e.g., labs, X-rays, dentistry, durable medical equipment, etc.

National organizations have also been instrumental in proposing several descriptions of what constitutes ideal transition of care service. The American Geriatrics Society has identified four best practices in transition of care: clinical care needs, policy needs, education needs, and research needs. In their report, they emphasize communication between the providers involved and unobstructed access to patient records containing problem lists, allergies, medications, advance directives, a baseline physical and cognitive assessment, and contact information for both professional care providers and a point of family contact [6]. Models, such as that described above, have taken root in places like Minnesota. The Reducing Avoidable Readmissions Effectively (RARE) campaign was a collaboration of 86 hospitals in the state of Minnesota [7]. Ultimately, more than 7000 readmissions were prevented through this campaign.

In Minnesota, there was a focus on five key areas during the transition of care:

- Comprehensive discharge planning
- Medication management
- Patient and family engagement
- Transition of care support
- Transition of care communications

It is a system like this that Medicare and larger health insurers should embrace. However, it's also the framework of this system which PCPs can strive to work within and create a practice around.

Other methodologies have also shown success. The Mathematica Policy report incorporated elements of care to reduce hospitalization. They concluded successful programs were more likely to provide the following six elements of care [8]:

- Face-to-face care coordinator contact with patients
- Face-to-face care coordinator contact with physicians
- Evidence-based patient education
- Management of care setting transitions
- Facilitation of communications across providers
- Medication management

The GRACE model, as described earlier, aspires to the following seven attributes [9]:

- NP/social work team assigned by physician and practice site
- Focus on geriatric conditions and medication management to complement primary care
- Provided recommendations for care and resources for implementation and follow-up
- Incorporated proven care transition strategies
- Provided home-based and proactive care management
- Integrated with community resources and social services
- Developed relationships through longitudinal care

What's important about the model isn't the number of items on the list, it's the concept of how to manage care throughout that continuum. Looking at how each neighborhood looks, and understanding it well, helps shape the way that primary care practice looks.

How Neighborhoods Differ

Independent Living Facilities

The setting itself is *currently* considered a completely independent setting, but it may be shifting giving the competitive nature of these communities. Currently, independent living facilities, at the very least, have included a service coordinator such as a social worker to navigate the dynamics of social services available to the aging population. The primary focus of these service coordinators is to identify those supportive services—housekeeping, transportation, meals, and socialization—and to create the "link" to service needs of the older adult. In some settings there are even nurses on staff during typical business hours to answer simple questions and provide health education, monitoring of basic vital signs like blood pressures, and coordination with the residents' physicians.

Assisted Living Facilities (ALF)

Assisted living facilities (ALFs) have literally proliferated with an estimated 1.4 million elderly adults currently residing in ALFs across the country [10]. To some extent, ALFs offer some potential advantages to PCPs in that geriatric adults are more collectively accessible. Developers too have marketed this residential option to the elderly as a place to go when they can't live independently in their own home. In 1999, research was done to evaluate the community at large in an ALF. At that time, the study evaluated ALFs that had 11 or more beds and that either self-identified as an assisted living provider or offered at least a basic level of service, including 24-h staff oversight, housekeeping, at least two meals a day, and personal assistance to include at least two of the following—managing medications, bathing, or dressing [11]. At that time, four out of five of the residents in these facilities were totally independent in all activities of daily living (ADLs), 13% needed help with one or two ADLs, and 8% needed help with three or more ADLs. It is obvious to see these findings indicate the assisted living population is significantly less impaired than the nursing home population. Additionally, only 44% of those ALFs had policies that would admit patients who needed assistance with transfers, and 47% would admit people with moderate cognitive impairment.

By 2002, that dynamic had already started to change. It was observed there was a shift, and even though ALF residents were still healthier than the nursing home population, they were older and required more services. Evidence suggested that ALFs were accepting less healthy people over time and that residents were also aging in place. The longitudinal analysis revealed an increase in the proportion of residents with significant functional disability [12]. Another additional dynamic was access to nursing services. In doing so, it significantly reduced the odds of individuals moving to a nursing home, and thereby ALFs could collect revenue that they would have otherwise lost. The conclusion is assisted living facilities had the potential to substitute for a nursing home.

By 2010, this dynamic has changed even more. More than half of ALF-admitted residents had considerable healthcare needs with roughly 40% of residents needing assistance with three of five basic ADLs. Additionally, they served more adults with dementia accounting for nearly 81% of residents in smaller-sized facilities and 63% of those in larger facilities [13].

Nursing Home Expansion into Assisted Living

Since that time, dropping occupancy rates and market competition have forced many traditional nursing homes to explore expansion into assisted living facilities. Some nursing home operators have transformed their building into makeshift ALFs, with nursing and service coordinators and an "in-house" team to support labs, X-rays, dentistry, podiatry, and even physician services across the spectrum of ALF to long-term care (LTC).

From a marketing standpoint, those facilities use terms like "aging in place" when in reality it's a tool for financial survival for these facilities. Although patients may never have intended to go to a nursing home, these individuals did have a sense of security of knowing that this higher level of care was right nearby.

The Evolved Continuing Care Retirement Communities (CCRC)

The concept of a continuing care retirement communities was initially established in the mid-1970s to address the demands and preferences of middle- to high-income individuals for a continuum of care that attempts to exemplify the "aging in place" concept. Findings from a series of regional workshops that invoked the thoughts of stakeholders suggested that many had mixed views about the role of independent apartments in helping their elderly tenants remain in the community and delay or avoid transfers to nursing homes [14]. Consequently, developers built a campus that included independent living settings (apartments and cottages), facilities similar to subacute care as precursors to assisted living when people couldn't go back to their independent environment, and nursing homes which might also include memory care if it was needed. And even though individuals could still transition from one setting to another, those who bought in, signed and purchased a life-care contract, understood they would be fully taken care of in the event of debilitating illness or disability. Forty-five years later, CCRCs still exist, and even though the signed contracts or the "buy-in dynamics" may have changed, many continue to provide this concept of aging in place.

This model more explicitly recognized ALFs as a residential and care setting designed to meet the needs of individuals who needed nursing and social services. For some residents, assisted living was the last stop along the continuum as hospice services were being provided in this setting. Consequently, what has followed has been an evolution of what the CCRC, or more specifically, what the ALF has become. It appears to be evolving into the "new nursing home" as has been demonstrated by Kindred who has sold all their "traditional" nursing homes in favor of focusing on their home health and hospice segments where revenue margins are better [15].

Given this perspective, the typical "primary care" model has shifted with it. A physician-led provider team of geriatric-trained physician assistants and nurse practitioners can literally bring the office to the patient. These teams have arrangements with service coordinators or property managers and have the ability to make house calls to chronically disabled older adults who have multiple chronic conditions, especially for those who find it difficult or impossible to go to a doctor's office or a clinic. The teams provide intensive chronic disease management (often using electronic health records, health information exchanges, and in part telemedicine) just as in a traditional clinic setting. These providers are reimbursed currently on a fee-for-service basis, but coordination with a service coordinator can provide that link to essentially turn an independent housing clinician into a comprehensive health- and long-term care model.

The Latest Model

Now integrated hospital and healthcare systems want to join in offering a "package" as part of their repertoire of services. Organizations such as IPC The Hospitalist Company have attempted to follow their patients along the continuum—or develop their own versions of facilities that span the continuum of care. This health system itself is attempting to manage the transitions between hospital and skilled nursing facilities and reach across the gap of coordinating care in assisted living to make efforts to avoid costly nursing home placement. It is important to note, however, comprehensive hospital, health, and long-term care systems that achieve administrative integration do not always achieve good service integration. The key word needs to be care management. Otherwise, assisted livings become just another production center of revenue and don't really achieve continuity of care nor do they achieve meaningful savings in the healthcare system.

How the Model Fits in the Current System

There is strong concern that our current system will not be able to supply an adequate amount of clinicians to meet the ever-increasing chronic care needs of the aging population. Countries that focus on cost containment also focus on having primary care as a centerpiece of their healthcare delivery system [16].

In 2008, the National Committee for Quality Assurance provided a road map to define the framework of what that primary care model might look like to improve patient outcomes. They even went so far as to define these homes as medical homes. The definition included a model of care that bolsters the clinician-patient relationship and replaces episodic care with coordinated care. Each patient developed a relationship with a primary care clinician and a team of PAs or NPs who collectively took responsibility for patient care along with the patients' healthcare needs and arrange for appropriate care with other qualified clinicians. This model was really intended to provide a more personalized touch that was both coordinated and efficient [17]. This model itself was also endorsed by the American Medical Association and 18 specialty healthcare organizations [18].

There are seven joint principles this model aspires to follow:

Personal physician: Each patient and their families have a relationship with a physician-led team who are all trained to provide continuous and comprehensive care. The intent being that patient-centered care is built on that foundation of a patient-provider relationship.

Physician-directed medical care: The physician leads a team of individuals that collectively take responsibility for ongoing patient care. The intent is meant to encourage physicians to adopt a team approach to care.

Whole-person care: The physician team is responsible for providing all the patient's healthcare needs and for arranging care with other qualified specialists if needed. The intent is again meant to encourage a team approach to care for a patient's acute, chronic, and preventive care needs.

Care is coordinated and integrated: Coordination occurs within the healthcare system but within the patient's community. The intent again is to foster a collaborative process where physical, occupational, and speech therapy and additional community-based services (i.e., pharmacists, podiatry, labs, imaging, dentistry, psychology) are providing a team approach to care.

Quality and safety: The model supports patient-supported disease management, but the information is shared through performance reporting, clinical decision support from clinicians, patient education, online communication, and ongoing quality improvement.

Enhanced access: Care is available not just during the workday but expanded hours of 24/7 access to the provider team using innovative techniques to communicate between patients, provider, and practice staff. The goal here is to constantly have access—whether it be in person and by telephone, secure email, or real-time video conferencing. Additionally, the care team gets secure text communication about the nature of a patient's concern and then decides when appropriate follow-up should take place.

Payment: To promote a sustainable model, reimbursement should be **rewarded** or given to those expanding services beyond just an actual patient encounter. The enhanced access demands and is deserving of a system that demonstrates value above the status quo, such as improved health outcomes and significant decreases in hospitalizations.

Bringing It to Fruition

By adopting those joint principles, primary care will be redefined, and those willing to embrace it will likely be rewarded. To facilitate that model though and create the multidisciplinary team as is described above, there is a need to include a physician who feels comfortable leading a team of PAs and NPs. And while the model certainly includes a physician seeing patients, it does not mean the patient needs to be seen for every acute, subacute, or chronic illness by the physician. In fact, the drivers of much of that care are led by a physician assistant or a nurse practitioner who is skilled in geriatric medicine. The physician is then called upon to carry out routine visits as mandated by law or limited to those situations where an additional knowledge base or skill set of the physician is required.

This multidisciplinary team must also include a nurse or well-trained medical assistant that runs the primary care practice. Much like an office-based setting, where office staff help facilitate labs, X-rays, and subspecialty visits, this person can do the same from a physical location. That physical location could be an office or it could be a person's home; this is the dynamic nature of this type of primary care model. Each primary care practice identifies the internal team to lead that medical home model whether that medical home be a nursing home, an assisted living facility, or an independent living setting. Ideally, a registered nurse or licensed practical nurse could coordinate all of this. However, a good medical assistant can also go a long way in providing quality care.

Advantages and Challenges

Being a primary care provider in these settings requires constant communication with the facility, a good relationship with nursing and non-nursing staff, and some real creativity. A patient's couch or bed, rather than an exam table, may be where a full assessment occurs. Improvisation is a prerequisite of this setting. All the while, productivity is the mainstay of success. Given most of the patients are housed in one environment though, this can be done very efficiently.

One challenge is being accustomed to mobile services as was discussed earlier. Blood draws, ultrasounds, EKGs, or X-rays will have delayed turnaround times. Providers need to rely more on their clinical skills while waiting for such tests to come back. Providers need to be patient with a variety of durable medical equipment (DME) companies so that equipment can be procured for their patients. Wound care, podiatric services, and audiology can be done onsite in many cases. And home health services—PT, OT, and ST—should and can all be done in this setting. Hospice care is also an integral part of this process and becomes an invaluable part of the medical care people receive.

As the practice grows, time efficiency and medication-related issues present two major obstacles. Documenting monthly medication lists can be time-consuming, and finding patients can sometimes be challenging as well. Additionally, a provider may have several facilities to travel to in 1 day. Therefore, "windshield time" needs to be accounted for. Furthermore, each facility is different. Some ALF facilities have licensed caregivers administering medications, and others do not. Some permit nurses to receive verbal orders, while others require a handwritten and signed order. Providers need to know the nuances between facilities and morph around the needs of the buildings and not require the buildings morph around their needs.

Where to Start

It needs to be stressed that although a practice needs an MD at the helm for oversight, and perhaps for those difficult cases, the initials following the providers' names, such as MD, DO, NP, and PA, matter little to most older patients [19]. Older adults want to know someone cares for them and has their best interest in mind. The advanced practice provider should be comfortable understanding when more specialist engagement is needed.

To create an effective practice, all providers need to feel supported. Allow them adequate time to evaluate and treat older complicated adults. Practices not allowing sufficient time for initial or follow-up visits will find themselves with frustrated providers which can lead to attrition and dissatisfied patients or families.

A team approach is also necessary in settings like assisted living facilities and skilled nursing facilities. Providers should have relationships with nursing, social work, pharmacy, and therapy. This sounds difficult, but something as simple as saying hello to any of these professionals goes a long way in setting the tone of approachability. The team approach is also perceived as having continuity centered around it. Providers who are enthusiastic about their work will naturally build a mini-practice within the buildings they frequent and build that practice from within. Naturally, too, their familiarity with those patients goes a long way in being able to be more productive.

Compensation Strategies for Providers

Practices can be successful and provide good geriatric care if their providers see 13 to 15 patient visits in an 8-h day. This time reflects a typical visit, extended visits (whether it be a new patient history/physical or complicated follow-up visit), and windshield time. In any practice, whether it be Medicare-managed care or traditional fee for service, a practice cannot expect a provider to render quality geriatric care if the bar is set too high. Stick within that "sweet spot" of 13 to 15 patients, and providers will likely stick around rather than leave the practice. There are also those providers who see considerably less than that volume of patients but who build the volume of patients and facilities within the practice. They are appropriately called "builders" rather than "producers," and they too hold their weight in the practice. Keeping this in mind allows a practice grows at a steady pace.

There are mechanisms to ensure attractive compensation. They include salary, productivity bonuses in the form of payment and vacation, and considering how part-time providers can balance the ebbs and flows of a practice. A competitive salary allows a provider to focus on quality of geriatric services without pressuring them to focus solely on the quantity of visits. Incentives, based on volume, can also be instrumental for those providers that desire to work harder and add to that competitive salary. Finally, the use of part-time employees with a prorated salary or productivity-only salary will allow a float to cover those providers who are out on vacation or whose facilities have a high number of patients during periods of time, e.g., more influenza cases in the winter months versus the summer or more elective surgeries in the summer months. The risks associated with that discussed above include a provider that may not be as productive as he or she should be to build the practice. It needs to be emphasized that some providers produce numbers under the expectation, while others produce volume over it. Successful practices find the right balance between salary and volume expectations.

One mechanism to account for this is a relative value unit (RVU) plan. Practices can design RVUs that reflect the time needed for various visits. For example, if a geriatric provider spent longer time with patients and families and it takes them one hour to complete this task, they get three RVUs for spending that time with a complex patient and family. On the other hand, a provider's colleague who is seeing three follow-up visits in one hour would get the same three RVUs. Therefore, each geriatric provider is not being penalized for the time needed to provide good geriatric care. RVUs make compensation fair regardless of how much time a provider devotes to geriatric services. However, it can be time-consuming for those in the accounting and human resource departments, and they need to calculate this weekly.

The Concept of Continuity of Care

In the leading paragraphs of this chapter, the importance of continuity of care was discussed. It is a selling point with ALFs and skilled nursing facilities (SNF) alike when they hear how a practice can drive volume into their buildings. It is not uncommon that patients take ill in their ALFs and end up hospitalized. A good geriatrician will serve the patient by trying to get them back home. To do so though means there may need to be a conduit—such as a skilled nursing facility—in the interim to get them back home. That continuity speaks volumes to the ALFs—knowing they're going to get their patient back—but it also improves overall care and makes the patient feel like they are literally being cared for by their "doctor" along that journey. For managed care, a 3-day hospitalization can oftentimes be bypassed; it equates to cost savings by not having that expensive hospital stay. Extending that geriatric arm is priceless and will ensure a practices success given it's managed correctly. To do that, a practice manager needs to maximize a geographic grouping of visits to make it convenient. For example, an advanced practicing provider should keep windshield time to a minimum and group facilities around one another.

Most importantly, the geriatric provider must know how to capture their work. This applies more to a nursing home than an assisted living. It is difficult for a provider to bill on time in an ALF (it's all based on a face-to-face visit), whereas in a SNF, total floor time can be captured, and billing is reflective of all that floor time. It is imperative providers know and understand those nuances. Providers who know how to capture their work through good use of E/M and time-based billing will help a practice immensely.

And though practices will find nursing homes/SNFs to be more financially rewarding for a practice, since seeing a higher patient's volume is likely, it will create additional work for the practice. Three are worth noting:

- The volume of calls from nursing homes is exponentially higher than that of an assisted living. Since concerns can and will arise at any hour of the night, providers will need to take that call.
- The patient acuity is higher. Many of the patients as early as 5 years ago aren't nearly as sick as the patient in 2017. Shorter hospital stays contribute to that. More importantly, providers need to feel comfortable with that higher level of acuity.
- The third issue involves regulations in nursing homes. From the history and physical in subacute care to the mandated monthly visit in long-term care. Each state is different in what they require, but both timely physician and advanced practitioner follow-up can be stressful to a practice.

These constraints are lessened in a practice that only focuses on assisted living.

Expanding into the Home

Residential home visits can be very risky for any practice. The scheduling of appointments, the windshield time for providers, and the unexpected events all cost time and money for the practice. It can be done though when focus is placed on independent living settings such as senior housing or cooperatives where the population is only geriatric and concentrated. This allows for effective geographic grouping such as a nursing home or assisted living facilities. Another challenge is how to fairly compensate a person who decides only to take on home visits. Initially, practices should steer away from this model of care unless they predominantly go into senior housing centers.

Recruiting and Retention Strategies

Successful practices have considered the financial and emotional costs of replacing unfulfilled providers. Recruitment, training, delays in provider efficiency when they start, staff morale, and patient relationships are the mortar that hold the bricks of the practice together. An office manager who continuously keeps in touch with all their providers, to understand their concerns, can improve provider satisfaction.

A High-Touch/High-Tech Experience

A good geriatric practice weighs the benefits of high tech and high touch. To be able to view faxed orders or prescriptions, review labs or progress notes, and check imaging studies such as X-rays, is important; to do it all from your phone is the high tech part of it. The use of devices for real-time video conversations with staff, families, and patients is the world that we have evolved into; medicine must evolve with it. For example, CPT codes now exist—and can be billed and paid in the state of Minnesota—for video conferencing and/or assessments.

Most importantly, all of this needs to be done in real time so that at any time, any provider, anywhere in the world, has access to those records. Ultimately, to span across the barrier of a wall within a practice, it's recommended that health exchange of information also be a part of this high-tech experience. It will make the practice stand apart from their competitors.

While young providers may have that skill set, older providers may struggle. But it works both ways. Older providers may offer insight in their experience and confidence to make complex decisions where those "techy" tools may not be as effective. It is a balance, but technology and a sense of touch can be very effective. Practices that incorporate high tech with high touch tend to more successful.

What's Next

The trends in America suggest older adults will be left without an adequate supply of primary care providers. Consequently, more care of older adults will fall upon non-fellowship-trained family practitioners, internists, and advanced practice providers [19]. However, given the right environment, creative solutions do exist for quality care. Advances in medical technology and mobile health services can enable a team of providers to fully deliver primary care service at the convenience of patients and families. The vast difference is they are not bound by the traditional brick and mortar older practitioners were accustomed to. These evolving practices can be highly reimbursable, with essentially low overhead expenditure, which is ideal for changing the language of primary care.

References

1. Berg R. The evolution of nursing homes. http://www.mcknights.com/guest-columns/the-evolution-of-nursing-homes/article/525771/. Retrieved Feb 2017.
2. Counsell SR, Callahan CM, Clark DO, et al. Geriatric care management for low-income seniors: a randomized controlled trial. JAMA. 2007;298:2623–33.
3. Rochester-Eyeguokan CD, Pincus KJ, Patel RS, et al. Department the current landscape of transitions of care practice models: a scoping review. Pharmacotherapy. 2016;36(1):117–33.
4. Snow V, Beck D, Budnitz T, et al. Transitions of care consensus policy statement: American College of Physicians, Society of General Internal Medicine, Society of Hospital Medicine, American Geriatrics Society, American College of Emergency Physicians, and Society for Academic Emergency Medicine. J Hosp Med. 2009;4(6):364–70.
5. Kahn JH, Magauran BG, Olshaker JS, et al. Current trends in Geriatric Emergency Medicine. Emerg Med Clin North Am. 2016;34(3):435–52.
6. Coleman EA, Boult CE. On behalf of the American Geriatrics Society Health Care Systems Committee. Improving the quality of transitional care for persons with complex care needs. J Am Geriatr Soc. 2003;51(4):556–7.

7. McCoy KA, Bear-Pfaffendof K, Foreman JK, et al. Reducing avoidable hospital readmissions effectively: a statewide campaign. Jt Comm J Qual Patient Saf. 2014;40:198–204.
8. Schore J, Peikes D, Peterson G, et al. Fourth Report to Congress on the Evaluation Mathematica Policy Research of the Medicare Coordinated Care Demonstration. March 2011. p. 16.
9. Counsell SR, Callahan CM, Buttar AB, et al. Geriatric Resources for Assessment and Care of Elders (GRACE): a new model of primary care for low-income seniors. J Am Geriatr Soc. 2006;54(7):1136–41.
10. Ledbetter L. Developing an assisted living practice. Today Geriatr Med. 2015;8(2):8.
11. Hawes C, Rose M, Phillips CD. A national study of assisted living for the frail elderly: results of a national survey of facilities. Washington, DC: U.S. Department of Health and Human Services; 1999.
12. Spillman BC, Liu K, McGilliard C. Trends in residential long-term care: use of nursing home and assisted living and characteristics of facilities and residents. Washington, DC: U.S. Department of Health and Human Services, Assistant Secretary for Planning and Evaluation, Office of Disability, Aging and Long-Term; 2002.
13. Han K, Trinkoff AM, Storr CL, et al. Variation across U.S. assisted living facilities: admissions, resident care needs, and staffing. J Nurs Scholarsh. 2017;49(1):24–32.
14. Harahan M, Saners A, Stone R. Findings from the regional workshops on affordable housing plus services strategies for low- and moderate-income seniors. Washington, DC: American Association of Homes and Services for the Aging and the Institute for the Future of Aging Services; 2006.
15. Barkholz D. Kindred is exiting the skilled-nursing home business. http://www.modernhealthcare.com/article/20161108/NEWS/311089982. Retrieved Dec 2016.
16. Davis K, Schoen C, Stremikis K. Mirror, Mirror on the Wall, 2014 Update: How the U.S. Health Care System Compares Internationally, 2014 Report. New York, NY: The Commonwealth Fund. http://www.commonwealthfund.org/publications/fund-reports/2014/jun/mirror-mirror. Retrieved Jan 2017.
17. National Committee on Quality Assurance. NCQA patient-centered medical home. Health care that revolves around you. 2011. http://www.ncqa.org/portals/0/PCMH2011%20with-CAHPSInsert.pdf. Retrieved Jan 2017.
18. Bein B. AMA delegates adopt AAFP's joint principles of patient-centered medical home. Ann Fam Med. 2009;7(1):86–7.
19. Murphy D, Shirar LE, Tapia S, et al. Building from within: 5 strategies for growing a geriatrics practice. Today Geriatr Med. 2014;7(6):10.

Primary Care in the Nursing Home

Robert A. Zorowitz

Quality of Medical Care in the Nursing Home

The drive for quality primary care in nursing facilities arose in the last few decades in response to public concern about substandard medical services provided to nursing home residents. In his seminal, Pulitzer prize-winning book, *Why Survive? Being Old in America*, Dr. Robert N. Butler wrote in 1975:

> One can also list a grim catalogue of the medical deficiencies of the nursing-home industry and related facilities. Nursing homes, however financed, do not provide well-organized, comprehensive medical care. Care must be obtained from family physicians or private physicians assigned by a welfare agency or the home itself. Many states do not even require a principal physician, let alone a medical director, for a nursing home, and when they do there is no assurance that the physician regards himself as responsible for the patients. Doctors seldom conduct regular rounds. Winter flu shots are often not given. There is minimal preventive care… [1]

In response to the serious problems plaguing nursing home care brought to the public's attention by Butler's book, a series of reports by the Special Committee on Aging of the United States Senate [2] and subsequently by a landmark report by the Institute of Medicine, "Improving the Quality of Care in Nursing Homes [3]," Congress passed the Federal Nursing Home Reform Act as part of the Omnibus Budget Reconciliation Act of 1987 (OBRA-87). Under the regulations of OBRA-87, a skilled nursing facility "must provide services to attain or maintain the highest practicable physical, mental, and psychosocial well-being of each resident, in accordance with a written plan of care which…is initially prepared…by a team which includes the resident's attending physician [4]."

R.A. Zorowitz, MD, MBA, FACP, AGSF, CMD
Optum, Inc., New York, NY, USA
e-mail: bobzorowitz@yahoo.com

© Springer International Publishing AG 2018
M. Wasserman, J. Riopelle (eds.), *Primary Care for Older Adults*,
DOI 10.1007/978-3-319-61329-1_10

In addition to introducing a series of quality metrics to be reported in the Minimum Data Set (MDS), OBRA-87 established the right of nursing facility residents to choose a personal attending physician and to be fully informed in advance about care and treatment. In this chapter, we will examine the challenges of providing medical care to this complex and vulnerable elderly population and several approaches to medical management that have evolved since the passage of that landmark bill.

Nursing Home Residents

There are over 15,000 nursing (OBRA-87)facilities in the United States with approximately 1.7 million licensed beds [5]. Most nursing facilities are comprised of two related, though often comingled, services. Long-term residential care is provided for those individuals who live in the nursing facility, often their last place of residence. Skilled nursing and rehabilitation services or subacute care is provided to patients discharged from the hospital but who require additional short-term inpatient nursing and rehabilitation services prior to safely returning home. More recently, many nursing facilities are also providing palliative care and, in collaboration with certified agencies, hospice services for terminally ill residents.

Medicaid is the main source of payment for residential long-term care nursing home services followed by out-of-pocket payments [6], whereas Medicare is the main source of payment for short-term skilled care [7] as well as medical services by physicians and other healthcare providers to both long-term care residents and short-term subacute patients.

According to the Centers for Disease Control and Prevention, 41.6% of long-term nursing home residents are age 85 and over, 27.2% are ages 75–84, 16.1% are ages 65–74, and 15.1% are under age 65. Chronic diseases and multimorbidity are extremely common. Approximately 50% of long-term nursing home residents suffer from Alzheimer's disease or other dementias, just under 50% suffer from depression and nearly a third suffer from diabetes and its complications [8]. Adding to this complexity is the phenomenon of polypharmacy, the administration of multiple medications, resulting in frequent adverse drug reactions [9, 10].

According the Medicare Payment Advisory Commission (MedPAC), in 2014, about 15,000 Skilled Nursing Facilities (SNF) furnished 2.4 million Medicare-covered stays to 1.7 million fee-for-service (FFS) beneficiaries. Most post-acute SNF admissions are for patients treated in the hospital for joint replacement, septicemia, kidney and urinary tract infections, hip and femur procedures, pneumonia, heart failure, and shock. Many recipients of skilled services are long-term nursing home residents returning from hospitalizations back to the nursing home, where they become eligible for skilled services under Medicare Part A. Therefore, post-acute SNF patients are older, frailer and disproportionately female, disabled, living in an institution, and dually eligible for both Medicare and Medicaid. In 2014, 37.6% of recipients of skilled nursing facility care were discharged to the community, although the percentage of patients, who had been living in the community prior to hospitalization and skilled services and subsequently discharged to the community, is significantly higher [11].

Thus, individuals in nursing homes, for either long-term care or short-term post-acute care, are among the most complex, frail, and vulnerable elderly. Moreover, there is evidence that over the last 20–30 years, nursing home residents have become increasingly frail and complex [12, 13]. A recent review and meta-analysis found that as many as 50% of nursing home residents were frail and approximately 40% were prefrail [14].

A 2006 Kaiser study noted that the average length of stay for long-term residents in nursing homes is just over 2 years [15], but there is great variability, depending on age on admission, comorbidities, and other factors. A 2010 study of lengths of stay of nursing home decedents also demonstrated variable lengths of stay, depending on factors related to social supports, but found that median and mean length of stay before death were 5 months and 13.7 months respectively, with 53% dying within 6 months of placement [16]. This can be expected to have a significant influence on decisions regarding management of chronic disorders as well as preventive care, since such decisions are often dependent on the anticipated time for treatment effect.

The Role of the Attending Physician and Medical Director in the Nursing Home

The attending physician plays a critical role in the nursing home as part of a team, including the nursing staff, social worker, dietician, and other healthcare professionals. Yet, the federal regulations regarding the roles of the attending physician and medical director are relatively brief and vague. The resident has the right to choose a personal attending physician, who must personally approve in writing a recommendation that an individual be admitted to a facility and must supervise the medical care of each resident. The physician must see the resident at least once every 30 days for the first 90 days after admission and at least once every 60 days thereafter([17]). Table 10.1 lists the requirements for physician services by the nursing home and for the nursing home physician.

Table 10.1 From code of federal regulations, 42 CFR §483.30 physician services

Requirements for physician services by the nursing home	*Requirements for the nursing home physician*
1. A physician must personally approve in writing a recommendation that an individual be admitted to a facility	1. Must review the resident's total program of care, including medications and treatments, at each required visit
2. Each resident must remain under the care of a physician	2. Must write, sign and date progress notes at each visit
3. The medical care of each resident is supervised by a physician	3. Must sign and date all orders
4. Another supervises the medical care of residents when their attending physicians are unavailable	4. Must see the resident at least once every 30 days for the first 90 days after admission and at least once every 60 days thereafter

Table 10.2 Responsibilities of the attending physician in the nursing home

Clinical	Administrative
• Approve each resident's admission to the facility and complete medical history and physical examination, including a list of medical diagnoses, cognitive and functional status, rehabilitation potential, and review of laboratory and diagnostic data	• Be familiar with federal and state regulations and facility policies
• Provide admission orders until staff completes a comprehensive assessment and interdisciplinary plan of care	• Serve on process improvement committees when asked by the medical director
• Supervise medical care of each nursing home resident including participating in assessment and care planning process, monitoring changes in medical status and providing treatment	• Provide nursing home residents, caregivers, and facility staff contact information for calls regarding resident care, and provide on-call and emergency coverage when unavailable
• Ensure that the resident is afforded privacy and dignity, provide informed consent when appropriate, and preserve the right of the nursing home resident to select clinicians for medical and dental care	• Physician visit intervals
• Discuss advance care planning with the resident or designee as appropriate	– Admission visit: no later than 72 h after admission (except when examination was performed and documented within previous 5 days of admission)
• Attend to any emergency or significant change in condition	– Scheduled visit: at least once every 30 days for the first 90 days and at least once every 60 days thereafter (may delegate every other visit to APC)
• Obtain consultations when needed	– Interim visits: in the event of an emergency and whenever indicated
• Order laboratory and diagnostic tests when needed and act on results with documentation	Information was adapted from Diamant, Unwin et al., Centers for Medicare and Medicaid Services and Title 42 Requirements for Long-Term Care Facilities
• Prescribe, monitor, and reconcile all medications and respond in writing to consultant pharmacist review, deprescribing whenever possible	
• Provide orders for transfer and discharge	

Adapted from Zweig SC, Popejoy LL, Parker-Oliver D, Meadows SE. The physician's role in patients' nursing home care. JAMA. 2011;306(13):1468–1478

Additional roles and responsibilities for attending physicians have been outlined by professional societies such as AMDA-The Society for Post-Acute and Long-Term Care Medicine [18] and have been published in the literature [19, 20]. Table 10.2 lists the responsibilities for the attending physician in the nursing home. Individual states, such as New York, have augmented federal regulations by issuing additional regulations or guidelines for the role of the attending physician in the nursing home [21].

There are a number of different medical staff models in nursing homes. The closed staff model usually involves a small number of employed physicians with or without advanced practice clinicians, to which the residents are assigned according to their floors or units. The open staff model or voluntary model usually involves community physicians, who spend varying parts of their time in the nursing home, but may also have an office practice or manage hospitalized patients. More recently, there has been an increased presence of large group practices that contract with nursing facilities to provide physicians and advanced practice clinicians, including nurse practitioners and physician assistants, to the facility. These group practices may exclusively serve nursing homes or have mixed practices serving both nursing homes and hospitals or their own office practices.

Most physicians, who care for nursing home residents, are reimbursed under a fee-for-service system by either the Centers for Medicare and Medicaid Services for residents covered by traditional Medicare or Medicaid or by a variety of managed care organizations delegated to administer Medicare Advantage, Managed Medicaid programs, or combined Medicare/Medicaid ("dual eligible") programs. A small but growing number of physicians receive a fixed monthly fee per beneficiary or capitation to cover all necessary visits and management services provided during the coverage period. There are also alternative payment models combining either fee-for-service or capitated reimbursement with additional payments linked to a variety of quality metrics. In 2015, the US Department of Health and Human Services announced that it had set a goal to have 50% of Medicare payments in alternative payment models and 90% of Medicare fee-for-service payments linked to quality metrics by 2018 [22]. As of this writing, it remains to be seen how these goals will affect payment models for physicians caring for nursing home residents, but it is evident that the trend, increasingly, is to link payment to quality, rather than just volume.

A 1997 survey of medical practice in nursing homes revealed that most physicians reported spending no significant time caring for nursing home residents. A majority of physicians with a nursing home practice spent less than 2 h per week with patients [23]. A 2008 American Academy of Family Physicians survey reported that the average family physician supervises 9.6 nursing home residents and conducts 2.3 weekly nursing home visits [24].

To better determine the effect of medical staff organization on the quality of nursing home care, Katz and his colleagues validated the dimensions of a nursing home medical staff organization [25, 26]. Using this framework, a cross-sectional study of 202 freestanding US nursing homes demonstrated that 30-day rehospitalizations, one accepted measure of nursing home quality, were less likely in nursing homes with a more formal appointment process for physicians than in those with a more open and less restrictive staff [27]. This suggests that physicians spending a greater percentage of their time in the nursing home and, therefore, able to spend more time with residents and respond more quickly to changes in condition may provide a higher quality of care than physicians who spend little time caring for nursing home residents.

Although federal regulations do not delineate requirements for nursing home physicians to possess specific competencies, AMDA-The Society for Post-Acute and Long-Term Care Medicine released a position paper outlining the framework, principles, and scope of nursing home competencies. The foundation of nursing home competency rests on addressing ethical conflicts, providing care that is at least consistent with legal and regulatory requirements, appropriate communication, and interaction with staff, patient, and families, exhibiting respectful and culturally sensitive behavior, and addressing resident/patient care needs in an appropriate and timely fashion. The recommended competencies, listed in Table 10.3, address the medical care delivery process, systems management, a minimum list of medical knowledge, and competency in quality assurance and process improvement [28].

Table 10.3 Competencies for post-acute and long-term care

Foundation, which focuses on ethics, professionalism, and communication, establishes the following six competencies for the NH attending physician

1.1 Addresses conflicts that may arise in the provision of clinical care by applying principles of ethical decision-making

1.2 Provides and supports care that is consistent with (but not based exclusively on) legal and regulatory requirements

1.3 Interacts with staff, patients, and families effectively by using appropriate strategies to address sensory, language, health literacy, cognitive, and other limitations

1.4 Demonstrates communication skills that foster positive interpersonal relationships with residents, their families, and members of the interdisciplinary team (IDT)

1.5 Exhibits professional, respectful, and culturally sensitive behavior toward residents, their families, and members of the IDT

1.6 Addresses patient/resident care needs, visits, phone calls, and documentation in an appropriate and timely fashion

Medical care delivery process includes the following five competencies

2.1 Manages the care of all post-acute patients/LTC residents by consistently and effectively applying the medical care delivery process—including recognition, problem definition, diagnosis, goal identification, intervention, and monitoring of progress

2.2 Develops, in collaboration with the IDT, a person-centered, evidence-based medical care plan that strives to optimize quality of life and function within the limits of an individual's medical condition, prognosis, and wishes

2.3 Estimates prognosis based on a comprehensive patient/resident evaluation and available prognostic tools and discusses the conclusions with the patient/resident, their families (when appropriate), and staff

2.4 Identifies circumstances in which palliative and/or end-of-life care (e.g., hospice) may benefit the patient/resident and family

2.5 Develops and oversees, in collaboration with the IDT, an effective palliative care plan for patients/residents with pain and other significant acute or chronic symptoms or who are at the end of life

Systems include the following six competencies

3.1 Provides care that uses resources prudently and minimizes unnecessary discomfort and disruption for patients/residents (e.g., limited nonessential vital signs and blood glucose checks)

3.2 Can identify rationale for and uses of key patient/resident databases (e.g., the Minimum Data Set [MDS]), in care planning, facility reimbursement, and monitoring of quality

3.3 Guides determinations of appropriate levels of care for patients/residents, including identification of those who could benefit from a different level of care

3.4 Performs functions and tasks that support safe transitions of care

3.5 Works effectively with other members of the IDT, including the medical director, in providing care based on understanding and valuing the general roles, responsibilities, and levels of knowledge and training for those of various disciplines

3.6 Informs patients/residents and their families of their healthcare options and potential impact on personal finances by incorporating knowledge of payment models relevant to the post-acute and LTC setting

(continued)

Table 10.3 (continued)

Medical knowledge includes the following six competencies

4.1 Identifies, evaluates, and addresses significant symptoms associated with change of condition, based on knowledge of diagnosis in individuals with multiple comorbidities and risk factors

4.2 Formulates a pertinent and adequate differential diagnosis for all medical signs and symptoms, recognizing atypical presentation of disease, for post-acute patients and LTC residents

4.3 Identifies and develops a person-centered medical treatment plan for diseases and geriatric syndromes commonly found in post-acute patients and LTC residents

4.4 Identifies interventions to minimize risk factors and optimize patient/resident safety (e.g., prescribes antibiotics and antipsychotics prudently, assesses the risks and benefits of initiation or continuation of physical restraints, urinary catheters, and venous access catheters)

4.5 Manages pain effectively and without causing undue treatment complications

4.6 Prescribes and adjusts medications prudently, consistent with identified indications and known risks and warnings

Personal quality assessment and performance improvement (QAPI) includes the following three competencies

5.1 Develops a continuous professional development plan focused on post-acute and LTC medicine, utilizing relevant opportunities from professional organizations (AMDA, AGS, AAFP, ACP, SHM, American Academy of Hospice and Palliative Medicine), licensing requirements (state, national, province), and maintenance of certification programs

5.2 Utilizes data (e.g., Physician Quality Reporting System indicators, MDS data, patient satisfaction) to improve care of their patients/residents

5.3 Strives to improve personal practice and patient/resident results by evaluating patient/resident adverse events and outcomes (e.g., falls, medication errors, healthcare-acquired infections, dehydration, rehospitalization)

Katz PR, Wayne M, Evans J, et al. Examining the rationale and processes behind the development of AMDA's competencies for post-acute and long-term care. Annals of Long-Term Care: Clinical Care and Aging. 2014;22(11):36–39

The monthly visit is an opportunity not only to fulfill regulatory tasks but also to operationalize good geriatric care. This includes, but is not limited to:

- Assessing and proactively managing chronic conditions
- Rationalizing and streamlining the medication regimen, eliminating unnecessary medications ("deprescribing") as feasible [29–31]
- Reassessing function; assessing need for rehabilitative services
- Assessing appropriateness of preventive services and screening
- Reviewing the advance care plan and advance directives

In addition, the attending physician should be encouraged to attend the required quarterly care plan meetings whenever possible. Physician input is not only required but is an invaluable contribution to a quality plan of care.

According to federal regulations, each nursing facility must designate a physician to serve as medical director. The medical director is responsible for implementation of resident care policies and the coordination of medical care in the facility [32]. While the attending physicians are responsible for supervising and managing the care of individual residents, the medical director provides oversight for the medical care, providing clinical guidance regarding the implementation of resident care policies, and collaborates with the facility leadership and staff to develop policies and procedures reflecting current standards of practice [5, 8]. Therefore, together with the administrator and director of nursing services, the medical director is a key leader in the delivery of quality services in the nursing facility.

Since 1991, the American Board of Post-Acute and Long-Term Care Medicine (formerly the American Medical Directors Certification Program) has provided a certification process for nursing facility medical directors. At least one study demonstrated that the presence of a certified medical director independently predicted quality in US nursing homes [33]. Most states do not have specific certification requirements for the nursing facility medical director, but the state of Maryland is an exception requiring "that a medical director's qualifications shall include, but are not limited to 'successful completion of a curriculum in physician management or administration from the American Medical Directors Association or another curriculum approved by the Department or its designee [34].'" Most other states, such as New York, do not require certification but have issued general principles and detailed guidelines regarding the qualifications, roles, and responsibilities of the medical director [35].

As the role of the nursing facility medical director has evolved, AMDA-The Society for Post-Acute and Long-Term Care Medicine updated its 1991 document delineating the roles and responsibilities of the medical director to reflect the growing complexity of services provided by the contemporary nursing facility. This 2011 document describes the position of the nursing home medical director in terms of the roles, functions, and tasks hierarchy [36]. The recommended roles and functions of the nursing facility medical director are listed in Fig. 10.1.

Reducing Avoidable Hospital Transfers

It has been well established that hospitalizations of nursing facility residents are often unnecessary or potentially avoidable. A: study, using structured implicit review of hospital transfers, concluded that in 36% of emergency department transfers and 40% of hospital admissions, the transfer/admit was inappropriate [37]. A later study reported that 67% of hospitalizations were potentially avoidable. The reasons given were lack of available primary care clinicians, inability to obtain lab tests or intravenous fluids, and other issues with care delivery [38]. Unnecessary hospital transfers may be caused by multiple factors, including patient and family preferences, inappropriate hospital discharge, lack of advanced directives, polypharmacy, lack of heart failure protocols, under-recognition of early symptoms or over-recognition of acuity of patient, fear of litigation, and poor communication between the hospital and nursing home [39].

Based on these studies, it would appear that the reasons for avoidable nursing home transfers fall into several categories:

- Staff structure: In homes with open medical staffs and little physician presence, residents are more likely to be transferred to the hospital when a change in condition occurs outside regular hours or when a physician is not on the premises.

<table>
<tr><td align="center">Four Key Roles</td></tr>
</table>

1. Physician Leadership
   - Serves as physician responsible for the overall care and clinical practice carried out at the facility
2. Patient Care-Clinical Leadership
   - Applies clinical and administrative skills to guide the facility in providing care
3. Quality of Care
   - Helps the facility develop and manage both quality and safety initiatives, including risk management
4. Education, Information and Communication
   - Provides information that helps others (including facility staff, practitioners and those in the community) understand and provide care

Functions

1. Administrative
   - Participates in administrative decision making and recommends and approves relevant policies and procedures
2. Professional Services
   - Organizes and coordinates physician services and the services provided by other professionals as they relate to patient care
3. Quality Assurance and Performance Improvement
   - Participates in the process to ensure the quality of medical care and medically related care, including whether it is effective, efficient, safe, timely, patient-centered and equitable
4. Education
   - Participates in developing and disseminating key information and education
5. Employee Health
   - Participates in the surveillance and promotion of employee health, safety and welfare
6. Community
   - Helps articulate the post-acute and long-term care facility's mission to the community
7. Rights of Individuals
   - Participates in establishing policies and procedures for assuring that the rights of individuals (patients, staff, practitioners, and community) are respected
8. Social, Regulatory, Political and Economic Factors
   - Acquires and applies knowledge of social, regulatory, political and economic factors that relate to patient care and related services
9. Person-Directed Care
   - Supports and promotes person-directed care

Fig. 10.1 The nursing home medical director: leader and manager. Adapted from AMDA-The Society for Post-Acute and Long-Term Care Medicine. White Paper on the Nursing Home Medical Director: Leader and Manager. March 2011

- Clinical staff capability: In homes with fewer registered nurses, higher resident-to-staff ratios, and/or clinical staff inadequately trained to recognize and manage changes of condition, residents are more likely to be transferred to the hospital when a change of condition occurs.
- Lack of resources: Without adequate available intravenous fluids, antibiotics, and other clinical resources, residents are more likely to be transferred to the hospital.

To address the organizational, cultural, and clinical factors contributing to unnecessary hospital transfers, Ouslander and his colleagues developed a comprehensive, multipronged quality improvement program called Interventions to Reduce Acute Care Transfers (INTERACT). The premise underlying this program is twofold. First, the rate of avoidable transfers to the hospital is considered a proxy for the quality of care, so reduction of avoidable transfers equates to an improvement in the quality of care [40]. Second, effectively impacting the rate of avoidable transfers requires commitment from the leadership of the facility but must involve all employees of the facility, that is, a commitment from the top to the bottom of the organization but implementation from the bottom to the top. This essentially involves a change in organizational culture, focusing on the reduction of hospital transfers by emphasizing early identification of changes of condition, accurate communication of findings to the medical staff, improved advance care planning, and rapid, effective interventions thereafter [41].

There are three types of tools provided in the INTERACT intervention: communication tools, care paths or clinical tools, and advance care planning tools [42]. To engage the entire facility staff in recognizing and reporting changes of condition, the INTERACT program utilizes the "Stop and Watch" tool. This tool, shown in Fig. 10.2, is a simple form that may be utilized by nursing assistants, housekeeping staff or any other facility employees to report a potential change of condition to nursing staff. Based on an illness warning instrument developed specifically for nursing assistants [43], this validated and standardized form facilitates the communication of observed signs of possible acute illness to the nursing staff.

Stop and Watch
Early Warning Tool

INTERACT
Version 4.0 Tool

If you have identified a change while caring for or observing a resident, please circle the change and notify a nurse. Either give the nurse a copy of this tool or review it with her/him as soon as you can.

S	Seems different than usual
T	Talks or communicates less
O	Overall needs more help
P	Pain – new or worsening; Participated less in activities
a	Ate less
n	No bowel movement in 3 days; or diarrhea
d	Drank less
W	Weight change
A	Agitated or nervous more than usual
T	Tired, weak, confused, or drowsy
C	Change in skin color or condition
H	Help with walking, transferring, toileting more than usual

☐ Check here if no change noted while monitoring high risk patient

Patient/Resident

Your Name

Reported to *Date and Time (am/pm)*

Nurse Response *Date and Time (am/pm)*

Nurse's Name

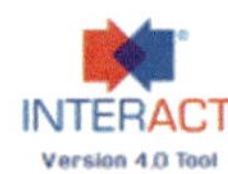

Fig. 10.2 The Stop and Watch early warning tool. http://interact2.net/docs/INTERACT%20Version%204.0%20Tools/INTERACT%204.0%20NH%20Tools%206_17_15/148604-Stop-and-Watch%20v4_0.pdf. Accessed 17 Dec 2016

Once a potential change in condition is either reported to nursing or observed by nursing, there are tools designed to facilitate the assessment and collection of appropriate clinical information and a form structured to encourage thorough and accurate documentation and communication of clinical findings. This SBAR ("Situation-Background-Appearance-Review") form, shown in Fig. 10.3, is based

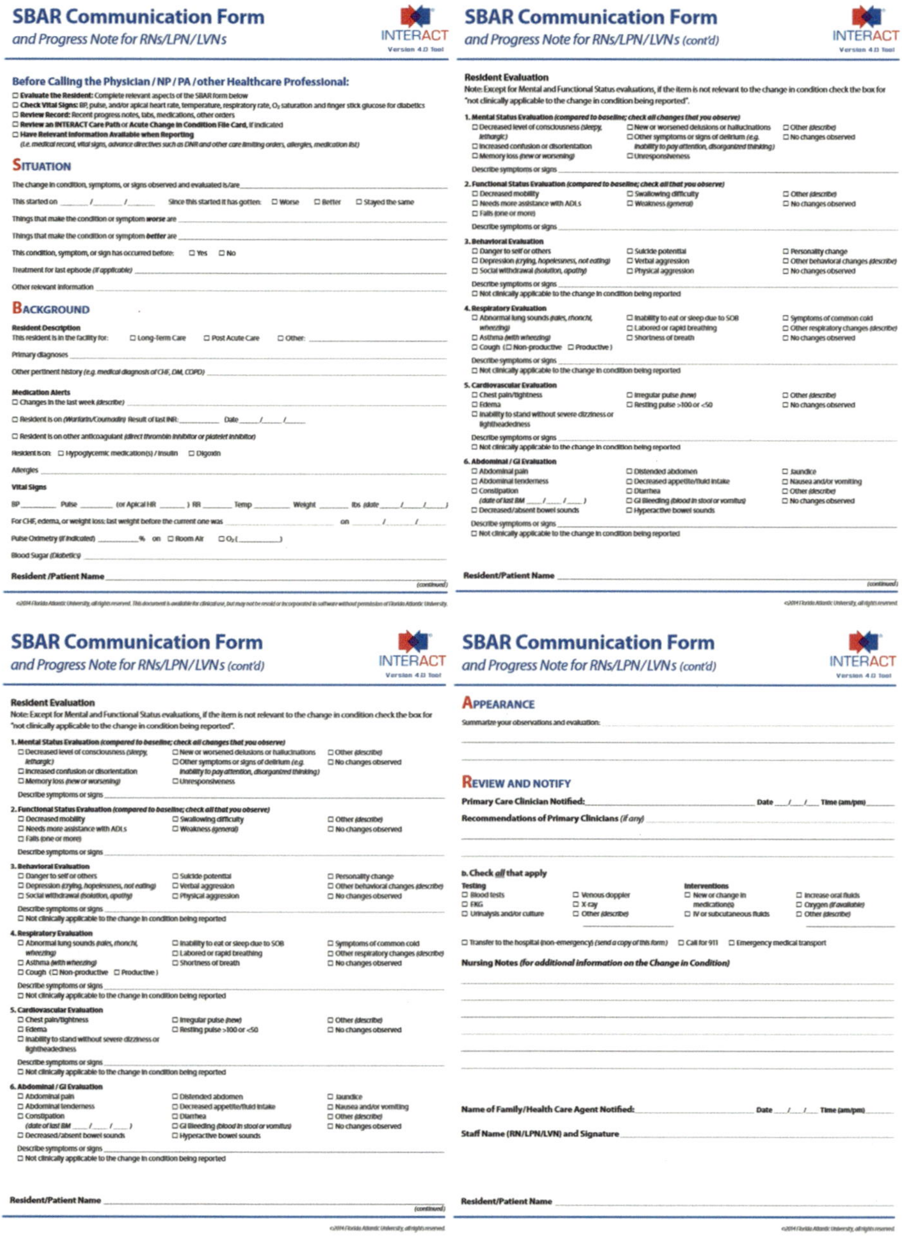

Fig. 10.3 The INTERACT SBAR communication form. http://interact2.net/docs/INTERACT%20Version%204.0%20Tools/INTERACT%20V4%20SBAR_Communication_Form%20Dec%2010. pdf. Accessed 17 Dec 2016

on similar forms utilized in nuclear submarines and provides a template for documenting and reporting clinical information to the covering physician. By allowing for efficient collection, organization, and presentation of clinical information, the SBAR process and form improves communication with the covering clinician and improves the timeliness and quality of clinical decision-making.

The cornerstone of INTERACT is its structure as a performance improvement program, based on the "Plan-Do-Study-Act" cycle [44]. The *sine qua non* of a quality improvement intervention is the process of root cause analysis ("study") allowing for identification of opportunities for further improvement ("act"). The INTERACT program requires that each hospital transfer undergoes root cause analysis, usually by a team consisting of the medical director, director of nursing, director of performance improvement, and other clinicians. By identifying root causes for each hospital transfer, particularly potentially avoidable hospital transfers, and implementing further process improvements, clinical quality is continuously monitored and improved, leading to fewer avoidable hospital transfers.

A partial implementation of the INTERACT quality improvement strategies resulted in a 50% reduction of hospitalizations and a 36% reduction in potentially avoidable hospitalizations [45]. A subsequent implementation of the INTERACT program in 30 New York nursing homes showed mixed results, depending on the level of engagement of facility leadership and staff. Whereas overall there was a nonsignificant 10.6% decrease in hospital admissions, there was a 14.3% reduction in nursing homes with the highest engagement and a 27.2% reduction in nursing homes in the highest tertile of baseline hospital admission rates [46]. This suggests that the INTERACT program requires a full commitment of leadership and complete engagement of staff to succeed [47]. It appears to work best in facilities with high baseline hospital transfer rates.

Continuing research on facilities implementing the INTERACT program has shed light on common root causes for potentially avoidable hospitalizations [48, 49]. Based on the lessons from this research, the INTERACT team developed order sets for common conditions associated with potentially avoidable hospitalizations [50]. As INTERACT has become increasingly adopted by nursing facilities across the country and elsewhere in the world, it is setting a standard for primary care in the nursing home.

Collaborative Physician/Advanced Practice Clinician Models

According to federal regulations, after the required first visit, the physician has the option of alternating subsequent visits with an advanced practice clinician (APC), such as a physician assistant or nurse practitioner ([17]). There are no other regulatory limits on the number of visits that may be provided by APCs. This has encouraged the development of collaborative models between physicians and APCs for a number of reasons, including augmenting the availability of medical care provided by physicians, providing a more rapid and proactive approach to preventive maintenance and changes of condition or simply to build a more lucrative business model.

Probably the most widespread and well-known impetus for a implementing collaborative model is to reduce unnecessary hospital transfers, thereby saving costs and improving the quality of care.

Most studies of collaborative care models examine the impact of nurse practitioners or advanced practice nurses (APN). In one review of the literature, five distinct APN roles were identified:

- Provider of primary care to long-term care residents
- Provider of acute care to both short-stay and long-stay residents
- Educator of residents, families, and staff
- Consultant for staff on system-wide patient care issues
- Consultant to organizations on improving facility-wide systems of care

The following outcomes of APN care were found:

- Management of chronic conditions
- Improved functional status
- Reduced hospitalization and emergency department use
- Reduced costs
- Reduced or equivalent mortality
- Increased time spent with residents
- Improved resident, family, and staff satisfaction [51]

The EverCare Model One of the earliest and well-studied models of collaborative care with APCs is the EverCare model. The EverCare model is a hybrid managed care plan and service model characterized by the delivery of care to long-term nursing home residents by advanced practice clinicians in collaboration with nursing facility attending physicians.

In the late 1980s, observing the frequency at which nursing home residents were transferred to the emergency room, the lack of adequate medical supervision, and the need for more coordinated care, two nurse practitioners in Minnesota, Jeannine Bayard, MPH, APRN, and Ruthann Jacobson, MPH, APRN, proposed a capitated, managed care model, in which nurse practitioners employed by the payer would collaborate with the facility's attending physicians to provide care to a panel of residents. By paying the facility a higher rate to manage sick residents in house, avoiding unnecessary hospitalizations, and sharing the resulting savings with the facility, the goal was to provide higher-quality, coordinated care at a lower cost to the plan [52].

Initially established in the Twin cities, the EverCare program was subsequently replicated as a Medicare demonstration program in six cities [53]. Studies at the time demonstrated that nurse practitioners spent about 35% of their working day on direct patient care and another 26% in indirect care activities. Of the latter, 46% was spent interacting with staff, 26% with families and 15% with physicians [54]. Early findings indicated that residents enrolled in the EverCare program were hospitalized at half the frequency of control residents, with significant savings in hospital costs per nurse practitioner [55]. When hospital admissions and in-house treatment days (known then as "intensive service days") were combined, EverCare enrollees had significantly fewer events than controls [56], suggesting that this collaborative model might have resulted in earlier detection and/or treatment of changes in condition. Family members of EverCare enrollees expressed greater satisfaction with some aspects of medical care than did controls, although satisfaction of EverCare enrollees, themselves, was more comparable with controls [57]. In addition, there is evidence that the EverCare model had higher completion of advance directives compared to controls [58].

In its current form, the EverCare model, now known as OptumCare CarePlus, continues to utilize a collaborative model partnering attending physicians with nurse practitioners or physician assistants. In a Medicare Advantage Institutional Special Needs Plan, eligible nursing home residents must be beneficiaries of Medicare A and Medicare B and be long-term nursing home residents. Prior participation in the Medicare End-Stage Renal Disease Dialysis benefit is an exclusion criterion, but enrollees subsequently requiring dialysis continue to be covered by the plan. A typical APC's panel includes approximately 80–90 enrolled nursing home residents. Depending on enrollment and facility size, the panel may be entirely in one facility or spread over two or more facilities. Depending on the staff model, an APC may collaborate with one or many attending physicians.

Recent studies confirm that the EverCare model successfully addresses important deficits in physician care for geriatric conditions [59]. Additional studies of Medicare managed care programs have shown that residents enrolled in managed care were more likely to have do-not-hospitalize orders, less likely to be transferred to the hospital for acute illness, and had more primary care visits per 90 days than those in traditional Medicare fee for service [60].

The OPTIMISTIC Model In 2012, the Centers for Medicare and Medicaid Services Innovation (CMMI) announced its Initiative to Reduce Avoidable Hospitalizations among Nursing Facility Residents, selecting seven organizations throughout the United States to participate [61, 62]. Participating organizations were located in Alabama, Nebraska, Nevada, Indiana, Missouri, Pennsylvania, and New York City. Here we look at one such project.

Using a similar collaborative approach to EverCare, the Indiana project, "Optimizing Patient Transfers, Impacting Medical Quality and Improving Symptoms: Transforming Institutional Care (OPTIMISTIC)" model, enlisted the participation of 19 nursing facilities. Unlike the EverCare model, OPTIMISTIC staff are not primary care providers. Rather, RNs and NPs work together in a more consultative fashion on collaborative care reviews, providing a structured interview and physical examination, with a focus on geriatric syndromes. Recommendations involving care areas including cognition, function, medication appropriateness, weight changes, skin problems, falls, vaccinations, and pain are discussed with a project geriatrician and finalized. Thereafter, the NP discusses the recommendations with the attending physician. Much like the EverCare model, the OPTIMISTIC model's aim is to improve in-house care and reduce avoidable hospital transfers [63, 64].

The RNs are placed in each facility full time, providing direct clinical support and education and training to the staff. In addition to identifying opportunities to reduce unavoidable hospital transfers, the OPTIMISTIC model has highlighted both the opportunity and difficulty in increasing and improving advance directives [65].

Another function of the OPTIMISTIC NPs is to provide transitional care to residents returning from the hospital. The NPs interventions included obtaining missing discharge summaries, obtaining additional information from the treatment team at the hospital, reconciling and adjusting medications, recommending modifications in treatment, and instituting monitoring and follow-up for existing problems. A majority of the visits required an intervention [66], consistent with prior studies demonstrating the need for improved transitional care between nursing homes and hospitals [67].

Other collaborative models combine the addition of APCs and/or RNs with the use of the INTERACT quality improvement program, telehealth technology, or some combination of the above. As more data is collected in the OPTIMISTIC project and other innovative collaborative models, additional best practices will undoubtedly be delineated. Nonetheless, there is increasing evidence that properly implemented, collaborative models utilizing APCs teamed with physicians can significantly improve the care of nursing facility residents and reduce unnecessary hospitalizations and control costs, while maintaining or improving patient and family satisfaction.

Telehealth in the Nursing Home

Telehealth or telemedicine may be defined as the remote management of patients using real-time electronic communication equipment. In the strictest definition of the term, telehealth has always played a role in nursing homes. As physicians or advance practice clinicians are not always present in the facility, much of the care is managed by telephone, particularly when a resident experiences a change of condition requiring immediate attention. A nurse would assess the resident and call the covering physician with the findings. Based on the information provided, the physician would devise a differential diagnosis and order appropriate diagnostic tests and treatment. If the physician determined that the resident required services not available at the nursing facility, the resident would be transferred to an emergency room, where additional diagnostic and therapeutic interventions could be implemented.

The success of managing residents' health by telephone is dependent on several factors, including the quality of the nursing assessment, the accuracy of the communication with the covering physician, the physician's diagnostic acumen, the quality of the execution of the new plan of care by the nursing home staff, and the willingness of the resident and family to accept the plan of care. Although there are no studies examining the quality of care delivery by telephone in the nursing home, programs such as INTERACT have attempted to improve the quality and success of telephonically delivered care by devising tools specifically designed to improve the thoroughness and accuracy of the nursing assessment as well as the communication and documentation thereof. There are also tools available to assist the nurse in

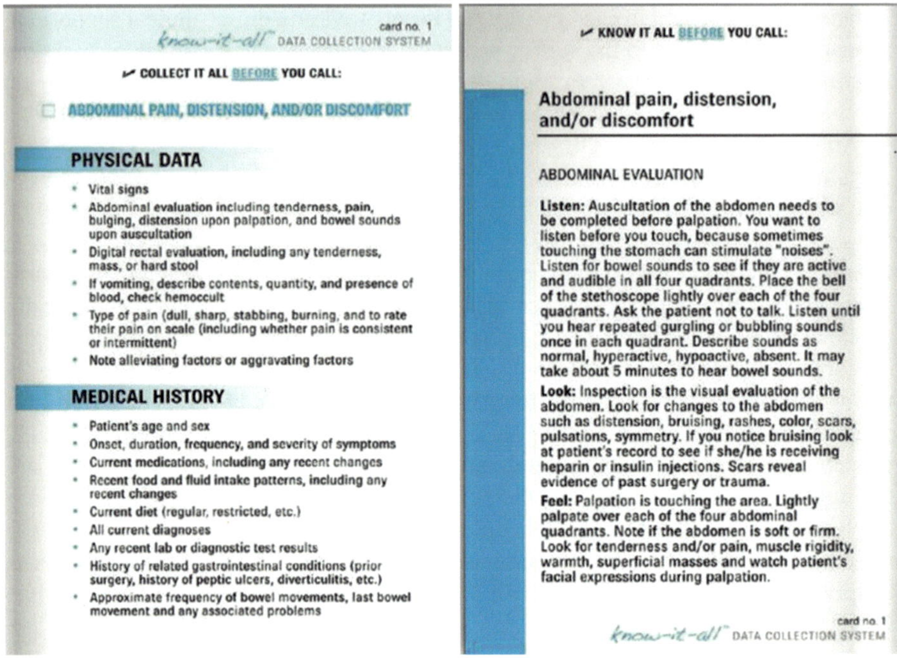

Fig. 10.4 Sample pages from "Know-it-all Before You Call". http://www.paltc.org/sample-know-it-all-when-youre-called-diagnosing-system. Accessed 17 Dec 2017

assessing and collecting appropriate information prior to calling the covering physician and to assist the covering physician in asking for appropriate clinical information, devising a differential diagnosis and care plan and determining whether a transfer to the emergency room is prudent [68, 69]. An example is shown in Fig. 10.4. Although these "Know-it-all" tools make sense as clinical decision aids, there is little published literature on the frequency of their use or efficacy.

Recent advances in internet technology coupled with increases in broadband width allow more sophisticated telemedicine devices to be introduced into the nursing home. These devices allow a greater amount of diagnostic data to be transmitted to the covering physician. For instance, telemedicine devices may include a camera to transmit real-time video of the resident, an electronic stethoscope to transmit real-time cardiac or lung sounds, an otoscope to visualize the ear, and an ophthalmoscope to visualize the retina. Machines may also transmit EKG or even ultrasounds. In most facilities, the machine is brought to the bedside and operated by a nurse, but in some programs, an emergency medical technician is stationed in the facility specifically to provide this service. In either case, the information is transmitted to the physician on call, who then uses the information to devise a plan of care or determine that the resident should be transferred to the hospital. Some of these technologies have been integrated into individual projects funded by CMS's Initiative to Reduce Avoidable Hospitalizations described above.

There is widespread agreement among nursing home healthcare providers that the use of advanced telehealth would improve timeliness of care, although there are varying opinions about who would be providing the remote oversight and consultative service [70]. Preliminary studies have shown that using telemedicine physician coverage during off-hours may reduce hospitalizations and generate Medicare cost savings [71]. Telemedicine may also be used to provide specialty services not otherwise available to the nursing facility. Obtaining the services of a dermatologist by telemedicine has been well accepted in the health system [72], and the use of telemedicine services to provide psychiatric and psychological services has grown and is under study [73].

As the enthusiasm for telemedicine services in the nursing home has grown [74], there is a need for continuing research to examine its effect on hospitalizations, costs, and other quality measures. The same may be said for the variety of nursing home primary care models being developed in today's evolving healthcare environment.

References

1. Butler RN. Why survive? Being old in America. New York: Harper & Row; 1975.
2. Subcommittee on Long-Term Care of the Special Committee on Aging. United States Senate. Nursing home care in the United States: failure in public policy. Washington: U.S. Government Printing Office; 1974.
3. Committee on Nursing Home Regulation, Institute of Medicine. Improving the quality of care in nursing homes. Washington: National Academies Press; 1986.
4. Omnibus Budget Reconciliation Act of 1987. https://www.gpo.gov/fdsys/pkg/STATUTE-101/pdf/STATUTE-101-Pg1330.pdf. Accessed 15 Oct 2016.
5. Centers for Disease Control and Prevention. National Center for Health Statistics. Long-term care providers and services users in the United States: data from the National Study of Long-Term Care Providers, 2013–2014. 2016.
6. The Kaiser Commission on Medicaid and the Uninsured. Medicaid and long-term services and supports: a primer. Kaiser Family Foundation. 2015.
7. Medicare Payment Advisory Commission (MedPAC). Report to the Congress: Medicare Payment Policy. Chapter 7: skilled nursing facility services. March 2016. http://www.medpac.gov/docs/default-source/reports/chapter-7-skilled-nursing-facility-services-march-2016-report-.pdf?sfvrsn=0. Accessed 8 Oct 2016.
8. Centers for Disease Control and Prevention. National Center for Health Statistics. Nursing home care. 2016. http://www.cdc.gov/nchs/fastats/nursing-home-care.htm. Accessed 8 Oct 2016.
9. Dwyer LL, Han B, Woodwell DA, et al. Polypharmacy in nursing home residents in the United States: results of the 2004 National Nursing Home Survey. Am J Geriatr Pharmacother. 2010;8:63–72.
10. Nguyen JK, Fouts MM, Kotabe SE, et al. Polypharmacy as a risk factor for adverse drug reactions in geriatric nursing home residents. Am J Geriatr Pharmacother. 2006;4:36–41.
11. Medicare Payment Advisory Commission (MedPAC). Skilled nursing facility services payment system. 2016. http://medpac.gov/docs/default-source/payment-basics/medpac_payment_basics_16_snf_final.pdf?sfvrsn=0. Accessed 11 Dec 2016.
12. Sahyoun NR, Pratt LA, Lentzner H, et al. Centers for Disease Control and Prevention. National Center for Health Statistics. The changing profile of nursing home residents: 1985–1997. 2001. https://www.cdc.gov/nchs/data/ahcd/agingtrends/04nursin.pdf. Accessed 8 Oct 2016.

13. Williams C, Rosen J, O'Malley M. Profiles of nursing home residents on Medicaid. Washington: The Kaiser Commission on Medicaid and the Uninsured; 2006.
14. Kojima G. Prevalence of frailty in nursing homes: a systematic review and meta-analysis. J Am Med Dir Assoc. 2015;16:940–5.
15. Kaiser Commission on Medicaid and the Uninsured. Private long-term care insurance: a viable option for low and middle-income seniors? 2006. http://www.kff.org/uninsured/upload/7459.pdf. Accessed 20 Nov 2016.
16. Kelly A, Conell-Price J, Covinsky K, et al. Length of stay for older adults residing in nursing homes at the end of life. J Am Geriatr Soc. 2010;58:1701–6.
17. Code of Federal Regulations, 42 CFR §483.30 Physician Services.
18. AMDA-The Society for Post-Acute and Long-Term Care Medicine. Role of the attending physician in the nursing home. 2003. http://www.paltc.org/amda-white-papers-and-resolution-position-statements/role-attending-physician-nursing-home. Accessed 16 Oct 2016.
19. Diamant J. Responsibilities of attending physicians in long-term care facilities. J Am Med Dir Assoc. 2002;3(4):254–8.
20. Diamant J. Roles and responsibilities of attending physicians in skilled nursing facilities. J Am Med Dir Assoc. 2003;4(4):231–43.
21. The Medical Direction and Medical Care Work Group, New York State Department of Health. Role of the attending physician in the nursing home. 2011. https://www.health.ny.gov/professionals/nursing_home_administrator/docs/11-13_att_phys_role.pdf. Accessed 16 Oct 2016.
22. Centers for Medicare & Medicaid Services. Better care. Smarter spending. Healthier people: paying providers for value, not volume. 2015. https://www.cms.gov/Newsroom/MediaReleaseDatabase/Fact-sheets/2015-Fact-sheets-items/2015-01-26-3.html. Accessed 10 Dec 2016.
23. Katz PR, Karuza J, Kolassa J, Hutson A. Medical practice with nursing home residents: results from the National Physician Professional Activities Census. J Am Geriatr Soc. 1997;45:911–7.
24. American Academy of Family Physicians. Practice profile I survey. 2008. http://www.aafp.org/about/the-aafp/family-medicine-facts.html. Accessed 20 Nov 2016.
25. Katz PR, Karuza J, Intrator O, et al. Medical staff organization in nursing homes: scale development and validation. J Am Med Dir Assoc. 2009;10:498–504.
26. Katz PR, Karuza J, Lima J, Intrator O. Nursing home medical staff organization: correlates with quality indicators. J Am Med Dir Assoc. 2011;12:655–9.
27. Lima JC, Intrator O, Karuza J, et al. Nursing home medical staff organization and 30-day rehospitalizations. J Am Med Dir Assoc. 2012;13:552–7.
28. Katz PR, Wayne M, Evans J, et al. Examining the rationale and processes behind the development of AMDA's competencies for post-acute and long-term care medicine. Ann Long-Term Care: Clin Care Aging. 2014;22(11):36–9.
29. Garfinkel D, Mangin D. Feasibility study of a systematic approach for discontinuation of multiple medications in older adults: addressing polypharmacy. Arch Intern Med. 2010;170(18):1648–54.
30. Newton PF, Levinson W, Masen D. The geriatric medication algorithm: a pilot study. J Gen Intern Med. 1994;9:164–7.
31. Scott IA, Hilmer SN, Reeve E, et al. Reducing inappropriate polypharmacy. The process of deprescribing. JAMA Intern Med. 2015;175(5):827–34.
32. Code of Federal Regulations, 42 CFR §483.75 Quality Assurance and Performance Improvement.
33. Rowland FN, Cowles M, Dickstein C, Katz PR. Impact of medical director certification on nursing home quality of care. J Am Med Dir Assoc. 2009;10:431–5.
34. Code of Maryland Regulations. Title 10 § 10.07.02.11 Medical Director Qualifications.
35. The Medical Direction and Medical Care Work Group, New York State Department of Health. Role of the Medical Director in the Nursing Home. 2011. https://www.health.ny.gov/professionals/nursing_home_administrator/docs/11-13_med_dir_role.pdf. Accessed 25 Nov 2016.
36. AMDA-The Society for Post-Acute and Long-Term Care Medicine. White paper on the nursing home medical director: leader and manager. 2011. http://www.paltc.org/sites/default/files/White%20Paper%20NH%20Medical%20Director%20Leader%20and%20Manager.pdf. Accessed 25 Nov 2016.

37. Saliba D, Kington R, Buchanan J, et al. Appropriateness of the decision to transfer nursing facility residents to the hospital. J Am Geriatr Soc. 2000;48:154–63.
38. Ouslander JG, Lamb G, Perloe M, et al. Potentially avoidable hospitalizations of nursing home residents: frequency, causes, and costs. J Am Geriatr Soc. 2010;58:627–35.
39. Morley JE. Opening Pandora's box: the reasons why reducing nursing home transfers to hospital are so difficult. J Am Med Dir Assoc. 2016;17:185–7.
40. Ouslander JG, Weinberg AD, Phillips V. Inappropriate hospitalization of nursing facility residents: a symptom of a sick system of care for frail older people. J Am Geriatr Soc. 2000;48:230–1.
41. Ouslander JG, Bonner A, Herndon L, Shutes J. The interventions to reduce acute care transfers (INTERACT) quality improvement program: an overview for medical directors and primary care clinicians in long term care. J Am Med Dir Assoc. 2014;15:162–70.
42. Interventions to Reduce Acute Care Transfers (INTERACT). 2016. www.intcract2.net/about.html. Accessed 3 Dec 2016.
43. Boockvar K, Brodie HD, Lachs M. Nursing assistants detect behavior changes in nursing home residents that precede acute illness: development and validation of an illness warning instrument. J Am Geriatr Soc. 2000;48:1086–91.
44. Langley GJ, Moen RD, Nolan KM, et al. The improvement guide: a practical approach to enhancing organizational performance. 2nd ed. San Francisco: Jossey-Bass; 2009.
45. Ouslander JG, Perloe M, Givens JH, et al. Reducing potentially avoidable hospitalizations of nursing home residents: results of a pilot quality improvement project. J Am Med Dir Assoc. 2009;10:644–52.
46. Tena-Nelson R, Santos K, Weingast E. Reducing potentially preventable hospital transfers: results from a thirty nursing home collaborative. J Am Med Dir Assoc. 2009;13:651–6.
47. Bonner A, Tappen R, Herndon L, Ouslander J. The INTERACT institute: observations on dissemination of the INTERACT quality improvement program using certified INTERACT trainers. Gerontologist. 2015;55:1050–7.
48. Ouslander JG, Naharci I, Engstrom G, et al. Lessons learned from root cause analyses of transfers of skilled nursing facility (SNF) patients to acute hospitals: transfers rated as preventable versus nonpreventable by SNF staff. J Am Med Dir Assoc. 2016;17:596–601.
49. Ouslander JG, Naharci I, Engstrom G, et al. Root cause analyses of transfers of skilled nursing facility patients to acute hospitals: lessons learned for reducing unnecessary hospitalizations. J Am Med Dir Assoc. 2016;17:256–62.
50. Ouslander JG, Handler SM. Consensus-derived interventions to reduce acute care transfer (INTERACT)—compatible order sets for common conditions associated with potentially avoidable hospitalizations. J Am Med Dir Assoc. 2015;16:524–6.
51. Bakerjian D. Care of nursing home residents by advanced practice nurses. Res Gerontol Nurs. 2008;1:177–85.
52. Bayard J, Jacobson R. How two NPs changed managed care: the birth of Evercare. Interview by Jill Rollet. Adv Nurse Pract. 2007;15(5):73–5.
53. Kane RL, Huck S. The implementation of the EverCare demonstration project. J Am Geriatr Soc. 2000;48:218–23.
54. Kane RL, Flood S, Keckhafer G, Rockwood T. How EverCare nurse practitioners spend their time. J Am Geriatr Soc. 2001;49:1530–4.
55. Kane RL, Keckhafer G, Flood S, et al. The effect of EverCare on hospital use. J Am Geriatr Soc. 2003;51:1427–34.
56. Kane RL, Flood S, Keckhafer BA, et al. Nursing home residents covered by Medicare risk contracts: early findings from the EverCare evaluation project. J Am Geriatr Soc. 2002;50:719–27.
57. Kane RL, Keckhafer G, Robst J. Evaluation of the Evercare demonstration program final report. Minneapolis: Division of Health Service Research and Policy, School of Public Health, University of Minnesota; 2002.
58. Lawrence JF. The advance directive prevalence in long-term care: a comparison of relationships between a nurse practitioner healthcare model and a traditional healthcare model. J Am Acad Nurse Pract. 2009;21(3):179–85.

59. Wenger NS, Roth CP, Martin D, et al. Quality of care provided in a special needs plan using a nurse care manager model. J Am Geriatr Soc. 2011;59:1810–22.
60. Goldfeld KS, Grabowski DC, Caudry DJ, Mitchell SL. Health insurance status and the care of nursing home residents with advanced dementia. JAMA Intern Med. 2013;173(22):2047–53.
61. Centers for Medicare & Medicaid Services. Initiative to reduce avoidable hospitalization among nursing facility residents. CMS Web Site. 2016. http://go.cms.gov/1QNwsfG. Accessed 10 Dec 2016.
62. Centers for Medicare & Medicaid Services. State operations manual. Appendix PP—guidance to surveyors for long term care facilities. (Rev 157, 06-10-16). 2016. https://www.cms.gov/Regulations-and-Guidance/Guidance/Manuals/downloads/som107ap_pp_guidelines_ltcf.pdf. Accessed 25 Nov 2016.
63. Holtz LR, Maurer H, Nazir A, et al. OPTIMISTIC: a program to improve nursing home care and reduce avoidable hospitalizations. In: Malone ML, Capezuti EA, Palmer RM, editors. Geriatrics models of care: bringing 'best practice' to an aging America. Cham: Springer International Publishing; 2015. p. 287–92.
64. Unroe KT, Nazir A, Holtz L, et al. The optimizing patient transfers, impacting medical quality, and improving symptoms: transforming institutional care approach: preliminary data from the implementation of a centers for Medicare and Medicaid services nursing facility demonstration project. J Am Geriatr Soc. 2015;63:165–9.
65. Hickman SE, Unroe KT, Ersek MT, et al. An interim analysis of an advance care planning intervention in the nursing home setting. J Am Geriatr Soc. 2016;64:2385–92.
66. Nazir A, Unroe KT, Buente B, et al. OPTIMISTIC transition visits: a model to improve hospital to nursing facility transfers. Ann Long-Term Care: Clin Care Aging. 2016;24(7):31–6.
67. LaMantia MA, Scheunemann LP, Viera AJ, et al. Interventions to improve transitional care between nursing homes and hospitals: a systematic review. J Am Geriatr Soc. 2010;58(4):777–82.
68. AMDA—The Society for Post-Acute and Long-Term Care. Know-it-all before you call: data collection system. Columbia: AMDA—The Society for Post-Acute and Long-Term Care; 2015.
69. AMDA—Society for Post-Acute and Long-Term Care. Know-it-all when you're called: diagnosing system. Columbia: AMDA—The Society for Post-Acute and Long-Term Care; 2015.
70. Driessen J, Bonhomme A, Chang W, et al. Nursing home provider perceptions of telemedicine for reducing potentially avoidable hospitalizations. J Am Med Dir Assoc. 2016;17:519–24.
71. Grabowski DC, O'Malley AJ. The use of telemedicine can reduce hospitalizations of nursing home residents and generate savings for Medicare. Health Aff. 2014;33(2):244–50.
72. Landow SM, DH O, Weinstock MA. Teledermatology within the Veterans Health Administration, 2002–2004. Telemed J E Health. 2015;21:769–73.
73. Volicer. Nursing home telepsychiatry. J Am Med Dir Assoc. 2015;16:7–8.
74. Morley JE. Telemedicine: coming to nursing homes in the near future. J Am Med Dir Assoc. 2016;17:1–3.

Primary Care in the Home: The Independence at Home Demonstration

George Taler, Peter Boling, and Bruce Kinosian

In the late spring of 2006, a small group of past presidents of the American Academy of Home Care Medicine met in the offices of the Academy's legal counsel, James Pyles, a prominent health law attorney in Washington, DC, with a particular interest in home healthcare. Drs. Peter Boling and George Taler were geriatricians with home-based primary care practices with a teaching focus, based in academic medical centers; Dr. C. Gresham Bayne was an emergency medicine physician who had become an entrepreneur in the home-based healthcare arena. It was clear that the Care Management for High-Cost Beneficiaries ("CMHCB") CMS Demonstration was unraveling and that there was an opportunity to create a new proposal based on a small-practice design with care centered in the home and coordinated around the needs of the patient. Thus was born the concepts of the Independence at Home Demonstration.

The challenge was to transform the healthcare delivery system to be more patient oriented, safer, realistic in clinical expectations, and less expensive; we had come to consensus that interdisciplianry care in the home provided the right foundation for our clinical design. Second, we recognized that the fee-for-service payment mechanism was stifling innovation; capitation, as the industry had evolved, created the wrong incentives and required large capital investments. Therefore, we also needed to devise a new payment system. Any "new money" would have to come from sharing a portion of the savings that our programs generated. Finally, we also had to find a way to balance the incentives to assure a high-quality service delivery system without overburdening bureaucratic documentation and reporting requirements.

G. Taler, MD (✉) • P. Boling, MD • B. Kinosian, MD
Geriatrics and Long Term Care, Georgetown University School of Medicine,
Washington, DC, USA
e-mail: george.Taler@Medstar.net

© Springer International Publishing AG 2018
M. Wasserman, J. Riopelle (eds.), *Primary Care for Older Adults*,
DOI 10.1007/978-3-319-61329-1_11

The first part of this chapter deals with a discussion of the regulatory landscape and payment mechanisms that preceded the Affordable Care Act and MACRA and that shaped the incentives at that time. We then will review the underlying policy decisions that form the basis for the Independence at Home Demonstration. Finally, we will provide an update on the current legislative and regulatory efforts to bring these ideas to fruition as a national program.

Background

Vilfredo Pareto, an Italian economist in the 1800s, recognized that 20% of the population accounted for 80% of all of the wealth. This ratio has been applied to many other socioeconomic phenomena, including healthcare. As seen in the illustration, 18.5% of the population accounts for 80% of all healthcare expenditures (Fig. 11.1). Of note, the reverse is also true: 80% of the population consumes less than 20% of all healthcare dollars—the bottom 50% account for less than 3% of all spending. The upper 20% can be further parsed, such that 10% accounts for 65% of all healthcare dollars and the top 5% accounts for approximately 50%; the top 1%, often called the catastrophic illness category, accounts for over $35,000/year in spending and over 20% of all costs (http://archive.ahrq.gov/research/findings/factsheets/costs/exptiach1.html). The questions were whether there was opportunity for realizing savings by providing better care for a defined subpopulation that fit into the top 5–10% of the whole and how we might best identify those patients whose care could be amenable to improvement.

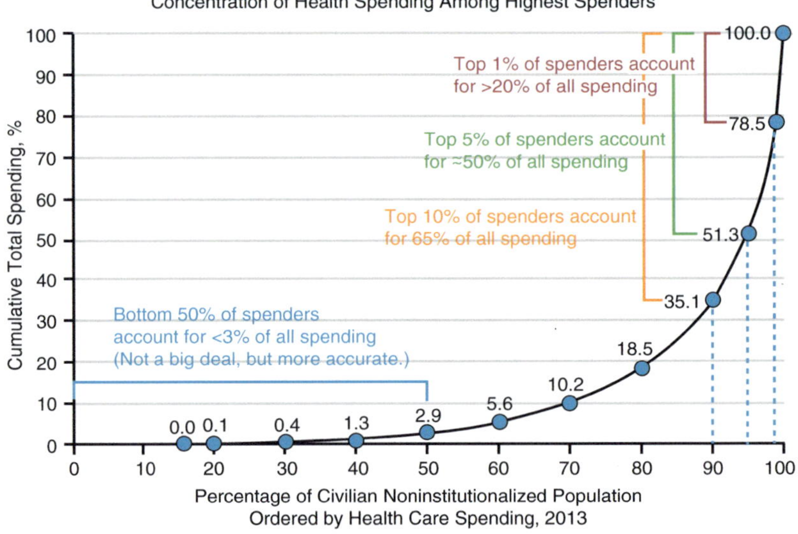

Fig. 11.1 https://newsatjama.jama.com/2016/08/25/jama-forum-why-are-private-health-insurers-losing-money-on-obamacare/

When one looks at those individuals with extraordinary costs in the course of a fiscal year, they divide into roughly two groups: those who have had the misfortune of a very bad year, but if not for bad luck would have been well, or reasonably so; the other half have multiple chronic illnesses with disability and their high costs were predictable and therefore potentially avoidable. The first group, the unlucky souls, may have had a serious injury, disabling heart disease, or the onset of cancer; others may have been ill but functional and finally become eligible for an organ transplant, or a chronic illness now requiring therapy with a high-cost biologic agent. This is why the average person buys health insurance. This is also where Medicine in America leads the world; except, perhaps, for certain high-priced pharmaceuticals, this is not where we should be looking for substantial savings. Our goal should be to restore health and productivity.

The second group, those with multiple chronic conditions and disability, do not share the same expectations. The goals of care are more aligned with those of palliative medicine, with a focus on symptom control and the preservation of functional independence. For those with impaired cognitive function or physical mobility, access to primary care becomes a hassle for both their caregivers and office-based physicians, prompting a reliance on emergency room visits for rescue from symptoms, with the associated repeated hospitalizations. The costs then escalate based on the use of post-acute services, such as a subacute rehabilitation, skilled nursing facilities, and home care [1]. Patients with five or more chronic conditions, on average, fill approximately 60 prescriptions per year, accounting for a disproportionate share of pharmaceutical spending, and the majority of the durable medical equipment and medical supplies. They also may receive care from six or more physicians [2]—most of whom do not communicate with one another. Eventually, without much forethought, these patients arrive in the ICU *in extremis*, where the costs skyrocket and the prognosis plummets. A remarkably consistent finding is that slightly over 25% of healthcare spending in one's lifetime occurs in the last year of life [3]. As a society, we are coming to realize that much of this is unwanted and likely without benefit [4, 5].

The challenge is that if we are to affect the outcomes, not only for costs but also for symptom management and meeting realistic expectations that give patients and their family peace of mind, we need to identify and engage these individuals as they cross some threshold that defines the last chapters of one's life. Usually that event is heralded through a hospitalization or the onset of disability [2, 6])—physical, cognitive, or both—that limits freedom of mobility. Epidemiologic research has shown that these events signal a decline in health and function, with associated increases in fragmentation and costs that define the last 4 years of life. Unfortunately, these are also the same factors that expose the worst of our healthcare delivery and payment systems. As Pogo famously said about pollution, "We have met the enemy and he is us."

In many ways, the current fee-for-service payment system and its implicit incentives explain the reasons that the beneficiaries who populate the top 5–10% tier experience such poor care. The first is in the evaluation and management system under which physicians are paid on the basis of documentation and coding, but sadly, not according to quality of care or outcomes. The ramifications were not lost on either the administrators or the clinicians. The administrators recognized that the more encounters, the more "economically productive" the clinician, without significant penalty if time constrained the quality of care and income was untethered from outcome for these patients. The fee-for-service system also failed to provide a funding source for other members of the interdisciplinary team, such as social workers, therapists and nutritionists, who are vital to chronic illness management. The clinicians found that they had fewer resources and less time to practice as they had been trained. Discouraged and economically disadvantaged, the primary care and non-procedural specialties quickly lost stature in academia, followed by a decline in trainees leading to a progressively diminished workforce.

The second is that procedures are by far more "productive," and the more interventions, the higher the income; facilitated documentation was built into most equipment. Observers both inside and outside of medicine were quick to point out that guidelines for care had lowered thresholds and called for more frequent scheduled interventions, and when similar procedures offered only marginal differences in benefits, they overwhelmingly favored the more remunerative approach [5, 7]. Although the opportunities for imaging escalated [8], most other procedures became too risky among the frail, and without procedures to offset inadequate reimbursement for office-based services, these patients also become less attractive to specialists.

The third is the irony that the most complex cases—those most in need of continuity, attention to disease management, and personalized goal setting—were the least attractive to both the specialists and the primary care enterprise: they took too much time, needed too many resources, and were too difficult to manage in the ambulatory setting. Eventually, these patients suffered from the overwhelming burden of their illness and required rescue through high-cost institutional services. Given the complexity of hospital care and the need for efficiency, the era of hospitalists arose, further fragmenting care from the perspective not only of the medical care plan but also between the hospital and the primary care provider in the community. Once the primary care physician was left out of the flow of information, the link to the community support system was also jeopardized.

The top 5–10% did not fare well under capitation either. Capitated healthcare systems were initially marketed with a simple premise: if the system can keep you healthy, both the provider and the patient win. However, primary preventive services for those who cost virtually nothing is hard to justify on an annual budget, since the return on the investment is decades off; managing chronic conditions is not easy and the rewards are most often delayed. On the other hand, it became readily apparent that avoiding the most compromised and disabled individuals paid by far the greatest dividend: if you were paid at the rate of 95% for the average cost of a population (the arrangement most programs had with Medicare, Medicaid, private insurance, and corporate health programs), discouraging enrollment of that small 5–10% segment that accounted for 50–65% of those costs—such recruiting office on the second floor of a building without elevators—avoided strains on the clinical systems and markedly reduced the medical losses. Before payers understood this, the capitated healthcare systems' profits could be enormous—and they were!

Eventually, the government tried to adjust the payments based on risk analyses, paying higher rates for those with higher risk scores and less for those who were healthy. But, as MedPAC showed, the government still overpays by 60% for the lowest 20% of the population, underpays by 14% for the highest 20% and underpays by 18% for the highest 5% (http://www.medpac.gov/docs/default-source/reports/jun14_ch02.pdf?sfvrsn=0 accessed 1/15/2017).

The urgency for addressing this issue stems from two demographic forces. The first is the surge of "baby boomers" joining the ranks of Medicare. According to the Social Security Trust Fund, approximately 10,000 beneficiaries are added to the rolls every day and this will continue for the next 5–10 years (https://www.ssa.gov/oact/tr/2014/tr2014.pdf accessed 1/15/2017). This cohort is also the longest lived in the history of humanity; the population turning 65 today has an average life expectancy of nearly 20 years (https://www.census.gov/prod/2014pubs/p25-1140.pdf accessed 1/15/2017). But age is only part of the reason for increasing healthcare costs. Although the rate of growth of the healthcare budget has begun to taper over the last few years, that growth is still multiples of the increase in inflation. We are using more diagnostic testing, more imaging, more pharmaceuticals, and more expensive drugs than ever before. Each patient's annual expenditures, as well as each encounter, continue to grow faster than our economy [9]. It is in this context that President Obama's warnings to Congress on September 9, 2009, have their greatest impact, "If we do nothing to slow these skyrocketing costs, we will eventually be spending more on Medicare and Medicaid than every other government program combined. Put simply, our health care problem is our deficit problem. Nothing else even comes close." If we do not find a way to control the rising healthcare costs per beneficiary, the rising numbers of beneficiaries will accelerate the national debt.

The second demographic factor is the change in the family and community structure, often due to financially motivated population shifts. Unfortunately, the millennial generation may be the first in the past century to be not as financially successful and socially integrated as their parents had been (http://money.howstuffworks.com/personal-finance/financial-planning/millennials-first-worse-parents1.htm accessed 1/15/2017). Social Security will be funded by a shrinking number of workers, further challenging the social fabric (https://www.ssa.gov/oact/tr/2014/tr2014.pdf accessed 1/15/2017). The dissolution of the family structure through lower rates of marriage, lower birth rates, and far more social mobility exacerbates these trends. This is especially acute among the lower socioeconomic classes, which affects minorities in great disproportion (https://www.census.gov/prod/2014pubs/p25-1140.pdf accessed 1/15/2017). As the need for "the village" becomes more acute, the healthcare system too often thwarts coordination and integration of social services.

Finally, at the same time that "baby boomers" are rapidly expanding the ranks of Medicare and caregivers become scarcer, the number of geriatricians continues to fall. Based on data from the Kaiser Family Foundation, over the past 7 years, we have lost on average five geriatricians per week (personal communications, Tricia Neuman)—as compared to adding 70,000 elders. This is the workforce trained specifically to manage these patients. Surveys of physician satisfaction show that geriatricians are among the most satisfied with their work and the most likely to "make the same choice of specialty." However, incomes remain in the lowest strata (http://www.medscape.com/viewarticle/737617). It is therefore not surprising that in the 2016 NRMP Fellowship Match, only 44% of geriatric fellowship positions filled, the lowest among all fellowship programs in the nation, and many of the graduating fellows go on to careers as hospitalists, where they can earn $40–60,000 more per year than in a primary care practice. The losses in the geriatric workforce can primarily be attributable to the design of the healthcare delivery system and to the model of payment.

The conclusion is clear: we need a new approach to healthcare delivery and a new approach to paying for it, which aligns incentives for the payer, the patient, and the provider. The payment system needs to reward value as measured by better disease management, better control of symptoms, and a better experience with the healthcare delivery system at a lower overall cost. Better care is achievable only through an approach that coordinates care across settings, over time, and with links to care in the community for medical, social, and mental health services. Coordinated care is both more effective and less expensive. If it also improves the health of the population, then society will have been well served.

The Independence at Home Demonstration

The Independence at Home Demonstration (https://innovation.cms.gov/initiatives/independence-at-home/) is built around three principles that include population targeting, healthcare delivery reform, and a shared savings methodology to augment fee-for-service income. Eligibility criteria need to be easy to identify and verifiable through readily available data sources, for the purpose of accurately defining beneficiaries most likely to be among the top 5–10% of costs for the population. For logistical reasons, the IAH Demonstration focuses on geriatrics patients in Medicare, but the design is applicable to similar populations with high-need and high-cost individuals in all age groups.

Eligibility

The first criterion is the presence of two or more persistent, chronic conditions that presents a significant risk for clinical exacerbation and disability. For the elderly, these are predominantly illnesses of the major organ systems and psychiatric disorders; most are progressive with an inexorable decline, either slowly or in a stair-step pattern, affecting both physiology and functional independence in activities of daily living. These conditions are readily verified through the ICD-10 diagnoses associated with CPT codes used for fee-for-service billing.

The second two criteria relate to utilization patterns: a nonelective admission to an acute care hospital, followed by referral to a post-acute service. This might include either a subacute rehabilitation stay in a skilled nursing facility, admission to an acute rehabilitation hospital, or a home health episode. Although referral is usually on discharge from the hospital, we wanted to capture those instances when a "post-acute" service failed to prevent a hospitalization. Therefore, order is not relevant, but both must have occurred within the previous 12 months. Utilization of each of these services is readily identifiable through billing codes submitted to Medicare and confirms eligibility.

A nonelective hospitalization is a readily identified milestone in the progression of chronic illness, [2, 6] differentiating a "condition" from a "severe condition," i.e., the point when a physiologic dysfunction that warrants a diagnosis now has an impact on the ability of the patient to care for him or herself, or to function in society. A single hospitalization confers a risk of a 30-day readmission for approximately 20% of these patients and more than 25% for those with advanced cardiopulmonary disease [10]. Little appreciated is that 30% are readmitted within 90 days and 50% are readmitted or dead within the year [10]. It became apparent that a further marker for advanced disease is if hospitalization did not restore functional independence, prompting referral to a post-acute service. Functional impairment in two or more ADLs is a very strong marker for added complexity, resource utilization, and costs and a predictor of mortality. The second reason that post-acute services were included is that each is associated with a mandatory functional assessment, either MDS, OASIS, or FIM, that includes a full functional assessment for activities of daily living. (Footnote: Minimum Data Set (MDS) is used in skilled nursing facilities; Outcome and Assessment Information Set (OASIS) is used in the home health industry and draws heavily from the MDS; the Functional Independence Measure (FIM) is used predominantly in the acute rehabilitation setting.) With the passage of the IMPACT Act (https://www.cms.gov/Medicare/Quality-Initiatives-Patient-Assessment-Instruments/Post-Acute-Care-Quality-Initiatives/IMPACT-Act-of-2014-and-Cross-Setting-Measures.html, accessed 1/21/2017), these forms will be combined in the future, but used in the same context. Regardless, these forms must be completed and submitted to Medicare as part of the documentation for reimbursement of services. This allows for corroboration of the fourth criterion, functional impairment in at least two activities of daily living requiring the assistance of another person.

Research has shown that these four criteria can define a cohort in each state representing 1.3–8.6% (average 6.6%) of the Medicare population, well within the 5–10% target [11]. An analysis of this population's utilization experience shows an average annual expenditure of approximately $54,000, which is 5× the per capita mean of $9900 [12]. Medicare-only IAH-Q beneficiaries had a mean monthly cost of $2827 (range, $2156–$3275 on a state-by-state analysis), and dual eligibles (Medicare and Medicaid) had a mean monthly cost of $3597 (range, $2059–$5246); overall the costs associated with IAH-Q beneficiaries accounted for approximately 30% of all spending. This population also accounts for 24% of all hospitalizations, 44% of all 30-day readmissions, and 23% of all nursing home admissions [11]. Therefore, these simple and readily available criteria have proven to be far more effective than much more complicated risk assessment tools.

Creating a Healthcare Delivery System Designed to Meet the Needs of the IAH Population

The second challenge was a redesign of the healthcare delivery system to best meet the needs of the targeted population, most of whom have significant mobility impairment. Several factors were clear. First it is far easier to bring the providers to the patients than the patients to the providers; second, psychosocial, functional, and environmental factors hold equal importance in stabilizing these patients as does the medical regimen; and, third, we could assume accountability for outcome in all settings and over time only if the practice was assigned an empanelled group of patients. Given these operational needs, the obvious approach was to organize care through a home-based primary care (HBPC) practice with an interdisciplinary team of healthcare providers. Given the high complexity of illness, we felt that the interdisciplinary teams should be led by either a physician or anurse practitioner with experience in providing healthcare in the home setting with physician collaboration, as per state regulations.

HBPC has several important characteristics that lend themselves to the management of this select cohort of patients. Most importantly is the ability to evaluate the patient in their natural environment, which provides a window into their lives. Compliance with the medical regimen is readily assessable: the medications are either present or not, and matching pill counts with fill dates provides an accurate accounting. The same is true for wound care and other disposable supplies. This perspective also allows the clinician to make better decisions in adjusting and streamlining the regimen. Second, a "kitchen biopsy" (done with permission) can provide a strong sense of compliance with dietary recommendations. Third, the presence of appropriate durable medical equipment and assistive devices should correlate with the patient's functional needs. Equally important is an observation of the patient and family interaction as an indication of support, or neglect, as well as caregiver burden. Finally, the functional assessment in light of environmental barriers highlights opportunities to maximize functional independence and reduce caregiver strain.

HBPC has other attributes that facilitate care and responsiveness. Patients can be seen only one at a time while they wait in their homes, which allow schedule adjustments on a day-to-day basis for more timely routine visits, or even on demand in coordination with central triage and dispatch personnel, for urgent care visits. Since these patients have a high prevalence of illness, the use of portable diagnostic and therapeutic technologies is easily justifiable and enhances the capabilities for both ongoing and urgent care.

The deep personal relationships that develop when the clinicians spend time with the patient in their home and with their family foster trust and a greater understanding of the patient's preferences and expectations, as well as those of their caregivers. These discussions result in more meaningful advance directives and better decision-making in both the chronic and acute phases of illness. The majority of people want to "age in place" and "die in my own bed" if they can be assured that their needs can be met. "Being there" sends a strong message of reassurance.

The team approach is a central theme of HBPC. In order to affect outcomes, it is crucial that all facets of illness be addressed contemporaneously, including the medical, social, and psychological and the ability to perform the activities of daily living; function is also dependent on environmental factors. "It takes a village" of professionals working with the patient and their caregivers to address each aspect of the plan of care. A highly functioning team has several key characteristics that can be illustrated through a semantic progression: *multidisciplinary* care conveys the idea that each professional adds to the regimen, while *interdisciplinary* conveys active coordination of these inputs, and *transdisciplinary* conveys a deeper understanding of what the other disciplines bring to the team and allows each to scout for opportunities for other members to tailor the team's recommendations to the individual. Each discipline "owns" the patient and family from their perspective and advocates for their needs among the other providers. To quote Norman S. Hidle, "A group becomes a team when each member is sure enough of himself and his contributions to praise the skill of the others." Therefore, team leadership shifts among the team members depending on the issues at hand, a situation that leads to a "flat" hierarchy, as opposed to the "command and control" hierarchy more often encountered among healthcare teams.

The Independence at Home Demonstration has shown that there is no set formula for successful team building. Unlike the Veterans Affairs HBPC Program, where the disciplines and time commitments are defined through a central administrative process, each IAH practice creates their own team through a combination of personnel, contract employees, and partnerships with community agencies. Various model programs have been established, both academic and private sector, with slightly different team designs, evolving organically based on available resources, local politics, finances, and needs. For example, social services can be addressed through hiring social workers; purchasing time or assigning social work services through an affiliated provider, such as a hospital or home care agency; contracting with private social workers and negotiating payments through fee-for-service and private billings; or, by partnering with a community social service agency under a shared mission. It has become an essential element for success that the practices be able to have the flexibility to bring the full range of services together through whatever formal or informal relationships are available through their local health and social services resources.

Assuring the Quality of Patient Care

The practices had to have in place an electronic medical record (EMR) and demonstrate the capacity to provide 24/7 access to a clinician who has access to the EMR and to be of sufficient size to be able to recruit more than 200 IAH eligible beneficiaries (smaller practices could band together to form a consortium to meet the threshold number, but would be treated as a single entity). The demonstration includes six quality metrics linked to payment and nine other performance metrics.

Quality Measures

1. Contact with patients within 48 h on admission to or discharge from the hospital, or an emergency department visit
2. Medication reconciliation in the home
3. Patient preferences documented in the medical record
4. Fewer than expected inpatient admissions for ambulatory care sensitive conditions
5. Fewer than expected readmissions within 30 days
6. Fewer than expected emergency department visits for ambulatory care sensitive conditions

The first three are self-reported with periodic chart audits to assure compliance and accuracy. For the latter three, the threshold must be equal to or less than the average utilization in a clinically similar population with case mix and geographic adjustments as determined by using Medicare claims analysis. In order to remain in the Demonstration, each practice needed to have achieved success on at least three of the six measures. If there were any savings attributed to their practice, they were eligible for their share in proportion to the number of quality metrics met.

The process measures include goals of care (not merely advance directives, but wishes and expectations), a depression screen, home safety, and falls assessment; cognitive screen; symptom interventions and control; self-management capabilities; and caregiver burden. These are monitored as an annual assessment of the quality, but do not determine savings shares. Their purpose is to assure that important factors of patient care are being addressed and the data is shared among the practice professionals as a means of improving care through peer support.

Shared Savings Methodology

The third component of the IAH demonstration is the ability to share in savings generated by the clinical care of each practice. The demonstration stipulates that the first 5% of savings in Medicare Parts A and B are to be returned to Medicare. Any savings beyond the first 5% would be shared with the practices with 80% going to the practice and 20% returning to Medicare. The intent is to create an incentive for these HBPC practices to seek out the most expensive beneficiaries in their region and then to provide better care to reduce their costs. The more complex and expensive the patient has been in the past, the greater the opportunity for savings. The problem of "regression to the mean" after an extreme swing in costs is managed by matching each case to an actuarial control population, so that the calculations are based on a difference in cost experience on a month-to-month basis, as opposed to an absolute difference in annual costs.

The challenge has been to accurately define the expected costs in the absence of the intervention and thus calculate the amount of savings by subtracting actual costs; this remains an ongoing effort. Several factors must be taken into account when making the comparison to beneficiaries who have met the IAH eligibility criteria, but who are not receiving primary medical care in the home. The most important is to control for mortality rate, which runs in the low to mid 20% range, which we found to be significantly higher in IAH-qualified enrolled persons than in the other Medicare beneficiary groups, likely reflecting more advanced disease burden. The death year is usually costly even if the patient is in HBPC, though less costly than if they are not in HBPC. Second, Medicare adjusts payments using a geographic index based on average costs in that region, otherwise known as "county rate adjustments." Interestingly, since IAH-qualified beneficiaries skew far to the highest end of the cost distribution, they are strikingly similar across regions, despite high variability in county rates attributed by Medicare for their geographic adjustment indices, so simple application of Medicare mean county costs in the prediction model works to the disadvantage of these programs. Third, many patients tend to enroll in IAH following an exacerbation or new onset of severe, chronic illnes resulting in a period of clinical instability. Experience has shown that this instability persists for approximately 3 months before the patient plateaues at their "new normal." The relative proportion of such "incident" cases in a given practice will increase its expected costs, compared with the costs for a program comprised of patients who have been stabilized, and an adjustment for population instability is needed. Finally, there are issues around high cost variances, extreme outliers, and confidence intervals for small programs. This potentially disadvantages smaller practices, which must meet a higher threshold beyond the 5% savings to assure that they have indeed been effective before they can participate in shared savings. Outlier protection can mitigate this challenge. Finally, the cost target model and savings calculation must be predictable at the practice level in order to have a sustainable business model. Work continues to hone the prediction model.

Despite some concerns over the methodology, CMS felt sufficiently assured that savings were being generated to release 2 years' worth of IAH data. In Year 1 (2012–2013) their analysis found that IAH practices served 8400 Medicare beneficiaries and saved over $25 million—an average of $3070 per participating beneficiary. CMS awarded incentive payments of $11.7 million to nine of the participating practices that reduced Medicare expenditures and met the designated quality goals. According to CMS' analysis, all 17 participating practices improved quality in at least three of the six quality measures; four practices met all six quality measures (https://www.cms.gov/Newsroom/MediaReleaseDatabase/Press-releases/2015-Press-releases-items/2015-06-18.html, accessed 1/21/2017). In Year 2 (2013–2014) the 15 remaining IAH practices served more than 10,000 Medicare beneficiaries and saved Medicare nearly $8M—an average of $746 per beneficiary. CMS awarded incentive payments of over $5M to seven participating practices that succeeded in reducing spending while improving quality (https://www.cms.gov/Newsrrom/MediaReleaseDatabase/Fact-Sheet-item/2017-01-19.html, accessed 1/21/2017). According to the original CMS Press Release, "On average, beneficiaries:

- Have follow-up contact from their provider within 48 h of a hospital admission, hospital discharge, or emergency room visit;
- Have fewer hospital readmissions within 30 days;

- Have their medication identified by their provider within 48 h of discharge from the hospital;
- Have their preferences documented by their provider;
- Use inpatient hospital and emergency room services less for conditions such as diabetes, high blood pressure, asthma, pneumonia, or urinary tract infection."

Year 3 (2014–2015) results are in process as CMS continues its work to improve the accuracy of the shared savings methodology.

Legislative History and Plans Going Forward

The Independence at Home Act was developed for the 2008 Congressional session and sponsored by Senators Ron Wyden (D-OR) and Richard Burr (R-NC) and Representatives Ed Markey (D-MA) and Michael Burgess (R-TX). As the Affordable Care Act of 2010 gained momentum, this bill was proposed as an amendment and endorsed with unanimous, bicameral support and incorporated into the ACA under Section 3024. The solicitation was offered through CMS in December 2011 and the Demonstration began in June 2012. Although the program was scheduled to be in effect for 3 years, it became evident to those in CMS and Congress that there was promise in the preliminary analysis for both savings and quality improvement. New, companion legislation in both the House and Senate was crafted in the summer of 2015 to extend the Demonstration for an additional 2 years, while the analysis continued on the original 3 years. In June, CMS reported their favorable results of Year 1 and the extension legislation, the Medicare Independence at Home Medical Practice Demonstration Improvement Act of 2015, was passed on a unanimous voice vote and signed into law in July 2015.

The Senate Finance Committee established the Chronic Care Work Group to highlight proposals to improve the care of frail populations. The first of their 24 recommendations was to expand the IAH Demonstration to a national program (https://www.finance.senate.gov/imo/media/doc/CCWG%20Policy%20 Options%20Paper1.pdf, accessed 1/23/2017). This continued to spur legislative initiatives.

In anticipation of a favorable analysis for Year 3, legislation has been crafted for a national expansion of the program. Senate bill 3130, the Independence at Home Act of 2016, was first introduced in the Senate in 2016, by Senators Markey (D-MA), Cornyn (R-TX), Bennet (D-CO), and Portman (R-OH) with four other co-sponsors (https://www.congress.gov/bill/114th-congress/senate-bill/3130). The Senate champions reintroduced the bill as S464 in the 2017 session. The House leadership is awaiting the Year 3 results and confirmation by CBO of the savings, but is primed to introduce a companion bill as soon as the timing is right.

In the meantime, meetings continue with the leadership of the Center for Medicare and Medicaid Innovation, who assumed administrative responsibility when the Office of Research and Demonstration Initiatives was subsumed, with the expectations of announcing the Year 3 results by early 2018. Leadership from the

IAH Learning Collaborative is working with CBO to lay the groundwork for their understanding of the program. Negotiations with the Senate Finance Committee to coordinate legislation and to update the House leadership are actively underway.

Research

There is a growing body of literature supporting the effectiveness of the home-based primary care model for frail elders. As might be expected from the Pareto Principle, the greater the need and the higher the costs, the greater the potential that a benefit can be shown for improving clinical quality and reducing utilization and costs. However, these benefits are largely dependent on direct involvement by the primary care physician, who is supported by an interdisciplinary team, and when access to care is available 24/7 [13].

Longitudinal chronic care provided by an interdisciplinary team, with active participation of the primary care physician or nurse practitioner, appears to be a universal component [13–15]. Models of care on which the Independence at Home Demonstration was developed rely strongly on a team approach [16, 17]. For example, The Veterans Affairs Home-Based Primary Care Model includes the primary care physician or nurse practitioner, who is held responsible for the care and accountable for the costs, supported by nurses, pharmacists, therapists, social workers, and mental health providers. Each practice has an empanelled group of patients who are managed in their homes for nearly all services and monitored by the team when hospitalized and for short-term institutional care [18]. As a whole the 141 programs showed lower hospital and nurse home use, 30-day hospital readmission rates, and lower overall costs of care without shifting costs to Medicare [17]. In Medicare fee-for-service, all home-based primary care practices are led by a physician (85%) or nurse practitioner and have a wide variety of additional team members, depending on the organization supporting the practice [15]. In another example, The home-based primary care practice at the MedStar Washington Hospital Center employs a team of geriatricians, nurse practitioners, and social workers, supported by an office-licensed practical nurse for triage and support personnel; mental health and pharmacy services are engaged on an ad hoc basis. During a mean 2-year follow-up, cases had 17% lower Medicare costs, averaging $8477 less per beneficiary ($P = 0.003$), with significant reductions in hospital utilization and nursing facility care. Although the home healthcare and hospice costs were higher, these lower cost services acted as substitutes for higher-cost services and were better aligned with the goals and expectations of care in this population.

The question remains about the ability of the workforce to respond to the need [19]. An analysis using the 2012 5% Medicare Beneficiary file identified approximately 2.2 M beneficiaries with characteristics that strongly correlate with eligibility for the IAH Demonstration. These were screened for having had at least one physician visit in their home, assisted living facility or group home by NPI numbers and identified approximately 150,000 patients. Approximately 60% of these were seen by physicians who billed for visits to 40 or more patients in their place of residence in that calendar year, which identified nearly 4000 practices and nearly 6000 providers; nearly 1000 practices had at least 160 patients. Several patterns of growth were used to estimate the potential of the workforce to respond to the societal need, should the reimbursement as suggested by the Year 1 results of the IAH demonstration materialize. The growth rate attributed to the hospitalist movement would meet the needs for 35% of eligible beneficiaries; using the higher growth rate of successful programs in the IAH Demonstration suggests that 64% of the need could be met within 10 years [20]. Generally, the greater the savings the greater the growth, as practice income is a function of savings share.

As important as growth may be for those in need, it is equally important to maintain the quality of care. There is a burgeoning literature on defining the parameters of quality in this highly skewed population, since the usual intermediate measures of disease state, adherence to guidelines, screening tests, and mortality rates have little relevance as illness burden increases and prognosis is diminished [21]. As previously noted, IAH has six quality metrics and nine process measures, but research in this area has offered additional elements that might be considered [22]. The National Home-Based Primary Care and Palliative care Network is field testing metrics focused on patient and caregiver experience [23] and will have a registry available to Advanced Alternative Payment Models under the new MACRA initiatives.

References

1. Newhouse JP, Garber AM. Geographic variation in medicare services. N Engl J Med. 2013;368:1465–8.
2. Anderson G, et al. Partnership for solutions: chronic conditions: making the case for ongoing care. Baltimore, MD: Johns Hopkins University; 2004.
3. Riley GF, Lubitz JD. Long-term trends in medicare payments in the last year of life. Health Serv Res. 2010;45(2):565–76.
4. Brawley OW, Goldberg P. How we do harm. New York: St Martin's Griffin; 2012.
5. Welch GH, Schwartz L, Woloshin S. Overdiagnosed: making people sick in the pursuit of health. Boston, MA: Beacon Press; 2011.
6. Lubitz JD, Riley GF. Trends in medicare payments in the last year of life. N Engl J Med. 1993;328(15):1092–6.
7. Brownlee S. Overtreated: why too much medicine is making us sicker and poorer. New York: Bloomsbury Publishing; 2007.
8. Smith-Bindman R, Miglioretti DL, Johnson E, Lee C, Feigelson HS, Flynn M, et al. Use of diagnostic imaging studies and associated radiation exposure for patients enrolled in large integrated health care systems, 1996–2010. JAMA. 2012;307(22):2400–9.
9. Martin AB, Hartman M, Washington B, Catlin A, The National Health Expenditure Accounts Team. National health spending: faster growth in 2015 as coverage expands and utilization increases. Health Aff. 2016;10:1377.
10. Jencks SF, Williams MV, Coleman EA. Rehospitalizations among patients in the medicare fee-for-service program. N Engl J Med. 2009;360:1418–28.
11. Kinosian B, Taler G, Boling P, Gilden D. The Willie Sutton effect in health care: independence at home qualifying (IAH-Q) criteria identify high, need, high cost Medicare beneficiaries. Abstract American Geriatrics Society Annual Meeting, May 2016.

12. Taler G, Kinosian B, Boling P. Editorial: a bipartisan approach to better care and smarter spending for elderly adults with advanced chronic illness. J Am Geriatr Soc. 2016;64(8):1537–9. doi:10.1111/jgs.14177. (Version of Record online: 31 May 2016)
13. Stall N, Nowaczynski M, Sinha SK. Systematic review of outcomes from home-based primary care programs for homebound older adults. J Am Geriatr Soc. 2014;62:2243–51.
14. Boling PA, Leff B. Comprehensive longitudinal health care in the home for high-cost beneficiaries: a critical strategy for population health management. J Am Geriatr Soc. 2014;62(10):1974–6.
15. Leff B, Weston CM, Garrigues S, Patel K, Ritchie C. Home-based primary care practices in the United States: current state and quality improvement approaches. J Am Geriatr Soc. 2015;63:963–9.
16. DeJonge KE, Jamshed N, Gilden D, Kubusiak J, Bruce SR, Taler G. Effects of home-based primary care on Medicare costs in high-risk elders. J Am Geriatr Soc. 2014;62(10):1825–31.
17. Edes T, Kinosian B, Vuckovic NH, Nichols LO, Becker MM, Hossain M. Better access, quality, and cost for clinically complex veterans with home-based primary care. J Am Geriatr Soc. 2014;62(10):1954–61.
18. Beales JL, Edes T. Veteran's affairs home-based primary care. Clin Geriatr Med. 2009;25:149–54. viii-ix
19. DeCherrie LV, Soriano T, Hayashi J. Home-based primary care: a needed primary-care model for vulnerable populations. Mt Sinai J Med. 2012;79(4):425–32.
20. Kinosian B, Taler G, Boling P, Gilden D, Independence at Home Learning Collaborative Writing Group. Projected savings and workforce transformation from converting independence at home to a medicare benefit. J Am Geriatr Soc. 2016).(Version of Record online: 31 May 2016);64(8):1531–6. doi:10.1111/jgs.14176.
21. DuGoff EH, Dy S, Giovannetti ER, Leff B, Boyd CM. Setting standards at the forefront of delivery system reform: aligning care coordination quality measures for multiple chronic conditions. J Healthc Qual. 2013;35(5):58–69.
22. Leff B, Ritchie C. Quality-of-care standards missing for the vulnerable homebound. Mod Healthc. 2015;45(4):25.
23. Leff B, Carlson CM, Saliba D, Ritchie C. The invisible homebound: setting quality-of-care standards for home-based primary and palliative care. Health Aff. 2015;34:21–9.

Nurse Practitioners and Primary Care for Older Adults

12

Debra Bakerjian

This chapter focuses on the role of nurse practitioners in providing primary care services to older adults. While the chapter focuses on nurse practitioners, it is important to keep in mind the potential role of physician assistants (PAs) and other advanced practice nurses in meeting the primary care shortages as well. Unfortunately, very few physician assistants have specialized in the care of older adults, and the physician assistant profession has not made significant strides in encouraging PAs to pursue this specialty. In contrast, nursing has made specific efforts to educate and train more nurses and advanced practice nurses in the care of older adults [1, 2]. The first part of this chapter will describe nurse practitioners in the US healthcare system followed by a discussion of the nurse practitioner role in various health delivery models and end with policy challenges surrounding NP care.

Nurse Practitioners in Primary Care in the United States

About Nurse Practitioners (NPs)

The American Association of Nurse Practitioners[1] defines NPs as a type of advanced practice nurse who complete a master's and/or a doctoral degree that includes advanced clinical training beyond their education and clinical preparation as a registered nurse. The didactic and clinical course work prepares nurses with specialized clinical knowledge and clinical competencies to work within primary care, acute care, and long-term care settings. Nurse practitioners provide a range of

---

[1]American Association of Nurse Practitioners—NP Facts https://www.aanp.org/all-about-nps/what-is-an-np.

D. Bakerjian, PhD, APRN, FAAN, FAANP
Betty Irene Moore School of Nursing, University of CA, Davis, CA, USA
e-mail: dbakerjian@ucdavis.edu

© Springer International Publishing AG 2018
M. Wasserman, J. Riopelle (eds.), *Primary Care for Older Adults*,
DOI 10.1007/978-3-319-61329-1_12

primary, acute, and specialty healthcare in a variety of different settings to include obtaining patient histories; ordering, performing, and interpreting diagnostic tests; diagnosing and treating acute and chronic conditions; prescribing medications; ordering treatments; and counseling and education of patients and families. Nurse practitioners may operate autonomously or in a collaborative practice, dependent upon the state in which they are licensed.

Types of Nurse Practitioners

As of 2016, there are approximately 222,000 NPs licensed in the United States with the majority of NPs practicing in a primary care settings (see footnote 1). Nurse practitioners are typically educated, licensed, and nationally certified to provide care to a specific population such as pediatrics, family, women's health, mental health, or adult-gerontological. They may also be setting specific such as primary or acute care.

Who Provides Care to Older Adults?

The most common type of NP providing care to older adults is family nurse practitioners (see Table 12.1). They are prepared to provide care to people across the age continuum and are the most prevalent type of NP accounting for 55% of all NPs. Gerontological nurse practitioners (GNPs) receive the highest degree of specialized preparation to care for older adults.

Unfortunately, similar to geriatricians, there are very few (<3%) certified gerontological NPs. To expand the numbers of NPs who received specialized education and training to care for older adults, nursing leaders made decisions through the APRN Consensus Model[2] process to combine the education of adult NPs and gerontological NPs with a goal of increasing the numbers of NPs qualified to care for older adults. Forty-one different nursing organizations endorsed the Consensus Model (Fig. 12.1), which provides agreed upon definitions, describes roles and population foci, and presents strategies for implementation of the model.

The APRN Consensus Model includes uniform guidelines for licensure, accreditation, certification, and education (LACE) to align the relationships across the various roles and population foci of advanced practice nursing. As a result, the specialty role of gerontological nurse practitioners (GNPs) and adult nurse practitioners (ANPs) combined into the new specialty of AGNP. When the numbers of ANPs were added to GNPs, the numbers of geriatric-trained NPs more than doubled. The most current information from the 2016 National NP Sample Survey[3] indicates that

---

[2] The Consensus Model for APRN Regulations: Licensure, Accreditation, Certification, and Education at http://www.nursingworld.org/consensusmodel.

[3] https://www.aanp.org/images/documents/research/2016%20np%20sample%20survey%20report_final.pdf.

Table 12.1 Distribution, top practice setting, and clinical focus area by area of NP certification[a]

Population	Percent of NPs	Top practice setting	Top clinical foci
Acute care	7.7	Hospital inpatient clinic (27.3%)	Cardiology (20.8%)
Adult[b]	16.8	Hospital outpatient clinic (16.3%)	Primary care (32.6%)
Adult-gerontology primary care[b]	4.0	Hospital outpatient clinic (14.5%)	Primary care (40.5%)
Family[b]	55.1	Private group practice (13.9%)	Primary care (47.6%)
Gerontology[b]	2.7	Long-term care facility (20.7%)	Primary care (51.8%)
Neonatal	1.7	Hospital inpatient clinic (44.9%)	Primary care (15.3%)
Pediatric—primary care[b]	6.4	Hospital outpatient clinic (25.4%)	Primary care (57.8%)
Psychiatric/ mental health—adult	2.4	Private NP practice (19.5%)	Psychiatric (96.1%)
Psychiatric/ mental health—family	3.0	Psych/mental health facility (20.5%)	Psychiatric (89.5%)
Women's health[b]	5.8	Private group practice (26.0%)	OB/GYN (72.6%)

[a]AANP Fact Sheet copied with permission from the AANP website—https://www.aanp.org/all-about-nps/np-fact-sheet
[b]Six of the ten population focused NPs are primary care providers with most of the primary care NPs practicing in outpatient clinics, private practice, or long-term care settings

8.1% of NPs have specialty preparation in gerontology. This is still a very small percentage, considering that the oldest old (>85 years) are the fastest growing segment of our population.[4]

The inability to attract a strong geriatric workforce has been a challenge for the last two decades [3–6]. A variety of barriers have been identified including lack of exposure to geriatric training [7], lack of perceived value by students given poor reimbursement when compared with other specialties [8], and an overall negative perception of the industry [6], all contributing to the shortage of geriatric providers.

Settings of Care

In general, there has been an increasing demand for nurse practitioners (and physician assistants) [9–11]. According to one of the top physician recruiters, Merritt Hawkins, in 2016, nurse practitioners are now the fifth most requested searches nationally.[5] The

---

[4] US Census Bureau (2016).

[5] http://www.forbes.com/sites/brucejapsen/2015/07/15/nurse-practitioners-physician-assistants-more-in-demand-than-most-doctors/#59f8c20a3610.

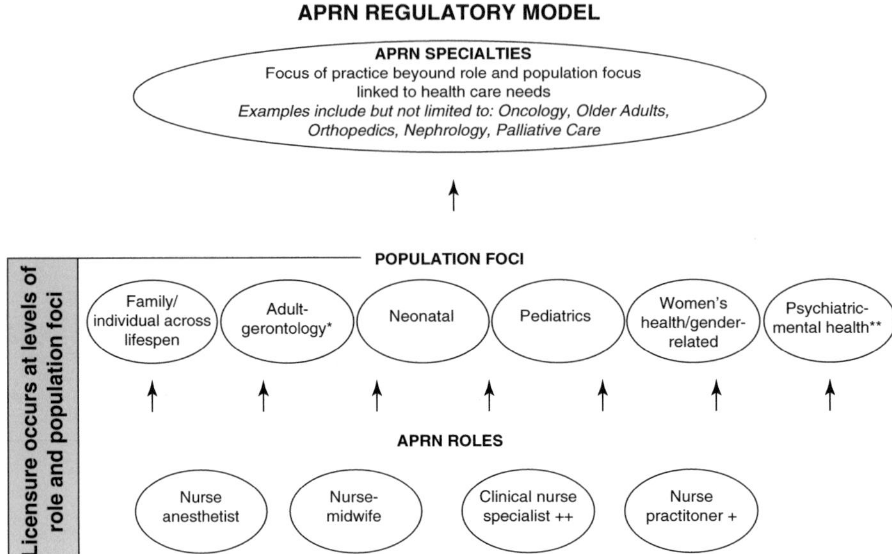

Fig. 12.1 The APRN Consensus Model (cite AANP)

demands come from many different types of healthcare organizations as well as from academic institutions.

Because of their foundation as a registered nurse that educates to work in a variety of settings and with multiple populations, NPs are well versed in both acute care, long-term care, community care, and home care and are familiar with the entire population span. Many NPs have had specialized experiences as an RN in areas such as pain management, women's health, long-term care, or home health, which may lead to their specialization as an NP.

Currently, nurse practitioners are employed in several different practice settings ranging from ambulatory clinics, emergency departments, acute care hospitals, long-term care hospitals, skilled nursing homes, palliative care, hospice, and industry. The most common practice settings include hospital outpatient clinics (14.5%), private group practice (14%), private physician offices (8.5%), hospital inpatient clinics (8.1%), and emergency room/urgent care (4.7%).[6] In most cases, these NPs provide primary care services and are working collaboratively with other healthcare professionals, but in some cases, they practice in a consulting model. The consulting model is common in acute care hospitals, where an NP or a clinical nurse specialist may advise physicians who are not geriatric certified in how to best manage the care of older adults. A significant number of nurse practitioners work as educators in various colleges and universities. They may also be employed in a variety of different research settings, although this is less common. A third of NPs work in rural settings or lower population areas.

---

[6] https://www.aanp.org/images/documents/research/2016%20np%20sample%20survey%20report_final.pdf.

Nurse Practitioners' Roles

As previously discussed, nurse practitioners play a variety of roles in the care of older adults and practice in several different types of settings. The most common roles and settings include:

1. Providing primary care services to older adults in ambulatory care settings such as outpatient clinics and private offices
2. Providing acute and chronic care services to older adults in institutions such as acute care hospitals, skilled nursing facilities, and residential care facilities
3. Providing patient education to patients and families
4. Consulting with organizations on quality of care, patient safety, and quality improvement

Depending on the practice environment, nurse practitioners may collaborate with various healthcare providers including physicians, registered nurses, licensed vocational nurses, medical assistants, social workers, pharmacists, and others. This effort to collaborate comes naturally from a long history of registered nurses working to coordinate care for patients. This also provides a strong foundation for nurse practitioners to work within an interprofessional team, which has been shown to improve the overall quality of care.

One of the advantages that nurse practitioners bring to any practice environment is that they are registered nurses and can incorporate the roles, responsibilities, and functions of the registered nurse into the care that they provide to patients and their families. For example, a nurse practitioner that goes out to visit an elderly patient in their home can assess their chronic diseases, order treatments, write prescriptions, and also provide comprehensive wound care as needed. In the nursing home, they can order pain medications for residents in pain and work directly with the nursing's staff to develop a comprehensive care plan for pain management. The ability of nurse practitioners to integrate the role of the registered nurse into their daily work greatly enhances the value of the care that they provide.

Challenges in Primary Care Services

With the passage of the Affordable Care Act and the aging population, the demand for primary care services has been on the rise.[7] This growth in demand is made more critical by decades of primary care physician shortages, both general internal medicine and family physicians. Additionally, there are a disproportionate number of medical schools and physician graduates concentrated in the northeastern portion of the United States that makes the shortage far worse in the western states. While the physician workforce overall has grown over several decades, there are far fewer

---

[7] http://kff.org/medicaid/issue-brief/tapping-nurse-practitioners-to-meet-rising-demand-for-primary-care/.

physicians entering primary care practice and even fewer who are prepared to care for older adults as mentioned previously.

These shortages are more critical in the face of a fast-growing older population who are living longer with more chronic diseases, significantly increasing the complexity of care. Overall, this higher complexity of care means that clinicians who care for older adults need more time to provide that care, making the shortages of geriatric-trained clinicians an even greater challenge. Nurse practitioners have historically filled that gap of physician shortages; however, the most recent shortages of physicians, the ever-increasing aging population, and the increased complexity of care provided the impetus for significant investments within the Affordable Care Act to expand the role of NPs in primary care [10, 12–15].

The next section describes several newer healthcare delivery models that incorporate nurse practitioners. Several of these new models have shown early success in improving access to care with a long-term goal of mitigating the shortage of geriatricians and geriatric-trained nurse practitioners by employing a team approach to care that incorporates other geriatric-trained health professionals such as pharmacists and social workers [15].

Healthcare Delivery Models and Nurse Practitioners

A variety of innovative healthcare delivery models have arisen in the past decade [16]. Many grew out of the Affordable Care Act, many were in response to the CMS Innovation Center grants and demonstration projects, and others grew directly from organizational innovations. While these models have been described in other chapters in this book, they are discussed briefly in this chapter because most of these models include nurse practitioner care.

One of the most well-known models is the *patient-centered medical home (PCMH)*, which focuses on primary care redesign and espouses a team-based approach to care, historically led by a personal physician, although nurse practitioners are recognized as PCMH leaders by the National Committee for Quality Assurance (NCQA), the committee that accredits PCMHs.[8]

Key components of the PCMH are patient-centeredness, coordinated team-based care, technology, and improving patient experiences of care. This model of care includes physicians, nurse practitioners, physician assistants, pharmacists, social workers, and others to provide comprehensive primary care (see Chap. 2 for further detail). PCMH clinics can be led by NPs in many states, and those NP-led practices have been shown to have similar or in some cases better (breast cancer screening and blood pressure control) outcomes compared with physician-led PCMH clinics [17].

Nurse-managed health clinics (NMHCs) were established through the Affordable Care Act to provide comprehensive primary care health and wellness services to underserved and vulnerable populations [18, 19]. These clinics must be led by an

---

[8]NCQA accreditation programs at http://www.ncqa.org/programs/recognition/practices/patient-centered-medical-home-pcmh.

advanced practice nurse and associated with a school, college, university, or department of nursing, a federally qualified health center, or an independent not-for-profit social services or healthcare agency. Studies of NMHCs have shown positive outcomes such as reduced cost, equivalent or better health outcomes, and improved patient satisfaction ([20]—health affairs [21, 22]).

Accountable care organizations (ACOs) are shared savings models designed to create incentives for institutional and individual healthcare providers to collaborate and share resources while providing coordinated care to patients. To be recognized as an ACO, a group of providers and suppliers of patient services must serve at least 5000 patients in a coordinated fashion and agree to participate in the program for at least 3 years (see Chap. 6 for more detail). Nurse practitioners were initially authorized to be ACO professionals; however, a last-minute change in the regulation precluded the assignment of patients in the program to nurse practitioners. It is hoped that future legislative changes will reverse the exclusion of nurse practitioners; as can be seen from the previous paragraphs, there are many NP-owned or NP-led practices that would benefit from participation in the ACO process.

Retail clinics are another innovation that, while sparking some controversy originally, have become more mainstream in recent years. Retail clinics were designed to provide basic healthcare services in a retail environment, where patients do not need appointments to obtain these services. Retail clinics provide basic services such as immunizations, diagnosis, and initial management of acute illnesses and are covered by many insurances including Medicare and Medicaid. Nurse practitioners and physician assistants typically provide the healthcare.

An interesting study comparing retail clinic, primary care physician office, and emergency department visits found that retail clinics provided primary care services to a greater number of underserved patients, many of whom did not have a primary care provider (Mehrotra et al.). Most of the reasons for visits included upper respiratory complaints, immunizations, ear and eye infections, and urinary tract infections. The authors of this study suggest that these retail clinics are functioning as a safety net for patients who previously sought care in the emergency department. That being said, there are concerns about care provided in retail clinics instead of a primary care office including potential disruption of primary care relationships, the ability to provide consistent chronic care delivery, and reduction in care coordination. More research is needed to better understand the long-term effects of retail clinics. In the meantime, these clinics are meeting the needs of some patients who may not have full access to care for basic services.

Independence at home is a CMS demonstration project currently being evaluated in the US medical practices. Both practices led by a physician or a nurse practitioner have participated in this demonstration project (see Chap. 11 for more detail). The purpose of the project is to provide comprehensive home-based primary care services to a frail elder population with a goal to reduce hospitalizations and emergency department visits for this group of frail elders. Advanced practitioners, including nurse practitioners and physician assistants, have played an important role in the independence at home practices whether led by a physician or a nurse practitioner. NPs and PAs are often the clinicians who make the home visit to homebound seniors in this model. The collaboration between physicians, NPs and PAs, nurses, social workers, pharmacists, and other health professionals is critical in the success of the model. This leads us into a discussion of interprofessional models of care.

Interprofessional Models of Care

While there is an ongoing discussion and debate about the full practice authority for nurse practitioners, there is little debate about the value of nurse practitioners in the care of older adults. In most cases, nurse practitioners work in a collaborative care environment that includes, at minimum, a physician collaborator. Some of the best models also include other health professionals such as geriatric pharmacists, geropsychiatrists, geriatric-trained social workers, and others who work collaboratively to provide comprehensive care to older adults in a variety of different institutional, community, and home settings.

The GRACE model (GRACE stands for geriatric resources for assessment and care of elders) is focused on care of older adults with care provided by a nurse practitioner and social worker in collaboration with an expanded GRACE team that includes a geriatrician, geriatric pharmacist, physical therapist, and mental health case worker [23]. This is an integrated care model that targets mostly dual-eligible (Medicare and Medicaid) patients with chronic diseases. Care begins with a comprehensive in-home assessment by an NP and social worker, who then consult with the expanded team (see Chap. 2 for more details).

A randomized controlled trial that studied the model found that patients enrolled in GRACE had fewer emergency room visits, hospitalizations, readmissions, and lower costs compared with a control group [24]. In this model, one of the highest values of nurse practitioners is that they can function both as a registered nurse and as an advanced practice nurse. Their knowledge of nursing care is instrumental in helping with a holistic assessment of patients in their home environment and with ongoing care coordination. This is particularly effective in caring for older adults with multiple chronic diseases and mental health and psychosocial challenges. Many of these patients have conditions that can be well managed by nurses such as common geriatric syndromes including pressure ulcers, incontinence, and functional decline. Nurse practitioners fully represent nursing in this interdisciplinary team-based collaborative model [24, 25].

Home-based primary care (HBPC) is a model that provides primary care to homebound older adults. This program focuses on transitional care for older adults recently discharged from the acute care hospital. The goal of care is to reduce re-hospitalizations and emergency department visits as well as to improve coordination and continuity of care. In many cases, the care is provided by a nurse practitioner who may be collaborating with a geriatrician and other health professionals such as a geriatric pharmacist and/or social worker (see Chap. 13 for more detail). Again, the fact that nurse practitioners function as both advanced practice and registered nurses contributes highly to the success of this model of care. Nurse practitioners can not only assess, diagnose, and prescribe treatments for these frail older adults, they can also carry out complex nursing care in the home such as wound care, medication reconciliation, and other nursing procedures that might be needed.

PACE or program of all-inclusive care for the elderly provides comprehensive medical and social services to an identified group of community-dwelling frail elders [26]. PACE programs are funded through Medicare and Medicaid with a goal of preventing older adults from being admitted to a nursing home. Medicare and/or Medicaid beneficiaries can join a PACE program if offered in their state. PACE programs are responsible for providing all necessary health services including outpatient, inpatient, and long-term care services as needed. In addition, PACE programs cover Medicare Part D, social services, transportation, occupational and physical therapy, and nutritional counseling. The original PACE program, On Lok, started as a CMS Demonstration Project led by a registered nurse. Within the PACE Program, primary care services are provided by a physician, physician assistant, or nurse practitioner who work within a collaborative team model. Studies of PACE model have shown that the use of team-based care in the PACE model improves healthcare outcomes for older adults [27].

The collaborative care model has been developed to provide care for patients with complex medical and psychiatric conditions. This model combines primary care and mental health services in an integrated fashion. Primary care services are provided by a physician, physician assistant, or nurse practitioner who collaborates with a mental health professional. Studies of this model have shown that this integrated care model provides better outcomes and greater satisfaction for both patients and providers [28, 29].

While not a specific model, much attention has been paid to Care Transitions and the role of nurse practitioners in improved outcomes [30, 31]. Nurse practitioners have had a significant impact on improving transitional care from the hospital to skilled nursing homes and home health settings, and in the care of older adults in general [32–35]. The Transitional Care Model is led by nurses, often advanced practice nurses (including nurse practitioners), and provides team-based health care that is designed to deliver person centered care for high-risk patients (often the elderly). In a randomized control trial of older adults with heart failure, advanced practice nurses improved patient-provider communication, educated patients on the meaning of their symptom and taught them self-care strategies, improving their quality of life [36].

Nurse Practitioners and Quality of Care

There have been numerous studies and systematic reviews over the years that have examined the quality of nurse practitioner care providing both primary care services to the general population and primary care to older adults [20, 37, 38]. While it is not the intent of this book chapter to review the literature related to quality of care, positive outcomes have been well documented and generally include improved health outcomes particularly in chronic care management, such as hypertension, heart failure, and diabetes improvements and functional status, and high levels of patient and family satisfaction [39, 40]. There is extensive evidence showing that nurse practitioners generally provide care equivalent to that of physicians. Moreover, the evidence of improved outcomes from nurse practitioners and physicians in collaboration is even stronger [38, 41] indicating that continued focus on collaborative care is warranted.

Regulatory Issues Related to Nurse Practitioner Practice

Based on the numerous studies demonstrating that nurse practitioners provide care equivalent to that of physicians, several states have granted nurse practitioners authority to practice fully within the scope of their education and training. These efforts have been partially driven by the shortage of physicians across the United States and the need for greater numbers of primary care providers. Unfortunately, despite the evidence that nurse practitioners provide high-quality care and increased patient satisfaction, controversies surrounding NP practice remain. Organized physician groups such as the American Medical Association and the American College of Physicians have lobbied extensively against nurse practitioners having full practice authority, and this has resulted in a wide variation in the scope of nurse practitioner practice between states, variations in access to care in different states, and confusion among consumers related to nurse practitioner practice.

Additionally, there are differences in the federal guidelines for what NPs are allowed to do in nursing homes that conflict with states that have full practice authority. Social Security regulations require that patients who are admitted to a nursing home on Medicare Part A must have a physician complete the comprehensive admission visit. This is a requirement that physicians cannot delegate to either a nurse practitioner or physician assistant. This conflicts with state regulations that allow nurse practitioners to function independently and is another source of confusion for Medicare beneficiaries as well as the physicians and nurse practitioners providing care. Nurse practitioners who are unsure about current regulations should look for the most recent version of the "Evaluation and Management Services" guide from the Medicare Learning Network; the 2016 guide is available online.[9] A specific guide for nursing facility service coding is also available online, the most recent of which is MM4246 (Oct 23, 2012)[10]; please note that these guides are updated periodically. Two other sources are available for up-to-date information on appropriate documentation, billing, and coding: (1) Gerontological Advanced Practice Nurses Association (GAPNA) at https://www.gapna.org/ and (2) American Medical Directors Association (AMDA) at http://www.paltc.org/. Both of these professional organizations provide up-to-date information.

---

[9] https://www.cms.gov/Outreach-and-Education/Medicare-Learning-Network-MLN/MLNProducts/Downloads/eval-mgmt-serv-guide-ICN006764.pdf.

[10] https://www.cms.gov/Outreach-and-Education/Medicare-Learning-Network-MLN/MLNMattersArticles/downloads/mm4246.pdf.

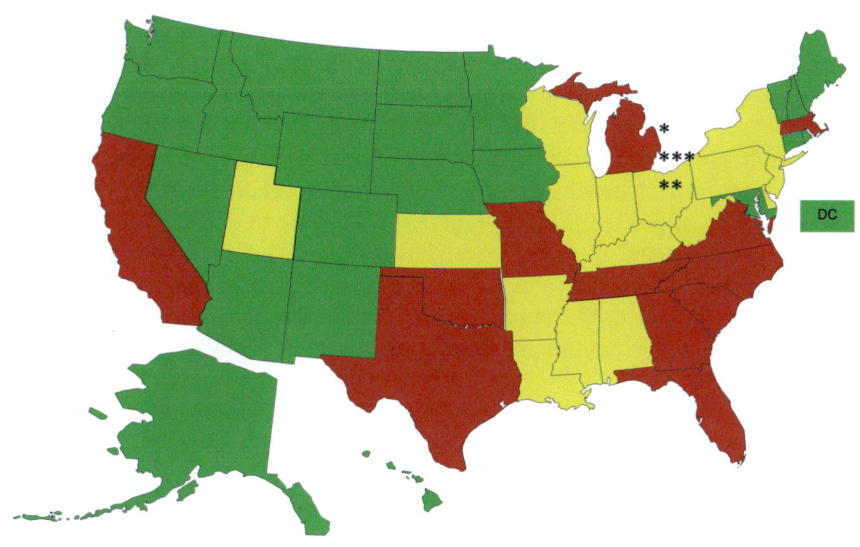

Fig. 12.2 The state practice environment—2017 AANP (https://www.aanp.org/legislation-regulation/state-legislation/state-practice-environment)

Regulation of NP Practice

In general, nurse practitioners are regulated at the state level through nurse practice acts. Unfortunately, the variability in how states regulate NP practice is problematic and continues to be a barrier to full practice authority in many states. The American Association of Nurse Practitioners (AANP) has published a map of state practice environments that is updated regularly. Figure 12.2 shows the current map with an "at-a-glance" view as to whether the state allows for full practice, reduced practice, or restricted practice and includes definitions of those terms. Two particularly important studies have been published recently that have advocated that all states passed legislation to enable all nurse practitioners to have full practice authority to evaluate, diagnose, order diagnostic tests, initiate treatments, and prescribe medications under the exclusive licensure authority of the state board of registered nursing.

The National Governors Association conducted a literature review of state regulations and quality of care related to nurse practitioner scope of practice. They wanted to understand the extent to which scope of practice rules and licensure vary across the states, to what extent state rules and regulations deviate from evidence-based research, and, given the current evidence, how would changes in state scope of practice laws impact healthcare access and quality. Their findings, consistent with other studies, indicated that nurse practitioners provided comparable care to physicians and suggested that NPs may provide improved access to care. Their association recommended that states consider reducing restrictions on scope of practice and ensuring adequate reimbursement for services to encourage and incentivize greater NP involvement in primary healthcare (Schiff—National Governor's Association, 2012).

In 2010, the Institute of Medicine (IOM) released a landmark report, "The Future of Nursing: Leading Change, Advancing Health," which strongly advocated for effective utilization of nurses to address the nation's most challenging healthcare issues. Significant improvements have been made in some areas; however, it has been recognized and reported that one major area that has not improved significantly is the ability of advanced practice registered nurses to practice to the full extent of their education and training due to scope of practice barriers at the state level (Fineberg and Lavizzo-Mourey 2013). The IOM report included recommendations to congress, state legislatures, the centers for Medicare and Medicaid services, and other regulatory agencies to remove barriers to full practice authority. Fineberg and Lavizzo-Mourey have since advocated that this become a reality, not just a recommendation. Subsequently, some states passed legislation to remove these barriers; however, as of January, 2017, there are only 21 states and Washington DC that have granted full practice authority for nurse practitioners. Significant policy work needs to be done to remove scope of practice barriers in the remaining states so that older adults have access to high-quality primary care services [10, 13, 42].

Conclusion

This chapter has focused on describing the role of nurse practitioners in a variety of practice models and settings in the United States. In addition, an effort was made to describe the environmental factors impacting healthcare including the shortage of primary care providers in general and particularly in geriatrics in the face of a rapidly expanding population of older adults. Recommendations have been made that nurse practitioners may fill this gap and provide care to older adults in a variety of settings. Evidence has been provided as to the high quality of the care provided by nurse practitioners as well as clinical nurse specialist and physician assistants, who also provide primary care services to older adults. And while both nurse practitioners and physicians can provide high quality of care independently, there is a growing body of evidence that healthcare outcomes are even better when clinicians work collaboratively in a team-based practice.

References

1. Bednash G, Mezey M, Tagliareni E. The Hartford geriatric nursing initiative experience in geriatric nursing education: looking back, looking forward. Nurs Outlook. 2011;59(4):228–35.
2. Wilson LD. The American Association of Colleges of Nursing's geriatric nursing education consortium. J Gerontol Nurs. 2010;36(7):14.
3. Kovner CT, Mezey M, Harrington C. Who cares for older adults? Workforce implications of an aging society. Health Aff. 2002;21(5):78–89.
4. Laurant MG, Hermens RP, Braspenning JC, Sibbald B, Grol RP. Impact of nurse practitioners on workload of general practitioners: randomised controlled trial. BMJ. 2004; 328(7445):927.
5. Poghosyan L, Lucero R, Rauch L, Berkowitz B. Nurse practitioner workforce: a substantial supply of primary care providers. Nurs Econ. 2012;30(5):268.
6. Stone R, Harahan MF. Improving the long-term care workforce serving older adults. Health Aff. 2010;29(1):109–15.
7. Curran MA, Black M, Depp CA, Iglewicz A, Reichstadt J, Palinkas L, Jeste DV. Perceived barriers and facilitators for an academic career in geriatrics: medical students' perspectives. Acad Psychiatry. 2015;39(3):253–8.
8. Bragg E, Hansen JC. A revelation of numbers: will America's eldercare workforce be ready to care for an aging America? Generations. 2010;34(4):11–9.
9. Colwill JM, Cultice JM, Kruse RL. Will generalist physician supply meet demands of an increasing and aging population? Health Aff. 2008;27(3):w232–41.
10. Institute of Medicine (US). Committee on the Robert Wood Johnson Foundation Initiative on the Future of Nursing. The future of nursing: leading change, advancing health. Washington, DC: National Academies Press; 2011.
11. Oliver GM, Pennington L, Revelle S, Rantz M. Impact of nurse practitioners on health outcomes of medicare and medicaid patients. Nurs Outlook. 2014;62(6):440–7.
12. Gilman DJ, Koslov TI. Policy perspectives: competition and the regulation of advanced practice nurses. Federal Trade Commission Report. 2014.
13. Hain D, Fleck L. Barriers to nurse practitioner practice that impact healthcare redesign. OJIN: Online J Issues Nurs. 2014;19(2)
14. Van Vleet A, Paradise J. Tapping nurse practitioners to meet rising demand for primary care. http://kff. org/medicaid/issue-brief/tapping-nurse-practitioners-to-meet-rising-demand-for-primary-care/.
15. Zwarenstein M, Goldman J, Reeves S. Interprofessional collaboration: effects of practice-based interventions on professional practice and healthcare outcomes. Cochrane Database Syst Rev. 2009;3(3):CD000072.
16. Boult C, Green AF, Boult LB, Pacala JT, Snyder C, Leff B. Successful models of comprehensive care for older adults with chronic conditions: evidence for the Institute of Medicine's "retooling for an aging America" report. J Am Geriatr Soc. 2009;57(12):2328–37.
17. Barkauskas VH, Pohl JM, Tanner C, Onifade TJ, Pilon B. Quality of care in nurse-managed health centers. Nurs Adm Q. 2011;35(1):34–43.
18. Auerbach DI, Chen PG, Friedberg MW, Reid R, Lau C, Buerhaus PI, Mehrotra A. Nurse-managed health centers and patient-centered medical homes could mitigate expected primary care physician shortage. Health Aff. 2013;32(11):1933–41.
19. Hansen-Turton T, Bailey DN, Torres N, Ritter A. Nurse-managed health centers. AJN: Am J Nurs. 2010;110(9):23–6.
20. Naylor MD, Kurtzman ET. The role of nurse practitioners in reinventing primary care. Health Aff. 2010;29(5):893–9.
21. Pohl JM, Vonderheid SC, Barkauskas VH, Nagelkerk J. The safety net: academic nurse-managed centers' role. Pol Polit Nurs Pract. 2004;5(2):84–94.
22. Scudder L. Nurse-led medical homes: current status and future plans May 27, 2011. Accessed at http://www.medscape.com/viewarticle/743197_2.

23. Counsell SR, Callahan CM, Buttar AB, Clark DO, Frank KI. Geriatric resources for assessment and care of elders (GRACE): a new model of primary care for low-income seniors. J Am Geriatr Soc. 2006;54(7):1136–41.
24. Boult C, Wieland GD. Comprehensive primary care for older patients with multiple chronic conditions: "Nobody rushes you through". JAMA. 2010;304(17):1936–43.
25. Bielaszka-DuVernay C. The 'GRACE' model: in-home assessments lead to better care for dual eligibles. Health Aff. 2011;30(3):431–4.
26. Kodner DL, Kyriacou CK. Fully integrated care for frail elderly: two American models. Int J Integr Care. 2000;1:e08.
27. Mukamel DB, Peterson DR, Temkin-Greener HE, Delavan R, Gross D, Kunitz SJ, Williams TF. Program characteristics and enrollees' outcomes in the program of all-inclusive care for the elderly (PACE). Milbank Q. 2007;85(3):499–531.
28. Callahan CM, Boustani MA, Unverzagt FW, Austrom MG, Damush TM, Perkins AJ, Fultz BA, Hui SL, Counsell SR, Hendrie HC. Effectiveness of collaborative care for older adults with Alzheimer disease in primary care: a randomized controlled trial. JAMA. 2006;295(18):2148–57.
29. Gilbody S, Bower P, Fletcher J, Richards D, Sutton AJ. Collaborative care for depression: a cumulative meta-analysis and review of longer-term outcomes. Arch Intern Med. 2006;166(21):2314–21.
30. Coleman EA, Parry C, Chalmers S, Min SJ. The care transitions intervention: results of a randomized controlled trial. Arch Intern Med. 2006;166(17):1822–8.
31. Ouslander JG, Lamb G, Tappen R, Herndon L, Diaz S, Roos BA, Grabowski DC, Bonner A. Interventions to reduce hospitalizations from nursing homes: evaluation of the INTERACT II collaborative quality improvement project. J Am Geriatr Soc. 2011;59(4):745–53.
32. Naylor MD. Transitional care: a critical dimension of the home healthcare quality agenda. J Healthc Qual. 2006;28(1):48–54.
33. Naylor MD. Transitional care of older adults. Annu Rev Nurs Res. 2002;20(1):127–47.
34. Naylor MD, Kurtzman ET, Pauly MV. Transitions of elders between long-term care and hospitals. Policy Polit Nurs Pract. 2009;10(3):187–94.
35. Bixby MB, Naylor MD. The transitional care model (TCM): hospital discharge screening criteria for high risk older adults. Medsurg Nurs. 2010;19(1):62–4.
36. McCauley KM, Bixby MB, Naylor MD. Advanced practice nurse strategies to improve outcomes and reduce cost in elders with heart failure. Dis Manag. 2006;9(5):302–10.
37. Bakerjian D. Care of nursing home residents by advanced practice nurses: a review of the literature. Res Gerontol Nurs. 2008;1(3):177–85.
38. Stanik-Hutt J, Newhouse RP, White KM, Johantgen M, Bass EB, Zangaro G, Wilson R, Fountain L, Steinwachs DM, Heindel L, Weiner JP. The quality and effectiveness of care provided by nurse practitioners. J Nurse Pract. 2013;9(8):492–500.
39. Horrocks S, Anderson E, Salisbury C. Systematic review of whether nurse practitioners working in primary care can provide equivalent care to doctors. BMJ. 2002;324(7341):819–23.
40. Newhouse RP, Stanik-Hutt J, White KM, Johantgen M, Bass EB, Zangaro G, Wilson RF, Fountain L, Steinwachs DM, Heindel L, Weiner JP. Advanced practice nurse outcomes 1990–2008: a systematic review. Nurs Econ. 2011;29(5):230.
41. Bakerjian D, Harrington C. Factors associated with the use of advanced practice nurses/physician assistants in a fee-for-service nursing home practice: a comparison with primary care physicians. Res Gerontol Nurs. 2012;5(3):163–73.
42. Golden AG, Tewary S, Dang S, Roos BA. Care management's challenges and opportunities to reduce the rapid rehospitalization of frail community-dwelling older adults. Gerontologist. 2010;50(4):451–8:gnq015

Collaboration with a Geriatric Pharmacist

13

Janice Hoffman

With the exponential growth expected over the next decade in the geriatric population, healthcare professionals will be challenged to match the demands to adequately treat this cohort [1–3]. Much of the care will default to primary care providers who will benefit from the resources of an interdisciplinary team to assist with assessments and treatment options [4]. The certified geriatric pharmacist is one such interdisciplinary team resource [5].

The certified geriatric pharmacist can help to manage many chronic disease states and assist with assessment and monitoring of the medication regimen in collaboration with the primary care provider [3, 5]. Trained geriatric pharmacists look at the patient as a "whole" and are not in a silo of one disease arena [6, 7]. Considering alternative therapy choices, titration of medications and adjustments of dose due to renal impairment are key roles the pharmacist can play [7, 8]. Drug information is another resource the certified geriatric pharmacist can provide with sufficient evidence-based medicine references that can assist in pharmacotherapy decision-making [9, 10].

A certified geriatric pharmacist has at least 2 years of practice with geriatric patients or a general pharmacy residency for 1 year and 1 year of practice [11]. In addition, the certified geriatric pharmacist has taken a written exam and passed [11]. The certification is good for 5 years and needs to be maintained with specific continuing education requirements set by the Commission for Certification in Geriatric Pharmacy (CCGP) [12]. Unlike other board certification programs, the CCGP is an internationally accepted certification [13]. Through the training process to become a certified geriatric pharmacist, the development in the expertise of the physiologic, pharmacokinetic, polypharmacy, and misuse, abuse, and compliance aberrations that occur with the aging process is achieved [14].

J. Hoffman, Pharm.D, CGP, FASCP
Western University of Health Sciences, College of Pharmacy,
309 East Second Street, Pomona, CA 91766, USA
e-mail: jhoffman@westernu.edu

© Springer International Publishing AG 2018
M. Wasserman, J. Riopelle (eds.), *Primary Care for Older Adults*,
DOI 10.1007/978-3-319-61329-1_13

Many changes in the aging process can affect the use of medications [15]. For example, as people age the gastrointestinal tract, particularly the stomach, becomes more basic from the traditional acidic environment of a pH less than 5 [15, 16]. This change in acidity can affect how a tablet might be dissolved in the stomach or a drug is absorbed [16]. Another example is wrinkling of the skin [17]. With wrinkles the skin is less smooth, is less hydrated, and has decreased surface lipids [17]. The use of a transdermal patch may be affected by the impact wrinkles have on the absorption of the drug getting through the skin as well as the patch adherence to the skin [15, 18]. There is also an increased potential for skin tears and skin complications [15]. A transdermal patch may be valuable to decrease systemic adverse effects; however, they may have an increased cost and potential risks of their own [15, 18].

Socioeconomic value of medication therapy may also play a role in compliance with the medication regimen [19]. At times new medications or those medications that do not have generics available can have high costs associated with their use [20]. Financial burden can contribute to nonadherence if the geriatric patient cannot afford the medication [20]. This can also be affected by third-party payor's refusal to share cost or when the shared cost is too much for the patient on a fixed monthly income [20]. On the other hand, some patients will struggle to pay the high costs and then take the medication every other day to make the medication last longer [19, 20]. Either scenario presents compliance issues [20]. The certified geriatric pharmacist can sometimes help the patient change to a different Medicare Part D plan (prescription coverage program) that better covers the costs of their individual medications or even look for pharmaceutical company financial assistance programs and lastly, the pharmacist can recommend an alternative medication that is covered by the insurance plan [21].

When a pharmacist reviews the medication regimen with the patient, there are situations where misuse and abuse can be detected [22]. Misuse may include, for example, overuse of an inhaler for chronic obstructive pulmonary disease or that the inhaler is not being orally inhaled but the patient is spraying on their chest or inhaling through their nose [23, 24]. This type of misuse can come from low health literacy or poor patient education [25]. Another area of misuse can be seen with pain medications, specifically opioids with abuse potential [26]. Even with elderly patients, abuse with the opioids is common [27]. The patient develops dependence on the opioid to get up every day [27]. This is a helpful "need" however, what can transpire is the transition to demands for pain medication and addiction from this dependent situation [27]. This can be followed by complications of the narcotic analgesic agents such as confusion, delirium, and the increased risk of fractures due to a mechanical fall [28].

There can be value in having collaborative agreements with certified geriatric pharmacists [29]. Pharmacists can assist with the assessment and monitoring of medication regimens, especially in regard to pain management, Diabetes, and cardiovascular conditions [29]. The remainder of this chapter focuses on the services and value of having a consultant pharmacist embedded in your interdisciplinary team.

The consultant pharmacist can also be of great value with transitions of care and medication reconciliation [5, 30]. When a patient goes to the acute care hospital, the medication regimen will likely change [30]. As an example, consider an 87-year-old female having an aortic valve replacement who is sent home with at least five new medications. The discharge medication list may have some of the previous medications she was taking at home missing [30]. The pharmacist can review the home medications and the discharge medications and devise a medication regimen that covers all her medications [31]. Additionally the pharmacist can define a monitoring plan for the medication regimen including monitoring of the new warfarin added at the hospital [31]. With a specific protocol approved by the physician providers, the pharmacist can be delegated for the anticoagulation therapy lab monitoring and dose adjustments for the warfarin [32]. The need to review all medications, determine duplications, unnecessary agents on the return to home, and the need to simplify the medication regimen are all responsibilities that can be designated to the pharmacist for patients experiencing a transition of care [5, 30, 32].

As our 87-year-old patient transitions back to home and starts to make her follow-up visits to her many specialists such as the cardiologist, nephrologist, neurologist, and psychiatrist. There is a greater risk of polypharmacy as the number of specialists increases [33]. Continued visits with the geriatric pharmacist can benefit the patient. The pharmacist can communicate with the variety of specialists, simplify the medication regimen, as well as monitor for adverse effects of the medication regimen [31]. While medications may be started in the acute hospital, if the hospitalist started at a low dose, the medication may need to be titrated upward [30–32]. As a medication is titrated, always consider "start low, go slow, but go" to reach the individual therapeutic range [34].

The geriatric pharmacist is a vital resource in the therapeutic monitoring of medications [29]. The pharmacist can calculate the creatinine clearance (or GFR) and adjust the dose for renal impairment [29, 35, 36]. For example, our 87-year-old patient has been on memantine 10 mg twice daily for the past 6 months; however, during this last hospitalization, her kidneys take a turn for the worse. The pharmacist calculated her creatinine clearance to be 25 ml/min. The recommended dose for memantine when the renal function has declined to less than 30 ml/min is 5 mg twice a day [37]. This is a service the pharmacist can add to decrease accumulation of renally cleared medications and decrease the risk of adverse events [29, 35].

Psychoactive medications are another area that certified geriatric pharmacists can be delegated for monitoring [36]. For antipsychotic medications, the pharmacist can complete an Abnormal Involuntary Movement Scale (AIMS) and report the finding and recommendations for dose reductions [36, 38]. Additionally, the pharmacist can perform the Mini-Mental Status Exam or the Mini-Cog and the geriatric depression scale to assess cognition and depression [36, 38, 39]. The finding of these assessments can be reported to the provider with recommendations for changes in medication regimen as indicated [29]. Another service the pharmacist can provide is behavioral mapping [40, 41]. With a report form completed by the caregivers over 3 days, at 15-min intervals for the frequency of maladaptive behaviors, the pharmacist can plot the behaviors and assist the interdisciplinary team visualize at what times the behaviors are occurring and if the medication dosing is appropriate and if the behaviors are improving [40, 41]. This can identify that behaviors occur when the patient is hungry or having anxiety when a family member is scheduled to visit [40, 41]. When you can visually see the plot of the frequency of behaviors, it is much easier to consider non-pharmacologic interventions such as giving a snack if the patient is hungry or keeping the patient busy until the family member arrives [41]. Psychoactive medications can also contribute to countless therapy and disease state complications [42, 43]. Minimizing the use of psychoactive is fundamental to decreasing the risks and benefit ratio [44]. Especially in dementia, psychoactive medications can be useful and harmful at the same time [45]. We know that the antipsychotic agents are not FDA approved for use in dementia, yet they are used for hallucinations and psychosis that may cause a danger to the patient with self-injurious behaviors or a danger to others such as staff when working closely with the patient and they are kicking, hitting, and spitting [46]. While non-pharmacologic interventions are always first line and are preferred by all involved parties including the patient, there are times that the patient can benefit from the use of psychoactive medication in relation to improved quality of life, caregiver burden, and safety issues [45].

Another area where the geriatric pharmacist can be advantageous is in the development of an antibiotic stewardship program and the empiric selection, renal dose adjustment, and frequency and duration of therapy for antibiotics [47, 48]. With the antibiotic development pipeline declining, the need to reduce resistance to current available antibiotics is increasing [47, 48]. Geriatric patients living within a facility may harbor multidrug-resistant organisms that can be transmitted to other patients [47]. Consider that our 87-year-old was admitted to the hospital for a community-acquired *Streptococcus pneumoniae* but her nasal swab tested positive for *Klebsiella pneumoniae* ESBL. This changed the regimen in the hospital from simply a macrolide to ertapenem [49]. Whether living in a facility or in the community, our frail geriatric patients are at risk for multidrug-resistant organisms [50]. We need to save antibiotics for when there are sufficient signs and symptoms of an infection before starting an antibiotic [49, 50]. If an antibiotic is not started, the provider might consider having the patient return to the office in 24–72 hours to ensure no new signs of infection have developed [49, 50]. Empiric therapy is key to appropriate antibiotic use and should be based on the antibiogram for the cohort of patients seen in your practice [49, 51]. The laboratory can provide the antibiogram, and the pharmacist can help design a plan for your antibiotic stewardship program [51]. Pharmacists have ample knowledge to be helpful with selection of the appropriate spectrum and best antibiotic regimen to reduce the risk of resistance [51]. In the community setting, there is a great need to reduce unnecessary antibiotic use to diminish microorganism resistance, and the pharmacist can be a key to your practice [52].

Another area that the geriatric pharmacist can be of value is in looking for drug-drug interactions [29]. For example, our patient was taking sertraline 50 mg daily and was started on tramadol 50 mg every 6 h as needed for pain in the hospital. She was very anxious on return from the hospital, and the pharmacist noted the possibility of mild serotoninergic syndrome [53]. The pharmacist recommended changing the tramadol back to acetaminophen since the patient had not taken any tramadol since discharge from the hospital.

Adverse drug events can contribute to a geriatric patient being readmitted to the hospital [54]. The difference between an adverse drug event and a side effect is that a side effect is anticipated and mild in nature, such as diphenhydramine causing drowsiness [55]. An adverse drug event can be detrimental to the patient's health [55], for example, blood in the urine with enoxaparin when bridging to warfarin. Our patient was also taking sertraline and the selective serotonin reuptake inhibitors (SSRI) as a class effect can decrease platelet aggregation and contribute to an increased risk of bleeding [56]. This can contribute to a longer hospital stay or a readmission. The pharmacist can play an important role in handling adverse events [57].

Adverse events can range from serotonin syndrome to QTc interval prolongation to medication-induced mechanical fall risk [57]. The certified geriatric pharmacist can remind the prescriber to consider an electrocardiogram to monitor for QTc interval prolongation to decrease the risk of a ventricular arrhythmia and a poor patient outcome [58].

In the setting of a mechanical fall, there are many factors that may contribute to the fall, and medications are one of them [59]. There are several medication fall risk predictors [59]. One of the easiest to use is the ASHP fall risk scoring system (Table 13.1). It looks at the classes of medication and quantifies the risk [60].

Another area that can be assessed by the pharmacist is anticholinergic burden, especially if signs and symptoms of anticholinergic adverse effects are noted such as dry mouth, dry eyes, urinary retention, constipation, or low blood pressure [61]. There are numerous medications such as furosemide and warfarin that have a low anticholinergic burden but when combined with multiple agents can contribute to adverse effects [62].

Dehydration and electrolyte imbalance are also common adverse events for the geriatric patient [63]. Many geriatric patients do not drink enough water [63]. Additionally, several medications can contribute to hyponatremia as an adverse effect, for example, the SSRIs, carbamazepine, and oxcarbazepine [63]. These adverse drug

Table 13.1 Medication fall risk scoring system[a]

AHFS pharmacologic-therapeutic classification	Risk for falls	Points	Mechanism for falls
Analgesics, antipsychotics, anticonvulsants, benzodiazepines	High	3	Sedation, dizziness, postural disturbances, altered gait and balance, impaired cognition
Antihypertensives, cardiac drugs, antiarrhythmics, antidepressants	Intermediate	2	Orthostasis, impaired cerebral perfusion, poor health status
Diuretics	Low	1	Increased ambulation, orthostasis

AHFS American hospital formulary service
Quality Improvement in a Medium-Sized Non-Academic Health System: Pharmacist Medication Profile Review to Decrease Hazardous Falls and Improve Patient Quality of Care. Date accessed: February (2011). American Society of Health-System Pharmacists Quality Improvement Initiative http://www.ashp.org/DocLibrary/Policy/QII/Quality-Success-Story-IssueBrief.pdf.
[a]A score of 6 or higher for a patient suggests an increased risk for falls and triggers evaluation of the patient (i.e., fall risk evaluation)

effects can be a factor in seizure risk and other negative patient outcomes [64]. Discussion of risk factors can help to avoid severe adverse events [63, 64].

Interdisciplinary team meetings can be a simple and effective use of time to get the more information about each patient [29]. The geriatric pharmacist can provide drug information and monitoring and suggest changes in the regimen with a verbal discussion of alternative therapy [29]. When the team members are present and interactive, the best pathway to positive outcomes for the patient can be devised [65]. Most interdisciplinary team meetings can take a few hours a week if done efficiently [66]. New patients can take more discussion to devise the care plan and should be dispersed over different meeting schedules to be efficient. Caregiver, patient, and family should be included when possible [67]. When a patient resides in a facility, the caregiver closest to the patient and the patient should at least attend virtually via teleconference or webinar [67].

While a patient is living within a facility, for example, an assisted living facility (ALF) compared to a skilled nursing facility (SNF), a prescriber should keep in mind the federal and state regulations that apply to medication use within these types of facilities [68]. For example, our patient has been taking sertraline for years and was recently placed in a SNF for rehabilitation after a bout of pneumonia. The facility staff completed the assessment for depression, and currently this patient is not displaying any signs or symptoms of depression. The consultant pharmacist cites the federal regulations that suggest that as the prescriber you should reassess the need for the sertraline and consider a slow downward taper [68]. The prescriber knows that the patient has a long history of depression and decides to keep the dose at the current 50 mg daily regimen. The consultant pharmacist's role in this scenario is to inform the prescriber of the guidelines and to obtain the documentation to support the fact that a dose reduction is clinically contraindicated [68].

Our patient is now being discharged home from the SNF, and the pharmacist is assessing her health literacy and understanding of her medication [29, 69]. Since she is now taking warfarin, the pharmacist asks if she can receive the medication education [69]. The pharmacist meets with the patient and reviews the diet, time to take the medication, and when to notify the prescriber if any symptoms of bruising or bleeding occur [69]. Pharmacists have value as medication education specialists and are often best suited to prepare and deliver this information [69]. Medical staff journal club organization or staff in-services about new uses of medications are additional valuable resources of the pharmacist [70].

Acknowledgments Elizabeth Akhparyan for her assistance with the references.

References

1. Yax, Population Division Laura K. Sixty-five plus in the United States. Sixty Five Plus in the United States. 03 Feb. 2017.
2. Lee W-C, Sumaya CV. Geriatric workforce capacity: a pending crisis for nursing home residents. Front Public Health. 2013;1:24.

3. Gray SL, Elliott D, Semla T. Implications for pharmacy from the Institute of Medicine's report on health care workforce and an aging America. Ann Pharmacother. 2009;43(6):1133–8.
4. Adams WL, Mcilvain HE, Lacy NL, Magsi H, Crabtree BF, Yenny SK, et al. Primary care for elderly people: why do doctors find it so hard? Gerontologist. 2002;42(6):835–42.
5. Keough ME, Field TS, Gurwitz JH. A model of community-based interdisciplinary team training in the care of the frail elderly. Acad Med. 2002;77(9):936.
6. Kasbekar R, Maples M, Bernacchi A, Duong L, Oramasionwu CU. The pharmacist's role in preventing medication errors in older adults. Consult Pharm. 2014;29(12):838–42.
7. Johnson A, Guirguis E, Grace Y. Preventing medication errors in transitions of care: a patient case approach. J Am Pharm Assoc. 2017;55(2):e264–74.
8. Berthe A, Fronteau C, Le Fur E, Morin C, Huon JF. Medication reconciliation: a tool to prevent adverse drug events in geriatrics medicine. Geriatr Psychol Neuropsychiatr Vieil. 2017;15(1):19–24.
9. Burkiewicz JS, Zgarrick DP. Evidence-based practice by pharmacists: utilization and barriers. Ann Pharmacother. 2005;39(7–8):1214–9.
10. Knoer S, Eck AR, Lucas A. A review of American pharmacy: education, training, technology, and practice. J Pharm Health Care Sci. 2016;9(2)
11. About the Certified Geriatric Pharmacist Examination | CCGP. N.p., n.d. 03 Feb. 2017.
12. About the Certified Geriatric Pharmacist Examination | CCGP. N.p., n.d. 03 Feb. 2017.
13. What Is a Certified Group Psychotherapist (CGP)? CGP Certification. N.p., n.d. 03 Feb. 2017.
14. ASCP Updates Introductory Modules on Geriatric Pharmacy Review | CCGP. N.p., n.d. 03 Feb. 2017.
15. Nkansah N. Boot Camp Biology of Aging. Biology of Aging. San Francisco: UCSF, n.d.
16. Feldman M, Cryer B, Mcarthur KE, Huet BA, Lee E. Effects of aging and gastritis on gastric acid and pepsin secretion in humans: a prospective study. Gastroenterology. 1996;110(4): 1043–52.
17. Why does skin wrinkle with age? What is the best way to slow or prevent this process? Scientific American. N.p., 23 Sept. 2005. 03 Feb. 2017.
18. Konda S, Meier-Davis S, Shudo B, Maibach J. Age-related percutaneous penetration part 2: effect of age on Dermatopharmacokinetics and overview of transdermal products. Skin Therapy Lett. 2012;17(6):5–7.
19. Alsabbagh MH, Wasem E, Lemstra M, Eurich D, Lix LM, Wilson TW, et al. Socioeconomic status and nonadherence to antihypertensive drugs: a systematic review and meta-analysis. Value Health. 2014;17(2):288–96.
20. Chan M. Reducing cost-related medication nonadherence in patients with diabetes. Physicians Practice. N.p., n.d. 03 Feb. 2017.
21. Bonner L. Annual medicare part D enrollment is here. American Pharmacists Association. N.p., 17 Oct. 2014. 03 Feb. 2017.
22. Silva C, Ramalho C, Luz I, Monteiro J, Fresco P. Drug-related problems in institutionalized, polymedicated elderly patients: opportunities for pharmacist intervention. Int J Clin Pharm. 2015;37(2):327–34.
23. Fan VS, Gylys-Colwell I, Locke E, Sumino K, Nguyen HQ, Thomas RM, et al. Overuse of short-acting beta-agonist bronchodilators in COPD during periods of clinical stability. Respir Med. 2016;116:100–6.
24. Takaku Y, Kurashima K, Ohta C, Ishiguro T, Kagiyama N, Yanagisawa T, et al. How many instructions are required to correct inhalation errors in patients with asthma and chronic obstructive pulmonary disease? Respir Med. 2017;123:110–5.
25. Rau JL. Practical problems with aerosol therapy in COPD. Respir Care. 2006;51(2):158–72.
26. Salinas GD, Susalka D, Burton S, Roepke N, Evanyo K, Biondi D, et al. Risk assessment and counseling behaviors of healthcare professionals managing patients with chronic pain: a National multifaceted assessment of physicians, pharmacists, and their patients. J Opioid Manag. 2012;8(5):273–84.
27. Chang Y-P, Compton P. Opioid misuse/abuse and quality persistent pain management in older adults. J Gerontol Nurs. 2016;42(12):21–30.

28. Krebs EE, Paudel M, Taylor BC, Bauer DC, Fink HA, Lane NE, et al. Association of opioids with falls, fractures, and physical performance among older men with persistent musculoskeletal pain. J Gen Intern Med. 2016;31(5):463–9.
29. Mcbane SE, Dopp AL, Abe A, Benavides S, Chester EA, Dixon DL, et al. Collaborative drug therapy management and comprehensive medication Management – 2015. Pharmacotherapy. 2015;35(4):e39–50.
30. Yvette C, Kripalani S. Medication use in the transition from hospital to home. Ann Acad Med Singap. 2008;37(2):136.
31. Carter MA, Amadio AL, Bruchet N. Should hospital pharmacists provide postdischarge follow-up care to high-risk patients? Can J Hosp Pharm. 2015;68(3):265–6.
32. Wilt V, Gums J, Ahmed O, Moore L. Outcome analysis of a pharmacist-managed anticoagulation service. Pharmacotherapy ACCP. 1995;15(6):732–9.
33. Veehof L, Schuling J. Polypharmacy in the elderly with chronic diseases: conflicting interests. Ned Tijdschr Geneeskd. 1997;141(4):177–9.
34. Pehlivan, Ozgur CoruhluSuleyman. "Worst Pills." Worst Pills. N.p., n.d. 03 Feb. 2017.
35. Hanlon JT, Lindblad CI, Gray SL. Can clinical pharmacy services have a positive impact on drug-related problems and health outcomes in community-based older adults? Am J Geriatr Pharmacother. 2004;2(1):3–13.
36. Page AT, Potter K, Clifford R, Mclachlan AJ, Etherton-Beer C. Medication appropriateness tool for co-morbid health conditions in dementia: consensus recommendations from a multidisciplinary expert panel. Intern Med J. 2016;46(10):1189–97.
37. Pumerantz Library Proxy Login. N.p., n.d. 03 Feb. 2017.
38. Rubio-Valera M, Chen T, O'reilly C. New roles for pharmacists in community mental health care: a narrative review. Int J Environ Res Public Health. 2014;11(10):10967–90.
39. Reinhold J, Earl G. Clinical therapeutics primer: link to the evidence for the ambulatory care pharmacist, first edition. Burlington: Jones & Bartlett Learning; 2017.
40. Wolf-Klein GP, Levy AP, Silverstone FA, Smith H, Papain P, Foley CJ. Psychiatric profile of the noncompliant geriatric patient in the community. Int Psychogeriatr. 1989;1(2):177–84.
41. Borson S. Geriatric psychiatry, an issue of clinics in geriatric medicine – 9780323320122 | US Elsevier Health Bookshop. N.p., 25 July 2014. 03 Feb. 2017.
42. American Geriatrics Society 2015 Beers Criteria Update Expert Panel. American geriatrics society 2015 updated beers criteria for potentially inappropriate medication use in older adults. J Am Geriatr Soc. 2015;63(11):2227–46.
43. Lin EH, Katon W, Von Korff M, Rutter C, Simon GE, Oliver M, et al. Relationship of depression and diabetes self-care, medication adherence, and preventive care. Diabetes Care. 2004;27(9):2154–60.
44. Gable R. 5.2 Altering consciousness with psychoactive drugs. Introduction to psychology. N.p.: Creative Commons, 2010. pp. 686–96.
45. Lindsey PL. Psychotropic medication use among older adults. J Gerontol Nurs. 2009;35(9):28–38.
46. Information for healthcare professionals: conventional antipsychotics. FDA information for healthcare professionals: conventional antipsychotics. N.p., n.d. 03 Feb. 2017.
47. Rhee SM, Stone ND. Antimicrobial stewardship in long-term care facilities. Infect Dis Clin N Am. 2014;28(2):237–46.
48. Dellit TH. Summary of the infectious diseases society of America and the society for healthcare epidemiology of America guidelines for developing an institutional program to enhance antimicrobial stewardship. Infect Dis Clin Pract. 2007;15(4):263–4.
49. IDSA Guidelines 2016: HAP, VAP & It's the End of HCAP as We Know It (And I Feel Fine). PulmCCM. PulmCCM, 31 July 2016. 03 Feb. 2017.
50. Bonomo RA. Multiple antibiotic resistant bacteria in long term care facilities: an emerging problem in the practice of infectious diseases. Clin Infect Dis. 2000;31(6):1414–22.
51. Joshi S. Hospital antibiogram: a necessity. Indian J Med Microbiol. 2010;28(4):277–80.

52. Lee VC. The antibiotic resistance crisis part 1: causes and threats. Pharm Ther. 2015;40(4):277–83.
53. Mayo Clinic Staff Print. "Serotonin Syndrome." Overview – Serotonin Syndrome – Mayo Clinic. N.p., 20 Jan. 2017. 03 Feb. 2017.
54. Dormann H, Neubert A, Criegee-Rieck M, Egger T, Radespiel-Troger M, Azaz-Livshits T, et al. Readmissions and adverse drug reactions in internal medicine: the economic impact. J Intern Med. 2004;255(6):653–63.
55. What is the difference between adverse drug reaction and side effect?? N.p., n.d. 03 Feb. 2017.
56. Mccloskey DJ, Postolache TT, Vittone BJ, Nghiem KL, Monsale JL, Wesley RA, et al. Selective serotonin reuptake inhibitors: measurement of effect on platelet function. Transl Res. 2008;151(3):168–72.
57. ASHP guidelines on adverse drug reaction monitoring and reporting. Medication Misadventures – Guidelines. N.p., n.d.
58. Mabasa VH, Yokoyama S, Man D, Martyn J. Analysis of orders for QTc-prolonging medication for intensive and cardiac care unit patients with pre-existing QTc prolongation (QTIPPP study). Can J Hosp Pharm. 2011;64(6):412–8.
59. Woolcott JC. Meta-analysis of the impact of 9 medication classes on falls in elderly persons. Arch Intern Med. 2009;169(21):1952.
60. Tool 3I: medication fall risk score and evaluation tools. Agency for Healthcare Research & Quality. U.S. HHS: Agency for Healthcare Research and Quality, 31 Jan. 2013. 03 Feb. 2017.
61. Hilmer SN. A drug burden index to define the functional burden of medications in older people. Arch Intern Med. 2007;167(8):781.
62. Drugs with possible anticholinergic effect. Anticholinergic cognitive burden scale drugs with possible anticholinergic effects (n.d.): http://www.agingbraincare.org/uploads/products/ACB_anticholinergic_possibles_Handout_040412.pdf.
63. Schlanger LE, Bailey JL, Sands JM. Electrolytes in the aging. Adv Chronic Kidney Dis. 2010;17(4):308–19.
64. Alomar MJ. Factors affecting the development of adverse drug reactions (review article). Saudi Pharm J. 2014;22(2):83–94.
65. Nancarrow SA, Booth A, Ariss S, Smith T, Enderby P, Roots A. Ten principles of good interdisciplinary team work. Hum Resour Health. 2013;11(1):19.
66. Kinship care wrap around services: eligibility and documentation requirements. PsycEXTRA Dataset (n.d.): n. pag. Center for Medicare and Medicaid Services.
67. Oliver Park D, Porock D, Demiris G, Courtney K. Patient and family involvement in hospice interdisciplinary teams. J Palliat Care. 2005;21(4):270–6.
68. CMS review of current standards of practice for long-term care pharmacy services long-term care pharmacy primer. Centers for Medicare and Medicaid Services (n.d.): n. pag.
69. Kaboli PJ, Hoth AB, Mcclimon BJ, Schnipper JL. Clinical pharmacists and inpatient medical care. Arch Intern Med. 2006;166(9):955.
70. Lamy PP, Westfall LK, Speedie SM. The effect of inservice education provided by consultant pharmacists on the behavior of nurses in long-term care facilities. Ann Pharmacother. 1981;15(10):777–81.

Peter A. Hollmann

Introduction

Primary care matters. It is associated with better health, better health-care quality, and lower costs [1–3]. It is also a field that has been under extreme stress due to the hard work of transformation of the delivery system and payment inadequacy. As in all of medicine, there is diversity of structure, process, and quality across the many sites of primary care. There is also great diversity and change underway in payment for primary care. This chapter seeks to define key attributes of effective primary care and to then discuss financial models to support the delivery of such care. A model can be evaluated from the perspective of the payer or the provider, but ultimately the different and sometimes conflicting views will need to be reconciled by evidence of the success or failure of any model based upon societal goals and realistic metrics. Additional chapters in this book provide details on specific programs and models of effective care—both in terms of cost and quality. In this chapter an attempt is made to set the stage for these more detailed presentations by providing more general information on finances and the lexicon of payment "reform." A principle that underlies any successful financial model is that it is sustainable and it supports and nurtures what matters and minimally stimulates what does not. Any model is also only as good as its implementation and no single approach or model will achieve all goals.

Defining Effective Primary Care

In 1996 the Institute of Medicine (IOM) defined primary care. "Primary care is the provision of integrated, accessible health care services by clinicians who are

P.A. Hollmann, MD
University Medicine-Geriatrics, Warren Alpert Medical School, Brown University, Providence, RI, USA
e-mail: phollmann@Lifespan.org

© Springer International Publishing AG 2018
M. Wasserman, J. Riopelle (eds.), *Primary Care for Older Adults*,
DOI 10.1007/978-3-319-61329-1_14

accountable for addressing a large majority of personal health care needs, developing a sustained partnership with patients, and practicing in the context of family and community." [4].

The IOM also defined quality care as addressing these six aims [5]:

- **Safe**: Avoiding harm to patients from the care that is intended to help them
- **Effective**: Providing services based on scientific knowledge to all who could benefit and refraining from providing services to those not likely to benefit (avoiding underuse and misuse, respectively)
- **Patient-centered**: Providing care that is respectful of and responsive to individual patient preferences, needs, and values and ensuring that patient values guide all clinical decisions
- **Timely**: Reducing waits and sometimes harmful delays for both those who receive and those who give care
- **Efficient**: Avoiding waste, including waste of equipment, supplies, ideas, and energy
- **Equitable**: Providing care that does not vary in quality because of personal characteristics such as gender, ethnicity, geographic location, and socioeconomic status

A defining concept in primary care is the patient-centered medical home (PCMH). In 2007 a coalition of primary care physician specialties adopted Joint Principles of the PCMH [6]. In summary the Principles state:

The patient-centered medical home (PCMH) is an approach to providing comprehensive primary care for children, youth, and adults. The PCMH is a health-care setting that facilitates partnerships between individual patients, and their personal physicians, and when appropriate, the patient's family.

Personal physician—each patient has an ongoing relationship with a personal physician trained to provide first contact, continuous, and comprehensive care.

Physician-directed medical practice—the personal physician leads a team of individuals at the practice level who collectively take responsibility for the ongoing care of patients.

Whole person orientation—the personal physician is responsible for providing for all the patient's health-care needs or taking responsibility for appropriately arranging care with other qualified professionals. This includes care for all stages of life, acute care, chronic care, preventive services, and end-of-life care.

Care is coordinated and/or integrated across all elements of the complex health-care system (e.g., subspecialty care, hospitals, home health agencies, nursing homes) and the patient's community (e.g., family, public, and private community-based services). Care is facilitated by registries, information technology, health information exchange, and other means to assure that patients get the indicated care when and where they need and want it in a culturally and linguistically appropriate manner.

Quality and Safety Are Hallmarks of the Medical Home
Evidence-based medicine and clinical decision-support tools guide decision-making.
Physicians in the practice accept accountability for continuous quality improvement
through voluntary engagement in performance measurement and improvement.
Patients actively participate in decision-making and feedback is sought to ensure
patients' expectations are being met.
Information technology is utilized appropriately to support optimal patient care,
performance measurement, patient education, and enhanced communication.
Practices go through a voluntary recognition process by an appropriate nongovern-
mental entity to demonstrate that they have the capabilities to provide patient-
centered services consistent with the medical home model.
Patients and families participate in quality improvement activities at the practice
level.
Enhanced access to care is available through systems such as open scheduling,
expanded hours, and new options for communication between patients, their personal physician, and practice staff.

It goes on to comment on payment principles necessary to sustain this model:
Payment appropriately recognizes the added value provided to patients who have
a patient-centered medical home. The payment structure should be based on the following framework:

- It should reflect the value of physician and non-physician staff patient-centered
  care management work that falls outside of the face-to-face visit.
- It should pay for services associated with coordination of care both within a
  given practice and between consultants, ancillary providers, and community
  resources.
- It should support adoption and use of health information technology for quality
  improvement.
- It should support provision of enhanced communication access such as secure
  e-mail and telephone consultation.
- It should recognize the value of physician work associated with remote monitoring of clinical data using technology.
- It should allow for separate fee-for-service payments for face-to face visits.
  (Payments for care management services that fall outside of the face-to-face
  visit, as described above, should not result in a reduction in the payments for
  face-to-face visits.)
- It should recognize case mix differences in the patient population being treated
  within the practice.
- It should allow physicians to share in savings from reduced hospitalizations
  associated with physician-guided care management in the office setting.
- It should allow for additional payments for achieving measurable and continuous
  quality improvements.

These are good principles and articulate important aspects of any financial model that will support effective primary care. However, there are many possible methods to implement these principles.

To individuals, effective primary care is care that meets their personal needs, regardless of how an expert may rate it. In today's world of value-based care goals, effective primary care in the eyes of payers and the public is the care that produces the highest possible quality result at the lowest cost. Additionally, it is the care that will reign in growth of national health-care expenditures to a sustainable rate.

Why Primary Care Matters and Where the Money Goes

The IOM asks primary care clinicians to practice in the context of family and community. The context of community can take many forms, from seeking to improve the public health infrastructure, to advocating for better schools and housing and to being a good steward of resources. Inevitably, there must be a limit on health-care spending, although historically America has spent an ever-increasing percentage of its gross domestic product on health care. Any limitation on spending will create a zero sum game where increases in one area must be offset by savings in another. On a larger social scale, America does this today. Compared to other economically advanced countries, we spend substantially more on health care in a presumed effort to achieve health. In turn, we spend less on social programs. Other nations spend a similar amount in the aggregate, but proportionally more on social programs, and achieve better health statistics than the United States [7].

It is likely that increased and sustained investment in primary care will be dependent on the ability of primary care to blunt spending trends. There is reasonably strong evidence that primary care supply, especially in relationship to specialist supply, is associated with improved quality and reduced cost [8]. Whether or not increased numbers of primary care providers will blunt cost spending trends is less clear [9].

It seems obvious that primary care capacity is central to achieving access to care and preventive services. Care coordination is generally a primary care function, even if some other disciplines do prominently coordinate care across the medical neighborhood, at least for select populations (e.g., dialysis patients) or on a time-limited basis (e.g., cancer treatment). If patients are to be cared for in lower cost settings than hospitals, inpatient and outpatient, there must be a primary care infrastructure for patients to get that care. Without other change, just spending more on primary care is unlikely to achieve the triple aim of better health, better health care, and lower cost. But without a strong primary care system, the aim is merely an imaginary dream. To attain the goals of the aim, primary care needs to transform. Many activities to create advanced centers of primary care are in progress. Today, although it varies by region and population of interest (e.g., children compared to the vulnerable elderly), approximately 6–8% of health-care spending is on primary care visits. These visits comprise roughly half of all patient visits, though the ratio of primary care to specialist visits is shrinking [2].

The financial models of greatest interest to geriatricians involve Medicare, though the dual-eligible population is very relevant, and models that combine Medicare and Medicaid expenditures such as the Program of All-Inclusive Care for the Elderly (PACE) are of great importance. A substantial portion of health-care expenditures is out of pocket and on services not covered by Medicare. That said, Medicare comprises the major source of payments to physicians and other geriatrics professionals. If Medicare Advantage (Part C) spending is removed and assumed to be spent in the same manner as the remaining funds, Medicare spends approximately 40% of its funds on hospitals, 16% on physicians and professionals, 15% on Part D drugs, 5% on skilled nursing, 3% on home health, and the rest on a variety of services such as durable medical equipment, hospice, and Part B drugs [10]. These proportions reflect the $597 billion spent in 2014. For hospitals, the 40% is split into 31% inpatient and 9% outpatient. In 2014, approximately $150 billion was spent on long-term care (nursing care facilities and continuing care retirement communities) [11], and Medicaid funded half of the nursing facility expenditures. The reason to understand these figures and sources of payment is because financial models will be designed to facilitate shifts in fund distribution with an overall net savings or better return on investment in terms of functional or health status.

Insurance Basics

It is important to understand some general principles of insurance and to have a working knowledge of health-care finance terminology in order to consider models of care. It is becoming even more essential as most of the newer models of finance are pushing insurance risk onto providers. Therefore, to a degree, provider entities are becoming quasi-insurance companies. Of course, historically there have been insurance companies that were also providers, merging financing and delivery, such as the staff model prepaid health plan represented by Kaiser and other staff model health maintenance organizations.

Risk Insurance is designed to pool risk across a group of people that contribute money (premiums), or have money contributed on their behalf, to pay for events that are generally predictable at the population level, but not at the individual level. The goal is to have enough money to pay for the cost of care of those persons who need care. Many individuals will have no costs and others will have very high costs. The law of averages keeps premiums affordable overall. By pooling resources, the risk is spread and no one person sustains financial calamity when a high-cost event occurs. This very basic principle is all too frequently forgotten. It is understandable that a fundamental concept can be overlooked when we use insurance to pay for predictable expenses such as preventive care. It also is the case that more and more high costs are not for random "events" such as leukemia or trauma; they are due to chronic high-cost conditions that will persist for years. Nonetheless, the implications of the basic principle of insurance are many. The first is that the risk pool needs to be large enough to blunt the effect of random events. Pooling the risk for 100 people together will not create financial protection from an expensive event, if one should occur. A one in a million very expensive event probably will not strike this small cohort, but if it does, the funds would never be enough, even if saved over many years of "dodging bullets." So a model of financing that expects a provider to accept risk needs to also require that the provider has a sufficiently large population to do so.

The next key point relates to the profile of people in the risk pool. Something bad *may* happen in a group of young healthy prevention-minded people. Something bad *will* happen in a group of frail elderly. If the premiums need to support the whole pool, they need to reflect the risk profile of the pool. Of course, we all know that the monthly health-care costs for the average working population are lower than the monthly costs for the average aged population. But the impact of a small subset of high-cost patients/insureds can be more significant than one might presume. It is the case that approximately 50% of health-care expenditures are generated by payments for care of 5% of the population [12, 13]. Let's label them "high-cost patients" and call this the 5/50 principle. Take two insurance companies, one has 5% high-risk patients, the other has 6% high-risk patients, a seemingly trivial difference. But, based on 5/50, 1% of the high-cost patients account for 10% of the plan cost, so the difference is not trivial. This is especially important to note because even excellent care management would be challenged to reduce overall costs of the entire population by 10%. To get back to the level of cost compared to the company that had 5% high-cost patients, medical management would need to reduce the cost on the extra 1% high-risk patients by 100% (an unlikely achievement) or on the 6% by 17% (one sixth). If that seems challenging, try finding the savings from a group of patients that already have no costs in a year or only costs related to appropriate preventive services. This is why there is a need for "risk adjustment" in premiums or risk assumption payment methodologies. Even with risk adjustment, there is usually still an incentive to "cherry pick" and engage in risk avoidance strategies, because the adjustment is partial or stated differently, undercompensates. A successful model will fairly risk adjust and not create incentives to avoid complex patients and the professionals who care for them.

Risk assumption can be modified. Even insurance companies often buy insurance, called "reinsurance" for extreme cost outliers. Sometimes special "high-risk pools" are funded to encourage people to be insured or to encourage insurance companies to enter a market place. One way this happens in payer contracts with risk-assuming provider groups is that the payer truncates the maximum per-patient per-year cost at a threshold number like $150 thousand. The payer retains the risk for any additional costs beyond the cap. The lower the cap, the lower the risk assumed by the provider group, but because high-cost patients generate most of the health-care costs, low truncation levels like $25 thousand are not used as essentially no risk is shared at that point. In primary care, the best example of modification is narrowing or broadening the type of risk. If a group of primary care providers is at risk for the total costs of care, their risk far exceeds (by almost 20:1) their typical primary care revenue, but the risk could be limited to primary care costs. For illustration simplicity, assume primary care is exactly 5% of the total cost of care and it is paid to a primary care provider group. Therefore, a mere 5% total cost overage would eliminate 100% of the gross income (i.e., before the practice expenses are even paid) of the primary care group. On the other hand, if the group was only at risk for an amount not to exceed 10% of *their* income, while the risk would be significant at 20% of take-home pay assuming 50% of revenue overhead costs, it would be feasible. The primary care group would be at risk for only 0.5% of the total cost of care, yet this financial model may well drive primary care clinicians to take measures that are likely to reduce the total cost of care by more than 0.5% of the total cost, as they have a huge share of their income on the line. A financial model for effective primary care will motivate primary care providers to improve access, to seek creative cost management solutions, and to be good stewards of resources, but not subject them to unacceptable risk levels.

Risk Adjustment   The focus above was on accepting financial risk and insurance by pooling risk. Besides cutting off risk acceptance at a dollar cap, it may be possible to otherwise adjust risk. Payment or the pool of dollars budgeted for care may be a risk-adjusted sum. For example, assume a large integrated health system is paid by a health plan every month (per month) for every assigned Medicare patient (per member or patient) an amount of money. We call this the PMPM (per member per month) payment. Assume that the average PMPM based on average historical costs of the Medicare population in that region is $1200. The plan will keep $200 dollars for administrative costs and for reserves and gives the providers a $1000 PMPM budget. This hypothetical integrated system is renowned for caring for complex patients and serves a large segment of people that lack supports and never had access to preventive care when younger, and it also has a large group of nursing homes in its system. Its patients are more complex, without question to all observers. In fact, in the year prior, the average cost for its patients was $1400 PMPM. Clearly the system will fail if it were to receive $1000 PMPM. So there is a need for risk adjustment. But how much? One might wonder if the expected costs in the region for such a more complex group of patients would be $1500 PMPM (i.e., the system was efficient relatively) or $1300 PMP (i.e., the system was relatively inefficient).

Age, gender, institutional status (as compared to residing in the community), functional capacity, social supports, and diagnoses all may be analyzed for their correlation with Medicare-covered medical costs. What Medicare has in large databases and for every beneficiary are costs and diagnoses in addition to age, gender, Medicaid eligibility, and institutional status. It uses this data to create the Hierarchical Condition Categories (HCC) methodology to risk adjust total costs. Diagnoses treated and reported in claims are used to create a risk score for every patient. Not every diagnosis matters (as an HCC) as one can imagine many have little to no impact on costs. An example would be allergic rhinitis. Some conditions when together in the same patient have a combined adjustment that is bigger than the sum of the individual factors as there is an interaction, consistent with the health risks clinicians well understand in patients with multiple interacting conditions. An example would be chronic kidney disease and heart failure. This HCC risk adjustment is used for total cost of care. There may be risk adjustors for other events that are structured differently, such as the risk for readmission to a hospital.

It is important to understand that these adjustments are based on modeling on large databases and are valid only for the intended use. So, a score that determines that a patient is likely going to cost 150% of the average does not mean that the chances of going to the ER are 150% more than average, even if they probably are higher. It is well known that factors such as health literacy, social supports, educational level, and income affect the probability of a patient receiving certain services or attaining certain clinical end points. It is obvious that financial impediments to obtaining insulin might affect glycemic control as an example. Risk adjustment is not generally used for quality measures. While this may seem unfair to a clinician being "graded" or paid based upon a quality metric in a pay for performance program, the general philosophy is that it is not a good social goal to set lower standards for disadvantaged populations. A cursory familiarity with the controversies in testing in education (e.g., "no child left behind") will serve to illustrate this conundrum.

Benefit Design The design of a health plan can affect costs by direct financial impacts or by behavioral alteration or both. Assume a benefit design where the patient pays 10% of all bills and there is no ceiling. If nothing else changes, 10% is saved by the plan over what it would have had to pay at the 100% benefit level. But, it is likely that behavioral effects will also occur. Some patients will not get unnecessary or low-value services, especially if they are costly, such as an MRI for a few weeks of low-risk back pain. But they may still seek inexpensive antibiotics for a viral respiratory illness. Others may not accept or be able to afford important, effective high-cost care. Some patients may forego important and generally cost-effective preventive care. While most preventive care still has a positive net cost (i.e., there is a cost per life year saved, not a net savings), this could result in higher medical costs for some, such as needing chemotherapy and radiation versus a lumpectomy, due to breast cancer being diagnosed at a later stage. Medications may be skipped and some medications do have a net cost savings, such as ACE inhibitors for patients with diabetes [14]. Professionals will become more conscious of costs and may change ordering behaviors. It is not always predictable what will occur. Beliefs that are not supported by evidence, fear of uncertainty, wealth, education level, confidence, entitlement, and perception of life expectancy are all factors relevant to the behavior of an individual. These may outweigh the effects of evidence-based decision-making. Nonetheless, design is attempted so as to promote good care and good patient behavior while reducing costs. Low primary care co-pays, high ER co-pays, and no preventive care co-pays would be examples of such design.

There are some limitations of benefit design that warrant mentioning. The first point is to not confuse saving money on one patient with saving on a population. In geriatrics the best example would be a state Medicaid agency saving nursing home costs by paying for in-home services. Assume that adequate in-home support costs one-third of the nursing home costs and that if available would allow a patient to return to the community from a nursing home. It seems a no-brainer to pay for the services. That is a 3 to 1 return on investment and most people would rather stay in the community. Win win. But if allowing payment for these services means that three people already in the community are now eligible for the service and use it, even if the one nursing home discharge was accomplished, it would still be a loss financially because now four people are receiving the service. The second point is that it is generally the case that benefit design is not targeted, or practical to be targeted in a way that optimizes behaviors or settings of care. It may be desirable to promote prevention and primary care and to seek to reduce discretionary specialty care or avoidable emergency department use by loading significant patient costs on these services. But the fact remains that the highest cost people, those who most need and use insurance, even when care and behavior is optimal, will still need specialty care and need the emergency room and hospital. They may need drugs for which there is no generic or lower cost alternative. A benefit design that seems to promote more efficient behaviors can actually become just a mechanism to shift the costs of care to the chronically ill.

Providers also need to understand, or accept, that not everything should be or can be paid for by insurance, no matter how useful the service may be. The most prominent example in geriatrics is long-term nursing home care. It could be an entitlement (i.e., available to all regardless of wealth status) like Medicare, but it is not. Society (as represented by government) has determined that preserving intergenerational transfer of wealth, even if modest, and reducing caregiver duties are of lesser import than reducing the cost to taxpayers. Any clinician who practiced prior to the creation of Part D recalls when Medicare beneficiaries assumed the full cost of their drugs and more senior clinicians recall a time when no preventive services, including influenza vaccinations and screening mammography, were covered. (As an aside, some benefit design can seem so illogical that it promotes cheating. Prior to screening mammography being covered, almost all women somehow had something of concern on breast exam and required diagnostic mammography, a covered service.)

Benefits should be tailored to the population served. This is not just for sales and marketing purposes to niche groups, but for meeting needs and promoting better care and health behaviors. For example, a nominal drug co-pay designed to lower monthly insurance premiums probably is irrelevant for most people with employer-based coverage. But that may not be the case for a Medicaid recipient. The same co-pay on a highly cost-effective prescription drug may be a true cost barrier to care. Many of the costs for younger women and children are preventive and maternity-related services. The main costs in employer-based coverage may be driven by specialty drugs for single chronic conditions and a nonrecurring cost such as cancer treatment for a year. The main costs in Medicare are for those with multiple chronic conditions. Those dually eligible for Medicare and Medicaid under 65 living in the community often have high mental health-care costs and needs.

A good benefit design will promote cost-effective care, be transparent about cost sharing, and allow for some level of alternative benefit delivery, such as paying for social supports only for a subset of patients for whom net savings are very probable and be tailored to the needs of the population for whom it is provided. A good benefit design will promote and support the provider type that can deliver the highest value care. A good benefit design may need to have the capacity to merge payment programs, such as what occurs in the Programs of All-Inclusive Care for the Elderly (PACE).

Attribution In order to care for or pay for the health-care cost of a population, there needs to be a mechanism to define the population. If an insurance company, it may be easy. It is everyone who has paid premiums. But if the population is a subset of all insureds, such as those assigned to a specific individual or group, it may be more complex. The process of matching patient to provider is called "attribution." One method of attributing a patient to a provider is for a patient to pick or be assigned to a specific provider or group. The patient's insurance card has a PCP (primary care provider) name right on it. Another method is to assign based on service utilization. The latter can be prospective, i.e., attribution is for the year ahead, based upon last year's usage patterns, or retrospective, i.e., attribution for the year is based on services obtained during the year and is only known after the year is over. Many programs in Medicare use a primary care physician-based methodology for attribution to the PCP or to a larger entity in which the PCP is a member. Traditional Medicare almost always allows the Medicare beneficiary to go to whomever the beneficiary chooses. Attribution methodologies need to match the intended usage. For example, if a program is about improving primary care, the attribution would logically be to a primary care clinician. If the program is about saving costs and improving quality over a 90-day episode of care for joint replacement, attribution would be more logically to a hospital or orthopedist. Attribution can seem simple until one recognizes the number of physicians/clinicians a patient may see in a year.

An example may illustrate. A patient has a regular primary care physician who does only outpatient care and who has a nurse practitioner on the care team. The goal is to assign the patient to this physician (PCP), using claims (billing/payment records). In February the patient goes to the PCP with a set of papers about how in January she got screened for dangerous hidden conditions at a van that came to her church with a nurse practitioner. A review of the papers indicates an EKG, heel ultrasound, limited carotid ultrasound, and blood tests were done. A sheet labeled "annual wellness visit" guides the patient to get her flu shot and mammogram every year and colorectal cancer screening (if by colonoscopy) every 10 years until age 75. The PCP sees her for her COPD, hypertension, osteoarthritis, obesity, and chronic low back pain. Despite vaccination efforts, in September the patient is admitted with pneumonia and an exacerbation of COPD. The patient has a long stay and steroids induce hyperglycemia requiring a new therapy of insulin. A team of general internal medicine hospitalists and various specialists care for her. With limited supports at home, the patient goes to a skilled nursing facility (SNF) for 3 weeks and is seen regularly (five times) by a physician/NP team there. The SNF physician also has an outpatient primary care practice. Once back to baseline function and off insulin, she is discharged. At discharge, the PCP performs transitional care services, but just billed an office visit because the office was not notified of the discharge, despite checking in with the facility during the stay, until 3 days after it occurred, so the transitional care CPT code could not be reported. The PCP office sees the patient two more times that year, both by the NP. Now consider the possible attribution methodologies. The PCP attribution could be based upon services that are hallmarks of good primary care, the annual wellness visit, and the transitional care management visit. But then a van NP is the PCP, as the transitional care was billed as a regular established patient visit. It could go by the greatest number of evaluation and management (E/M) visits by a provider tax ID/NPI combination for a provider/group with a primary care specialty, but then the hospitalist group is the PCP. Maybe a better way is to define primary care providers as people in a primary care specialty who have 40% of their total Medicare payments based on primary care services, like office visits and exclude hospital visits as counting. The primary care provider with the most E/M becomes the assigned PCP. Getting closer, but it still is the nursing home doctor who is the PCP, who, by the way, does not want her attributed to him as she was expensive that year. In order to not keep long-term care-focused providers from being PCPs, the new and improved method of using E/M by a primary care specialty provider *does* count nursing facility CPT codes (so long-term care patients may be attributed), but *not* if the site of care (site of service code) is the *skilled* nursing facility as compared to the nursing facility. Finally, now the actual PCP is the attributed PCP unless it is the NP in the PCP office. And what specialty are nurse practitioners and can they be PCPs, you might now ask? To sum up, an effective system will correctly attribute patients the large majority of times. It will never be perfect. Attribution is relevant as it determines patient assignments for payment, quality measurement, risk assumption—all the types of newer "value-based" payments.

Key Terms

Accountable care organization (ACO): An entity that is accountable for cost and quality of care for a population. "Accountable". generally means that there is financial risk at some level bourn by the ACO.

Allowance: The allowed fee or payment amount set by the payer for a participating or contracted provider. Amounts charged in excess of the allowance for a covered service cannot be charged to the patient.

Alternative payment model: A method of payment that entails upside and usually downside risk for the provider or provider organization. It could be for a population for comprehensive care or a set of services (such as joint replacement, breast cancer treatment, or management of diabetes over a year). The term has the potential to be used to describe such a wide variety of arrangements that there may not be a consistent definition at this point in time, except that it is an alternative to straight fee for service.

Beneficiary or member: The insured. ".Providers refer to them as patients.

Capitation: A payment per head ".or per member. It requires additional specificity to determine what service or services are being capitated or being paid on a per head basis.

Codes: When billing for care, it is necessary to use a procedure code and a diagnosis code. This is a terminology schema. CPT is Current Procedural Terminology and is the core of procedure (including office visits) coding. ".Medicare and other payers also use Healthcare Common Procedure Coding System (HCPCS) Level II codes like the G codes. Diagnosis codes are ICD-10-CM, the International Classification of Diseases series.

Cost sharing: Cost sharing is when the insured pays a sum when consuming services. It is in addition to the insurance premium. It may be a deductible (an amount that must be paid prior to the insurance paying anything), a coinsurance (a flat percent of the allowed amount), or a co-pay (a fixed sum paid for a service). The Affordable Care Act disallowed cost sharing for many preventive services. In Medicare there is significant cost sharing in Parts A and B. However, it is typically unseen as almost all patients have supplemental insurance (Medigap) or Medicaid.

Covered services: This a service that is a benefit of the plan. Participating providers must accept allowances for a covered service as payment in full (after collecting any member cost share). Plan rules do not dictate payment for non-covered services which would most likely be an out-of-pocket expense for the patient. There are often rules about notifying patients that a service is non-covered prior to provision and charge.

Hierarchical Condition Categories: This is the Medicare risk adjustor for payments to ACOs and Medicare Advantage Plans. It is based upon age, gender, institutional status, and billed diagnosis codes. It has major economic impacts, potentially many thousands of dollars per patient, which can be much more significant than the effects of medical management.

IPA: Independent practice association. This is a mechanism to form an entity that is of greater mass, while retaining independent practices. The IPA agreement governs the degree of independence and mutual obligations between practices and between practices and the administrative structure formed. There are costs associated with operating the IPA and any centralized services. An IPA may form to create greater contracting influence or to pool risk or to simply share costs and services by creating economies of scale.

Medicare Advantage/Medicare Part C: Medicare contracts with insurance companies to provide benefits to Medicare beneficiaries. The plans are called Medicare Advantage Plans. They must provide actuarially equivalent benefits and usually provide enhanced services such as annual physicals. They do not have to pay contracted or participating providers in the same manner that Medicare does. They can have limited networks, typically have a higher level of utilization review and prior authorizations, and take other actions to control costs. They are subject to risk-adjusted payments from the government based on HCC scores. They are also subject to substantial quality payment adjustments in the "Five-Star Quality Rating Program." Accordingly, they are very interested in providers meeting the quality metrics and advancing optimized risk adjustment.

Medicare Parts A, B, and D: Medicare has parts that are for different services and have different beneficiary enrollment and benefit rules. Part A includes inpatient hospital services and skilled nursing facility services, Part B is outpatient hospital and professional services, and Part D is for drugs. Parts A and B are sometimes called "Traditional Medicare."

Network: The set of contracted/participating providers. Some payers control costs by limiting networks, e.g., by capitating a subset of the community of providers and requiring all patients to use that subset or by having lower cost sharing for preferred providers. Providers could be preferred because they share financial risk with the payer or because they are judged to be better by some measure, usually an efficiency measure.

Participating provider: A provider that agrees to a contract. In Medicare the "contract" is essentially the rules of Medicare and the fee schedule or allowances. Professionals may "participate" and receive direct payment from Medicare. They may be "nonparticipating" and charge and collect from beneficiaries, but the final charges to the beneficiary are still limited by law. The beneficiary pays the provider and then receives reimbursement from Medicare. A third provider option is to "opt out" and privately contract with the patients. In this case the provider is ineligible for any Medicare payment for any service to any beneficiary. It is not a patient-by-patient option; the provider leaves Medicare completely. Patients are not allowed to collect from Medicare, though services ordered are covered when performed by providers that have not opted out, meaning tests, consults, drug prescriptions, etc., are unaffected.

PMPM: Per member per month. A payment or cost allocation method that allows correction for population size and time.

Value-based payment: The concept of paying providers differentially based on performance.

Payment Basics

There are a variety of ways to pay for primary care [15, 16]. Anyone of them, in isolation or in combination, can be effective. or ineffective depending on how they are executed and depending on the vantage point of the evaluation. The goals, behavior, and ethics of the payer, recipients of care, and providers can be factors. Each method has its pros and cons and risks. In many cases the methods are somewhat interrelated. For example, a PCP may have a salaried position, but the salary is fundamentally based on productivity using a fee-for-service payment methodology. At this point in history, payment methods are being used to change behavior and transform delivery systems. In theory, they are also designed to recognize high performance, but the transformation goals appear more significant than paying more for "the best." A first point to consider in evaluation is whether a payment model is relevant, available, or practical to the primary care practice. This could be because a provider elects to not accept any insurance, sets their own fees, and individually contracts with the patient. It could be because the payer has one method of payment that is not negotiable. It could be that the payer would like to have the providers manage populations and accept insurance risk, but the provider in question lacks sufficient numbers of patients or sophistication to be given the risk. It is useful to address some specific models and assess whether they promote effective primary care.

Productivity and RVUs Because so much of payment is based on some measure of productivity, it helps to understand how that may be measured. One method could just be number of visits. Another could be number of patients assigned to a provider without regard to how often the patient has a visit. Another could be hours worked. Another could be billed (not necessarily paid) services. Usually, productivity in primary care is based on visits that are adjusted for level of complexity or work. If the prices the practice charges are also based on that method, billings and work are equivalent. Every visit is assigned a "billing" code, a CPT (Current Procedural Terminology) code. Practitioners are familiar with these codes, such as 99214, an evaluation and management service in the office or other outpatient setting for an established patient that is of moderate complexity requiring a detailed history or exam. The specialty societies and the American Medical Association convene an expert body to help place services in a spectrum of *relative* work, and they make recommendations to Medicare. The recommendations are in units of work. The precise definition of a unit does not matter as all services are arrayed relative to one another, so an arbitrary service of 1.0 can be set and all services are a factor more (e.g., 1.74) or less (e.g., 0.68). Accordingly, these are called work relative value units or RVUs. Medicare sometimes sets the RVUs without advice and ultimately has authority to reject or accept any advice it receives. The methodology is inevitably imperfect, even if useful, and the code structure and fees/RVUs assigned are a source of debate. Though the word "value" is in the RVU term, it is important to understand that the term does not reflect utility, social value, or scientific value; it just reflects relative work. It is also very hard to effectively compare very different services such as an office visit, reading an MRI, and performing a total hip arthroplasty. But it is less difficult to compare different levels of office visits for established patients.

Salary A salary can be an effective. financial model. However, as noted, the money for the salary must come from somewhere. Therefore, there are usually productivity requirements, with or without other incentives. A salary can be particularly effective in promoting high-quality care when it pools revenue streams so as to create an ability to provide care for time-consuming complex patients or for a population subset that is lower in income. For example, a 20-person primary group has five locations. One location is in a part of the community with high poverty rates. The other locations serve a well-insured population. The per-visit and per-patient revenue is lower in the lower socioeconomic status practice, even though the work RVUs could be more. The socially conscious group sets the salary without regard to location and actual revenue. Another good example may be patient population/panel size in a staff model HMO that has working aged and senior populations. A general internist will have some complicated patients, old or young. A geriatrician will have more complex patients, on average, and the practice of the HMO may even be to transfer complex patients from the general internists to a specialized geriatric team. Accordingly, the geriatrician's panel size may be significantly smaller, if it is agreed that the internists and geriatricians all work at the same level of intensity, effort, and productivity. Therefore, the salaries may be the same. Salaries may not create a churn mentality of seeing more and more patients or performing marginally needed services. Conversely, there may be no productivity incentive. Of course, salaries can be coupled with incentives for retention, quality, productivity, and participation in activities that benefit the organization and its patients (sometimes labeled "citizenship").

Fee for Service (FFS) This is the "eat what you kill" financial model, though the terminology seems a little misplaced in health care. Like any business, revenue and expenses are key to having profit or take-home pay. They require careful monitoring and consideration. This model can be very successful financially and drive toward patient satisfaction as it is important to have satisfied customers to maintain business volume. There are many factors that determine the likelihood or ease of success. These include payer mix. A practice that is all Medicaid will be in dire condition. These include types of services. A practice that does everything, inpatient, nursing home, office, and occasional home care, may struggle with efficiency. In a given provider's hands, some otherwise RVU equivalent services may be easier or more difficult, efficient or less efficient, and profitable or less so. There also needs to be a definition of success. Is an income of $100, $200, $300, or $400 thousand in a year a success? Is success defined as independence and self-determination—being your own boss? Is success defined as financial security or time with friends or family? Are there key attributes of care that if unable to be provided will cause career dissatisfaction?

To make this more concrete, let's run some scenarios. In some cases, the scenario is somewhat artificial, but the overall example is valid.

Sample office practice: Goal income is $200,000 after expenses including health insurance, before reserves/savings, taxes, and retirement funding. 100% collection. Fee is 100% of the Medicare Physician Fee Schedule. 50% of visits coded 99213 ($74), 50% coded 99214 ($109). No other services are reported. Office overhead is 55% of gross revenue at a gross revenue of approximately $450,000. Because a large share is fixed costs like rent, utilities, staff (independent of volume), and professional liability and health insurance, a low patient volume will have a limited effect on reducing expenses.

Gross income will need to be $200,000/0.45 or $444,444.

The average visit is $91.5, so this will take 444,444/91.5 or 4860 visits annually.

The physician takes 4 weeks off a year for vacation, sick, and CME and works nine 4-hour sessions a week. This is 432 sessions annually. The number of patients seen each session must be (4860/432) or 11.25. The physician will book accordingly, considering cancelation rates.

That is a lot of hard work, but it may be possible. Alter any assumption and it can have a significant effect. Let's look at a few:

Case 1: Fee Allowance of the Payer

The payer pays better than Medicare and the average visit is $100. That is not the 10% bonus Medicare once paid, but almost. This means $8.50 × 4860 or $41,310 annually just came to the physician. Expenses did not increase at all. Of course, if the fee was $8.50 less than Medicare, the lost income would be the same amount.

Case 2: Volume Effects

The physician wants to work less hard. The choices are eight sessions a week or nine patients a session.

Nine patients a session is a loss of 2.25 × $91.5 × 432 or nearly $89,000 in lost revenue. Maybe expenses decreased minimally (fewer disposable gowns and less exam table paper). Going to eight sessions is 48 fewer sessions annually, and this is a loss of 48 × $91.5 × 11.25 or $49,400 in revenue, and again expenses really do not fall. This illustrates how volume-dependent fee for service is. At some point, reductions in patients seen may mean fewer staff and increases may require more staff, but this mostly occurs at extremes or when there are multiple providers in a practice all making the same changes.

Instead the physician decides to make life easier by hiring another medical assistant (MA) and delegating some tasks appropriately. The physician works nine sessions and sees 11.25 patients per session, the MA costs $35,000 including all benefits, and the physician is much happier. It feels like seeing nine patients a session.

Case 3: Complete and Accurate Coding

The physician (physician A) compares billing patterns with another colleague (physician B) and notes that the colleague does not split the services 50/50 between 99213 and 99214; most are the higher level service. Both see their patients once a year for an annual visit to make sure all the bases are covered. Physician A usually codes the annual with 99214 because the patients usually have a few problems, but are not high complexity. Physician B usually does the same for the same reason, but also reports a variety of preventive medicine codes, since the services are being performed.

Service	Dr. A	Dr. B
99214 established patient office visit	$109	$109
G0439 annual wellness visit		$118
G0442 annual alcohol misuse screening		$18
G0444 annual depression screening		$18
G0446 annual face-to-face behavioral therapy for cardiovascular disease		$26
99497 advance care planning		$83
99406 counseling to prevent tobacco use (3–10 min)		$15
Total	$109	$387

Physician B is very conscientious and knows all the requirements of each service. If a service is not medically necessary, it is not performed. For example, if the patient is not a smoker, 99406 is not reported, or if the physician asks if the patient is willing to discuss quitting and gets a quick negative response and stops there, the tobacco cessation counseling service is not reported. Physician A completes his annual in 30 min. Physician B takes 45 min and has a team-based system that involves a questionnaire and standardized instruments asking about depression, instrumental and other activities of daily living function, hearing, substance use, falls, physical activity, nutrition, use of preventive services, and advance care plans. His staff have been trained to do follow-up services such as a PHQ-9 if the PHQ-2 is positive and provide resources on a variety of items, like explaining the state-approved advance directive forms. They also complete a checklist for the doctor and patient on services already documented or needed such as colorectal cancer screening and immunizations. The physician reviews each item and provides assessments, advice, and arranges for needed assistance with the help of his staff. Aspirin and cardiac risk factor reduction is discussed. Of course, the usual medical treatment issues are addressed as well. The patient's values and understanding of prognosis with potential medical events are reviewed, and the doctor checks to determine if the patient has had such discussions with a surrogate decision-maker. One other thing physician B does is to use a medical record with alerts that help to correctly code the complexity of care by ICD-10 and also by prompts that a high-risk diagnosis was not included in the assessment and provisional claim even though it is on the problem list. Physician B said that the practice used to code like Physician A, but they had a compliance program that determined they were under-coding many of the 99213 visits and not even billing the preventive screening and counseling services they performed. The practice felt strongly about advanced care planning and created a system to make sure it was addressed annually. They got organized and not only is the care better, it is more efficient and the practice income is much improved.

Case 4: The Care Manager

The practice always thought it would be great to have a nurse that could do triage and education and follow some of the patients by phone to monitor them and provide self-management support. One of the private payers would pay an office for a nurse that did diabetes education, and then Medicare began to pay for transitional care management and chronic care management. The practice read an economic model article [17] that suggested after staff and opportunity costs, each Medicare member enrolled in chronic care management would actually net the practice over $300, so long as 131 Medicare patients per nurse were enrolled. The practice assessed the number of patients with chronic conditions that would potentially benefit. Some of the doctors thought the patient cost sharing would be an issue or that it was wrong to charge for something that was done all along. Others in the practice pointed out that it was not being done, because it was not paid for and none of the doctors had unlimited time to do this, not to mention that nurses might do a better job in many cases. The patients did not pay the cost share out of pocket as that amount was usually picked up by "Medigap" insurance or Medicaid. If they did have to pay a small amount, why was that wrong? The practice has to be financially viable, and the practice has no issue charging for all the other services it provides, they argued. So they set up a specific program to identify the patients, comprehensively assess them (if not already done), create care plans, and get consents. Then, if the patient needed such services, everything was ready to go. When Medicare began paying for complex chronic care management and paid additional sums to do the assessment, if extra work was required, it was an even better decision, in retrospect.

What these cases show is that optimizing revenue or RVU generation requires a systematic approach of assessing costs and revenue. The examples focused on office-based practice, but the principles apply to a home visit or nursing facility practice. Success requires knowledge of coverage, coding, and billing rules. It requires putting a system and workflows in place that makes the activity work. It may require an electronic record or other forms to be created. These forms or templates may be available from Medicare or a specialty society as resources for a practice. The last few years have seen significant enhancements in describing and paying for services for those with chronic illness, including behavioral health problems. Payment has facilitated and is intended to drive providers toward creating teams and integrating behavioral health into primary care. However, many feel that these adjustments are the wrong model of paying for primary care because they are still within a volume-driven payment system that inadequately addresses payment disparity based upon complexity being undervalued. In a treadmill day at the office, a complex patient is a disruption, whereas a minor acute illness is a pleasant break. Effective primary care should focus on the complex patients and make room in the daily schedule for them, while handling minor illness through a portal or phone call. Fee for service also motivates providers to generate income through such practices as the "annual EKG" and having an in-office lab for revenue rather than clinical care reasons.

Capitation for Primary Care Services Capitation for primary care services can be an effective model. Capitation is a payment per person (or head) for a defined period of time. A payer would want to be sure that a practice was not just creating access barriers or turfing every issue to the emergency department or a specialist, so it might be coupled with monitoring through quality measurement or service usage, i.e., encounter data may still need to be provided for tracking and to address cost-sharing issues. This type of capitation does not put the provider at risk for anything but their own time and overhead. While that is not inconsequential, it is to be distinguished from the total cost-of-care risk that an accountable care organization (ACO) may take on. It is critical to define what is primary care, however. Is it just office visits? Are vaccines included, which are a costly supply? Are any office labs, tests, and procedures bundled into the capitation? The capitation payment needs to have some level of risk adjustment, even if just age. A payment for a specific patient could be based upon historical costs for that patient. Payment by head requires attribution and assignment rules and these may affect adequacy of payment. In Medicare, fewer patients have no services than a population of young adult males, but the issue is still relevant. The payment for a population using an attribution method that is not based on service history, but is based upon selecting a PCP on enrollment, includes payment for persons who do not use services, whereas payment based upon patients attributed by service use history with a PCP does not include nonusers. If there is substantial cost sharing for primary care, the capitation can be complex. A fixed co-pay can be factored in with limited difficulty, but a deductible creates difficulty as it would vary based upon the timing of a primary care service in relation to other services. Capitation inherently allows payment for non-face-to-face care alternatives to the face-to-face visit. It may promote team-based services, such as care review and education by a team member such as a pharmacist, who otherwise could not be a billing provider. For this reason, the Comprehensive Primary Care Plus Medicare Innovation Center program has a track where payments are split capitation and fee for service [18, 19]. Primary care capitation is a form of population management, but for a specific set of services. It may promote a structure and skill set that promotes successful total cost of care population management. Capitation creates an incentive to manage more patients and grow panel size. As fewer physicians enter primary care, this may be an important societal goal. This may help drive the development of team-based care where every team member operates at the top of their license or skill set and efficiencies are created. A patient visit volume practice will need to adjust to this payment method, and it may be difficult to operate under capitation with one payer and visit volume system with another.

Capitation could also be for a subset of services or "infrastructure." Several PCMH programs have a PMPM for care management. This is a form of capitation that helps fund the PCMH and team-based care. Because this payment is often used to advance primary care, it is reasonably viewed as an effective financial model.

Fee for Service Linked to Quality and Value Medicare is now using this payment methodology with the onset of MACRA (Medicare Access and CHIP Reauthorization Act of 2015). This type of payment is FFS, but the fees are adjusted based upon performance. It could be a multiplier being applied to fees (less than or greater than 1.0). It typically would only be applied to certain fees, for example, payment for an administered chemotherapy drug that costs $1000 a dose would neither be cut nor enhanced. Different payers may use different criteria, but usually quality and cost are factors. The payment could be presented as a bonus, but if fees are held down so as to fund the bonus, then it really is just an opportunity to regain ground and possibly surpass what would have been otherwise paid. If it truly is new money to primary care, then it can help promote the discipline. It remains to be seen whether this is a good model for effective primary care. On the one hand, it promotes quality measurement and improvement, processes that were rare in most practices until the advent of meaningful use and PCMH programs. It rewards those who invest and succeed in improving primary care. On the other hand, the record of performance programs improving outcomes and health is uncertain [20]. Driving focus on specific measures may not drive overall health improvements and measures of member experience, while important may not correlate with professional assessment of technical quality [21]. It is also the case that performance on outcomes type measures is affected by patient socio-demographics [22] and that conclusions based on small numbers are suspect. For example, efficiency on total cost of care, even with risk adjustment, or efficiency based upon inpatient admission rates would be unreliable at the individual provider or small group level. Some primary care providers care for atypical populations and are more significantly affected either by lack of appropriate measures or by factors that skew results. There is also a significant cost for the practice and payer to collect, report, and assess data and then modify fees or process bonuses. This approach seems to address a desire to pay for performance, but it may also be so inherently random or unfair that what it does most of all is to stimulate practices to move on to alternative payment models.

Alternative Payment Models Built on Fee for Service These types of payments rely upon a fee-for-service event to trigger the payment model or population definition. It is more than an adjustment to the fees based on quality or efficiency. It usually requires downside risk, i.e., the potential for the provider to lose money and therefore be stimulated to manage the patient efficiently. This does not necessarily mean the provider is at risk for the total cost of care. An example of a more limited risk APM would be that the provider receives infrastructure support, such as a capitation payment for a nurse care manager. The provider also gets an advance on a quality and efficiency bonus. If the quality is inadequate or the costs do not suggest effective management, the funds for the nurse and prepaid bonus must be returned. Practices can do well in such an arrangement. In fact, primary care geriatrics may clamor for such arrangements as the Independence at Home and CPC+ demonstration. The model can drive and support effective primary care. The problem with any such risk or quality-based payment system is that it could also serve to drive a threatened provider segment into extinction. If the quality metrics and thresholds are not set properly, failure can be all but assured. Likewise for the financial targets. For this reason, it is important that any model have testing and protections for unexpected events. A basic example may serve to illustrate. Our goal is to design a payment system that promotes efficient high-quality care.

Approach A: A risk-adjusted budget for the population of concern is set, based upon national spending patterns for Medicare beneficiaries. There are corrections applied to account for payment amount differentials regionally, but not for regional utilization differences. In other words, if a DRG is paid more in New York City than in a rural Idaho hospital, that payment differential is accounted for, but no adjustment is made for the possibility that more New York City beneficiaries receive that DRG per thousand persons than is the case for the Idahoans. This system rewards efficient regions. It may even promote the redistribution of health-care providers to serve less urban areas which often use less services because profits are higher in Idaho than New York. There is still an impetus for the Idaho providers to be more efficient, though ironically if more providers were to move into the region, costs would predictably rise because provider supply has an enormous effect on service usage variation. This method is pay for performance with a lesser potential to be paid for improvement. A higher cost region would be at very significant risk for losses if it does not dramatically improve. If the threshold to break even after investment costs is too high, this essentially guarantees losses and is a funds redistribution program more than a program to drive performance. Urban safety net hospitals could be wiped out.

Approach B: This is the same as approach A, except the benchmark or goal is based upon historical costs for the region. In this case a very efficient region that has a year with higher costs is penalized, whereas the region that improves from ridiculously overly costly to just overly costly is rewarded. This method does reward improvement. It does account for factors in regional spending variation that may be beyond the control of any provider entity and take a generation to change.

As in all financial models, there are pros and cons and incentives and disincentives, so execution matters greatly. But, if the model is well designed, an APM can be very positive for primary care. It can stimulate better primary care and promote recognition (and thus proper payment) for primary care. If the existence of a home visit service and digital medicine will prevent usage of an emergency room and exacerbation of chronic disease due to inattention, then they will be built or sustained. These services are not being promoted in a FFS system. The geriatric hip fracture comanagement system with a coordinated post-acute care service will prevent readmissions and drive down the complications that are costly for the hospital. It is no longer a pilot research project, but becomes an essential care element. The palliative medicine team that helps assure patient-centered care and in doing so reduces readmissions is now more than a nice-to-have service. But, if the model is poorly designed, the pioneers in transformation will be burned and future innovation stifled.

An interesting feature of any payment system that puts providers at risk is that the providers tend to adopt many techniques that payers have long used and providers had railed against. However, it may not just be a different perspective that justifies this change of heart; the application may be considerably more deft.

Any payment system that has financial gainsharing must have quality metrics and other oversight programs. No payment system is without fraud or abuse. While most providers are of high integrity, not all issues are about gross misconduct. Hospitals need their beds filled to break even financially as they have huge fixed costs. That does not mean that the community-spirited members of a not-for-profit hospital board want their neighbors to be sick, but they do want margin for mission. So too will every system have some degree of perverse incentives. Accordingly, it is essential to have measures of quality of care, access, and patient experience. Public trust, common sense, and lessons learned demand this.

Alternative Payment Models of Population Management This is the attainment of providers being accountable to manage a population. There is no tie to a fee-for-service event. There is no disease-specific payment and silo by condition. Provider organizations must work together across specialties, professions, and institutions to achieve the triple aim. The promotion of or risk to effective primary care is essentially the same as in the APM based on FFS. Where the money goes matters even more in this model. A primary care capitation will go to primary care. A population payment could go to a provider organization that marginalizes primary care. While such an attitude may ultimately be an impediment to the long-term success of that organization, the short-term effects may be a complete loss of control by primary care. Protections could be applied, such as a minimum amount of payments being for primary care services or a requirement that organizational leadership must include a set percentage of primary care providers. It would be logical for Medicare programs to require organizational leadership by professionals with geriatric care competencies. Again, if well executed, this model can promote effective primary care and reward primary care providers.

Concierge Medicine While there is great discussion, policy, law, and regulation on increasingly complex financial models, some clinicians have turned back the clock to a time before insurance for primary care. These providers contract with their patients through a variety of mechanisms. They may be able to reduce overhead associated with billing or quality measurement that seems to miss the mark. Medicare allows some forms of concierge practice without opting out. This is typically by not having a retainer per se, but by having an annual fee for non-covered services. While a concierge provider may be more practical for an upper income patient, the model can allow for charitable care and should not be dismissed as socially unconscious. A concern about this model, beyond the major concern of equity, relates to keeping the customer satisfied. If the patients who elect a concierge practice have a sense of entitlement or the provider anticipates this situation, there is a risk that medically unnecessary services will proliferate. Every test will be done, and entry to the practices of the best specialist for whatever ails you will be facilitated, needed or not. This is a potential outcome that serves neither the patient nor society. On the other hand, this payment method can promote personalized service and time with the patient and caregiver for discussions that really matter. It was a mechanism to pay for chronic care management before such a benefit and payment were created in Medicare. It remains a mechanism to pay for case management, the additional nonmedical supports many patients or families need.

Practice/Provider Organization Size and Structure

There is no inherently ideal practice size or structure that promotes high-quality, efficient, and effective primary care [23]. A micropractice may have intense focus on access and patient empowerment and be highly conscious of cost [24]. They may deploy resources external to the practice, such as a community health team, and outperform groups and organizations. They may measure what really matters [25] and risk stratify their patients for effective management better than others. However, most providers benefit from a greater support structure and need scale to develop that structure. The present value-based payment system is also potentially averse to smaller practices. Medicare estimated that smaller practices would receive more penalties under MACRA [26]. This may relate to infrastructure needed to succeed in the measurement paradigm, e.g., smaller practices are more likely to also not use electronic records or to be able to measure quality, and not be due to actual performance on quality of care or efficiency. Where organizational size is legitimately critical is risk assumption and investment capacity. No single provider can assume total cost of care risk. It takes sufficient numbers of patients to make the basic principles of insurance work. Payment models that entail risk typically pay the reward (if achieved) more than a year after the investment period begins. Capitalizing an ACO requires millions of dollars of investment [27] in infrastructure and care managers. There must be an ability to withstand a loss of more than investment, but have an actual payback capacity. Therefore, the organization must have strong financial reserves. Organizational size does not require a common employer. It can be achieved with an independent practice association (IPA) or other mechanisms. Success in any payment model and success in delivering effective primary care do depend on shared mission, goals, and consistent processes. Success in newer models of payment requires more than is typically provided within the four walls of the primary care office. It requires planning, effective execution, maintenance, and support systems. It requires analytics and more sophisticated financial management structures. It requires an ability to invest in new services that may not immediately generate revenue. The ideal is to achieve the intense patient focus of the micropractice with the organizational support (clinical and administrative) and financial resilience of a larger organization.

Preparing for the Future

Predicting the future, especially in a chaotic political environment, is risky or hubris, but planning is important. It may make sense to seek to be prepared to meet the needs of our society and to keep fundamentals in mind. Health care is too costly. Quality is too variable. The solution does not lie in tweaking insurance company or Medicare rules, but in delivery system change. Providers know their patients and know the system best. Therefore, providers are the ones who can transform health care and address the needs of the population. They will be limited by a national focus on health care rather than health, but there is great opportunity within their locus of control. With this opportunity will come accountability. This means financial risk acceptance, quality measurement, and regulation. Primary care has been and will continue to be the cornerstone of any successful system of care. Therefore, any successful model will need to support effective primary care.

Summary

A small portion of total health-care expenditures goes to primary care, but primary care is an essential element to safe, timely, effective, equitable, efficient, and patient-centered care. In communities and countries where primary care is a higher proportion of resources and expenditures, care is of higher quality and lower cost. There are many ways to finance primary care and many business models for primary care providers. Some can operate simultaneously and be complementary; others may be in conflict and create confusion, such as simultaneous "value"- and "volume"-based payments. All models will depend upon the local environment (infrastructure, readiness, competing market forces) and the quality of execution. Productive and hard workers will always be needed. Providers and payers need to exist in the current world, while they prepare for and stimulate change to a more effective system of total care and improved primary care. Flexibility, creativity, self-assessment, big picture understanding, and preparation for change are required.

References

1. Chang C, Stukel T, Flood A, David G. Primary care workforce and Medicare beneficiaries' health outcomes. JAMA. 2011;25(20):2096–105, corrected June 7, 2011.
2. Phillips R, Bazemore A. Primary care and why it matters for U.S. health system reform. Health Aff (Millwood). 2009;29(5):806–10.
3. United Health Center for Health Reform and Modernization. Advancing primary care delivery: practical, proven and scalable approaches, September 2015. https://www.uhc.com/content/dam/uhcdotcom/en/ValueBasedCare/PDFs/UNH-Primary-Care-Report-Advancing-Primary-Care-Delivery.pdf. Accessed 19 Oct 2016.
4. Donaldson MS, Yordy KD, Lohr KN, Vanselow NA, editors. Primary care: America's health in a new era. Committee on the Future of Primary Care, Institute of Medicine; 1996.
5. Institute of Medicine (IOM). Crossing the quality chasm: a new health system for the 21st century. Washington: National Academy Press; 2001.
6. American Academy of Family Physicians (AAFP), American Academy of Pediatrics (AAP), American College of Physicians (ACP), American Osteopathic Association (AOA) Joint Principles of the Patient-Centered Medical Home, March 2007. https://www.acponline.org/system/files/documents/running_practice/delivery_and_payment_models/pcmh/demonstrations/jointprinc_05_17.pdf. Accessed 30 Oct 2016.
7. What do we know about social determinants of health in the U.S. and comparable countries? Peterson-Kaiser health system tracker measuring the performance of the U.S. health system. http://www.healthsystemtracker.org/chart-collection/what-do-we-know-about-social-determinants-of-health-in-the-u-s-and-comparable-countries/. Accessed 30 Oct 2016.
8. Baicker K, Chandra A. Medicare spending, the physician workforce, and beneficiaries' quality of care. Health Aff (Millwood). 2004;23:w184–97.
9. Chernew M, Sabik L, Chandra A, Newhouse J. Would having more primary care doctors cut health spending growth? Health Aff (Millwood). 2009;28(5):1327–35.
10. The facts on Medicare spending and financing Kaiser family foundation, July 2015. http://kff.org/medicare/fact-sheet/medicare-spending-and-financing-fact-sheet/. Accessed 30 Oct 2016.
11. National Health Expenditure Data Table 2. https://www.cms.gov/research-statistics-data-and-systems/statistics-trends-and-reports/nationalhealthexpenddata/nhe-fact-sheet.html. Accessed 30 Oct 2016.
12. Stanton MW, Rutherford MK. The high concentration of U.S. health care expenditures. Rockville: Agency for Healthcare Research and Quality; 2005. Research in Action Issue 19. AHRQ Pub. No. 06-0060. https://archive.ahrq.gov/research/findings/factsheets/costs/expri-ach/expendria.pdf. Accessed 5 Feb 2017.
13. Concentration of health care spending in the U.S. population, 2010. Kaiser Family Foundation Charts and Slides. http://kff.org/health-costs/slide/concentration-of-health-care-spending-in-the-u-s-population-2010/. Accessed 5 Feb 2017.
14. Rosen AB, et al. Cost-effectiveness of full Medicare coverage of angiotensin-converting enzyme inhibitors for beneficiaries with diabetes. Ann Intern Med. 2005;143:89–99.
15. Primary care payment models: draft white paper. The Primary Care Payment Model (PCPM) Work Group, Health Care Payment Learning & Action Network. October 2016. http://hcp-lan.org/workproducts/pcpm-whitepaper-draft.pdf. Accessed 30 Oct 2016.
16. Quinn K. The eight basic payment methods in health care. Ann Intern Med. 2015;163(4):300–6.
17. Basu S, Phillips R, Bitton A, Song Z, Landon B. Medicare chronic care management payments and financial returns to primary care practices: a modeling study. Ann Intern Med. 2015;163:580–8.
18. Comprehensive Primary Care Plus (CMS Webpage for program). https://innovation.cms.gov/initiatives/comprehensive-primary-care-plus. Accessed 30 Oct 2016.
19. CPC+ payment methodologies: beneficiary attribution, care management fee, performance-based incentive payment, and payment under the Medicare physician fee schedule, January 1, 2017. https://innovation.cms.gov/Files/x/cpcplus-methodology.pdf. Accessed 5 Feb 2017.

20. Mendelson A, Kondo K, Damberg C, Low A, Motúapuaka M, Freeman M, O'Neil M, Relevo R, Kansagara D. The effects of pay-for-performance programs on health, health care use, and processes of care: a systematic review. Ann Intern Med. doi:10.7326/M16-1881 (This article was published at www.annals.org on 10 January 2017).
21. Chang J, Hays R, Shekelle P, MacLean C, Solomon D, Reuben D, et al. Patients' global ratings of their health care are not associated with the technical quality of their care. Ann Intern Med. 2006;144:665–72.
22. Committee on Accounting for Socioeconomic Status in Medicare Payment Programs; Board on Population Health and Public Health Practice; Board on Health Care Services; Institute of Medicine; National Academies of Sciences, Engineering, and Medicine. Accounting for social risk factors in Medicare payment: identifying social risk factors. Washington: National Academies Press (US); 2016 Jan 12.1, Introduction. Available from: https://www.ncbi.nlm.nih.gov/books/NBK338757/.
23. Mehrotra A, Epstein A, Rosenthal M. Do integrated medical groups provide higher-quality medical care than individual practice associations? Ann Intern Med. 2006;145:826–33.
24. Wasson JH, Anders GS, Moore LG, Ho L, Nelson EC, Godfrey MM, et al. Clinical microsystems, part 2. Learning from micro practices about providing patients the care they want and need. Jt Comm J Qual Patient Saf. 2008;34:445–52.
25. How's Your Health Tools. https://howsyourhealth.org/hyhinfo1.html. Accessed 5 Feb 2017.
26. Table 64 in Centers for Medicare & Medicaid Services (CMS), HHS. Medicare Program; Merit-Based Incentive Payment System (MIPS) and Alternative Payment Model (APM) Incentive Under the Physician Fee Schedule, and Criteria for Physician-Focused Payment Models: Proposed Rule. Federal Register/Vol. 81, No. 89/Monday, May 9, 2016/Proposed Rules: 28375.
27. National ACO Survey Conducted November 2013 (Final January 21, 2014). National Association of ACOs. http://www.naacos.com/assets/docs/pdf/acosurveyfinal012114.pdf. Accessed 5 Feb 2017.

Incentivizing Primary Care Physicians: Opportunities and Challenges

15

Michael Wasserman and James Riopelle

Many healthcare business "experts" would say that there is one simple way to incentivize physicians. Give them money! We would respectfully disagree. While financial incentives are one way of impacting physician behavior, they are not the only way. Furthermore, in order to pass muster with both our profession and society as a whole, financial incentives must either maintain or improve the quality of care. This concept has led to the focus of moving from "volume to value." One of the problems in moving from "volume to value" in the care of older adults is that value has yet to be adequately defined. For example, in someone nearing the end of life, is not a comfortable death of greatest value? Maintaining a bed-bound, demented nursing home resident in a nonfunctional state is certainly not considered to be something of value. The challenge of defining value in the frail older population has significant implications for all ongoing attempts to move the Medicare program in this "value"-driven direction. And this is only one of the issues that we face when addressing this topic.

There are a number of fundamental problems with financial incentives. The first is the actual need for clinicians to be susceptible to such incentives. Granted, there are some physicians who do very well with volume-based incentives, particularly those that have gravitated to procedurally based specialties. On the other hand, there are those physicians that have landed in more cognitively based specialties, geriatric medicine being a prime example, who do not respond well to financial incentives. This, I would posit, has been one of the reasons for the lack of success demonstrated by geriatricians practicing in today's fee-for-service world!

Senior Care of Colorado, PC, was founded in 2001 by Dr. Don Murphy and myself (Michael Wasserman). We were founded as a primary care geriatric practice

M. Wasserman, MD, CMD (✉)
Rockport Healthcare Services, Los Angeles, CA, USA
e-mail: wassdoc@aol.com

J. Riopelle, MD
Physician Consultant Institute, Denver, CO, USA

© Springer International Publishing AG 2018
M. Wasserman, J. Riopelle (eds.), *Primary Care for Older Adults*,
DOI 10.1007/978-3-319-61329-1_15

functioning completely in a fee-for-service world. We started with six physicians and two physician assistants. When we sold our practice 10 years later, we had 30 physicians, 35 nurse practitioners and physician assistants, and 3 social workers. Over that period of time, we had extensive experience in what it took to incentivize our clinicians. Money was rarely at the top of the list for the majority of them. In fact, a focus on financial gain often turned off many of these dedicated professionals.

When Senior Care was founded, we originally developed contracts that paid our physicians a percentage of the revenue that they brought in. We quickly discovered that our doctors wanted security and didn't function well with this method. This was our first clue that geriatricians were different in relation to traditional volume-based incentives. We changed to a salaried system with incentives based on work value units. Similarly, we provided salaries for our nurse practitioners and physician assistants and developed a similar bonus system based on work value units. While there were a few clinicians who had no trouble focusing on productivity and worked diligently to gain bonuses based on their visit volume, we found that most of our clinicians were turned off by this approach. At the heart of our care model was the "geriatric approach to care." This person-centered approach often meant spending more time with patients and their families in order to provide the necessary care. That approach would certainly be at odds with a volume-driven productivity model, especially since the CPT coding system rewards clinicians for a higher number of shorter visits.

The practice struggled under this work value unit methodology. This led us to develop a metric called patient care units, or PCUs. PCUs were developed with the idea that clinicians would be rewarded for the total amount of care they delivered in a day. Hence, there was concomitant value awarded for spending more time with patients. The key to the success of the PCU system was that clinicians were encouraged to fully document all of the care they delivered over the course of a day and to properly code for that care. Hence, a nurse practitioner might only see eight patients in a day, and if they spent 1 h with each patient, their PCUs would reflect that. We also took the initiative to educate our clinicians on the proper use of "time-based coding," so that their time delivering care could be effectively captured. This was particularly critical as we had calculated that "time-based coding" provided an acceptable degree of revenue production for our practice to at least break even.

On the back end of the PCU system was a crosswalk to the revenue production that each PCU would generate. From a practice perspective, we could adjust PCUs to reflect certain needs for the practice, such as higher PCUs for time-consuming home visits. We also took great pains not to create disincentives to spending more time with patients. This ran counter to traditional CPT codes, which tend to pay less per minute for longer visits. Our number one priority was to assure that our clinicians received credit for all of their patient care time delivered over the course of a day. This system worked very well for the vast majority of our clinicians. We did have a few who worked very hard and endeavored to receive a higher number of PCUs in order to get a bonus. On the other hand, most of our clinicians were happy to find that the practice was quite satisfied if they were documenting that they actually spent 8 h caring for their patients. It is not in the realm of this chapter to quantify how we strategically adjusted PCUs in order for the practice to flourish overall. Nor is this chapter a treatise on the effective use of time-based coding. Both of these topics have been covered elsewhere [1].

In the frail older population, the population that drives the brunt of Medicare expenditures, reducing costs by reducing visits can be counterintuitive. On the other hand, reducing unnecessary care could be beneficial both from a quality and cost perspective. The devil is in the details. In taking a "high-touch, low-tech" geriatric approach to care, increased visit volume might prove to be helpful. At Senior Care of Colorado, we had a very robust house call program. We targeted patients with severe congestive heart failure for weekly home visits and had excellent results in reducing hospitalizations. Of the 30 physicians in our practice, over half were board certified and fellowship trained in geriatric medicine. The rest, as well as the nurse practitioners and physician assistants, were influenced by those of us with geriatric training. The practitioners tended to follow the core elements of the GeriMed philosophy of care (Table 15.1) [2].

On the other hand, clinicians following a "classic" internal medicine approach to care, diagnose, treat, and cure might easily coalesce around a more volume-driven type of practice. Recent literature has finally started to call the traditional internal medicine approach into question in the oldest old. A recent study from Britain questions the aggressive treatment of diabetics in relation to blood sugar, blood pressure, and cholesterol [3]. They found increased mortality in patients over the age of 80 who were treated most aggressively. Similarly, another recent study questioned the value of statins in older adults hospitalized for coronary events [4]. Evidence like this, in addition to previous studies such as one that questioned aggressive treatment of prostate cancer in older men, may be the tip of the iceberg [5].

This discussion brings us to the heart of a bigger issue. If we are to financially incentivize clinicians for value rather than volume, we have additional questions that must be answered. What is value? What is quality care? Do financial incentives work to drive value-based quality care? This approach requires that there is clear financial reward for well-defined outcomes and that there is clarity on how to achieve those outcomes. In a healthcare world where many clinicians still try to

Table 15.1 GeriMed philosophy of care

• Focus on function
• Focus on managing chronic disease(s) and developing chronic care treatment models
• Identify and manage psychological and social aspects of care
• Respect patient's dignity and autonomy
• Respect cultural and spiritual beliefs
• Be sensitive to the patient's financial condition
• Promote wellness
• Listen and communicate effectively
• Patient-centered approach to care, customer-focused approach to service
• Realistically promote optimism and hope
• Team approach to care

aggressively treat blood pressure, blood sugar, and cholesterol in older diabetics, it is difficult to see how this type of incentive system can work. Coupling that with the fact that many geriatricians and primary care physicians just want to "do the right thing," rather than focus on getting a bonus, creates a conundrum.

Let's pause and consider the latest focus of the Centers for Medicare and Medicaid. It has shone a light on the "quadruple aim," a concept first developed in 2007 by Dr. Donald Berwick and the Institute for Healthcare Improvement (IHI) as the "triple aim" [6, 7]. The four dimensions of the now "quadruple aim" are improving the patient experience of care (including quality and satisfaction), improving the health of populations, reducing the per capita cost of health care, and, now, the fourth goal of improving the work life of healthcare providers, including clinicians and staff. Partly in response to this approach, the new Medicare Access and CHIP Reauthorization Act (MACRA) of 2015 legislation endeavors to bring about a value-based model of care delivery. This sounds great, but one has to wonder what physicians have been trying to do for the past century. As professionals, do we not expect physicians to be working to provide quality care? Managed care organizations have presumably been trying to accomplish these same goals for the past 40 years. Unfortunately, the literature on the success of these types of incentives is mixed [8]. Why this "new" approach through MACRA is supposed to finally bring about such change is confusing, to say the least.

Calling something a "quality program," doesn't make it so. At the heart of MACRA is MIPS, or the Merit-based Incentive Payment System. This program will combine four areas: quality, improvement activities, advancing care information, and cost into some type of composite score. The data will be collected during a calendar year, and then the clinician will be bonused (or possibly penalized) over a year later. How this forms any type of effective incentive remains to be seen. There are also the challenges already alluded to. What type of quality metrics are truly pertinent in the frail older adult population? What type of clinical decisions truly impact the overall cost of care in this population? Clinicians can choose to avoid this approach by joining an "Advanced Alternative Payment Model." These models presently include the Comprehensive Primary Care Plus program, Next Generation ACOs, and Medicare Shared Saving Programs [https://qpp.cms.gov/docs/QPP_Advanced_APMs_in_2017.pdf]. The criteria for Advanced Alternative Payment Models have recently been defined by three criteria: require participants to use certified EHR technology, provide payment for covered professional services based on quality measures comparable to those used in the quality performance category of the Merit-based Incentive Payment System (MIPS), and either be a Medical Home Model expanded under CMS Innovation Center authority or require participating APM entities to bear more than a nominal amount of financial risk for monetary losses. At the heart of these programs is some type of shared risk [ibid]. These models tend to reward and penalize clinicians based on the overall cost of care.

There has been a push to add more advanced payment models so that physicians can avoid the MIPS program. In some ways, this could be looked at as a "bait and switch," insofar as CMS is aware that the advanced payment models are capitated, with the intent of limiting overall Medicare expenditures. Similarly, the MIPS program is intended to be a "zero-sum" program, which creates its own challenges, as bonuses will ultimately need to be evened out by penalties or cuts in reimbursement elsewhere. Solo practices, or small group practices, often run on very narrow margins. It remains to be seen how these programs will impact such practices, although the industry has clearly been moving toward consolidation of physician practices into larger groups or having physicians employed by hospitals and health systems [9].

There is also the question regarding the ethics of adding the cost of care to the equation of clinical decision-making. What are the implications of how a clinician will make decisions in such settings? Perhaps even more important is how effectively a clinician can predict the overall cost of care based on a particular approach. Trying to save money by not ordering tests or delaying treatment might ultimately be more costly. Similarly, aggressive initial treatment might ultimately save money. Is this what consumers really want their physicians to be thinking about when they make health care decisions? Furthermore, as the system is presently structured, physicians will not get feedback on the actual cost of care for well over a year after the end of the calendar year the care occurred. How this can possibly influence physician behavior in an effective manner remains to be seen.

Let's go back to our original question. What type of outcomes do physicians, nurse practitioners, and physician assistants want to provide for their patients? These answers are fairly clear in younger patients and in single system diseases that occur in the younger population. Clinicians are looking to make a diagnosis and develop a treatment plan in hopes of finding a cure or at least to significantly curtail the disease. In frail older adults, these questions become quite muddled. Geriatric medicine and the care of older adults are about function and quality of life. It would also appear that the primary goal should be to provide the highest-quality, evidence-based care. The irony of this, based on some of the aforementioned literature, is that the common principles of geriatric medicine appear to lead to a very cost-effective, person-centered approach to care.

There is presently a renaissance in regard to person-centered care. This leads us to a chicken and egg phenomenon. Will incentives drive a person-centered geriatric approach to care? Perhaps if the existing and growing evidence can be effectively shared with clinicians, they can be both educated and incentivized. On the other hand, it is clear that consumers are pushing for person-centered care, as they ought to be. Do we just allow traditional market forces to drive an approach that will turn out to be cost-effective in regard to Medicare and the frail older adult? These questions have led to attempts to describe the "value" of a person-centered approach to care based on traditional business principles. A recent publication from the SCAN Foundation set out to describe "the business case" for person-centered care [10]. They summarized that "Person-centered care is characterized by accounting for individuals' values and preferences and using them to guide all aspects of their health care. The provision of such care for older adults with multiple chronic conditions and functional limitations is widely regarded as being in the best interests of those served—the person and their families. There is also evidence that it can enhance provider satisfaction and reduce turnover…The business case for PCC turns on its capacity to avoid medical costs. Since the target population for PCC consists of high utilizers of the medical system, the resulting burden of medical costs presents a potentially strong basis for the business case" [ibid].

Let's go back to our assumption that physicians, nurse practitioners, and physician assistants want to do "the right thing" in regard to patient care. As professionals, their ultimate goal is providing quality care. The satisfaction of providing such care is their ultimate incentive. If we couple that with a person-centered geriatric approach to care, we have the potential for the best of all worlds. We find ourselves in the milieu of high-quality, cost-effective care. In such a setting, we can afford to provide excellent compensation and benefits to the dedicated professionals that care for many of our most complex patients. Is that not the incentive system that we really want in healthcare?

References

1. Wasserman MR. The business of geriatrics, Assisted Living: Healthcare or Real Estate, p. 83, Springer International Publishing; 2016.
2. Wasserman MR. Care management: from channeling to grace, healthcare changes and the affordable care act. In: Powers JS, editor. Springer International Publishing, p. 133–52, doi:10.1007/978-3-319-09510-3_8.
3. Hamada S, Gulliford M. Mortality in individuals age 80 and older with type 2 diabetes mellitus in relation to glycosylated hemoglobin, blood pressure, and total cholesterol. JAGS. 2016;64:1425–31.
4. Rothschild D, Novak E, Rich M. Effect of statin therapy on mortality in older adults hospitalized with coronary artery disease: A propensity-adjusted analysis. JAGS. 2016;64:1475–9.
5. Stangelberger A, Waldert M, Djavan B. Prostate cancer in elderly men. Rev Urol. 2008;10(2):111–9.
6. Berwick DM, Nolan TW, Whittington J. The triple aim: care, health, and cost. Health Aff. 2008;27(3):759–69.
7. Bodenheimer T, Sinsky C. From triple to quadruple aim: care of the patient requires care of the provider. Ann Fam Med. 2014;12:573–6.
8. Armour BS, et al. The effect of explicit financial incentives on physician behavior. Arch Int Med. 2001;161:1261–6.
9. Kane CK, Emmons DW. New data on physician practice arrangements: private practice remains strong despite shifts toward hospital employment, AMA Economic and Health Policy Research, September 2013.
10. Tabbush V, Coulourides Kogan A, Mosqueda L, Kominski GF. Person-centered care: the business case, June 2016. TheSCANfoundation.org.

The Future of Primary Care for Older Adults

16

Patrick P. Coll

Demographics

Like all developed nations, the United States is experiencing an increase in the number of its citizens who are older. People are living longer. The US Census estimates that there will be more than ten million Americans 90 years of age or older by 2050. Increasing life expectancy leads to an increase in the number of older patients who need primary care services. Increased longevity is frequently associated with an increase in the number of chronic diseases and associated disability, which further increases primary care needs for older patients. According to the Centers for Disease Control, 34% of Americans 75 years of age or older have three or more chronic medical conditions compared to 2.1% of Americans less than 45 years of age (http://www.cdc.gov/nchs/data/ahcd/namcs_summary/2012_namcs_web_tables.pdf). Most of us wish for a long, happy, fulfilling life, free of disease, pain, disability, and dependency. Though this is a laudable goal, many Americans do not achieve it. A healthy lifestyle throughout a lifetime may only postpone disease burden in old age [1]. Recent data show that women in particular are more likely to experience late-life disability [2]. For the foreseeable future, increasing numbers of older Americans, with an increasing number of chronic medical conditions, will require an increasing number of primary care providers.

Though the United States will experience an unprecedented increase in the number of older people over the next 30 years, because of a relatively high birth rate and because of net immigration, the percentage of seniors in the total population of the United States will be lower than many other developed nations. Italy and Japan are examples of nations with low birth rates and low levels of immigration. Unless birth rates increase or immigration policies change, they will have an even greater percentage of seniors in the future than the United States. Without a sufficient number of

P.P. Coll, MD, AGSF, CMD
Center on Aging, UConn Health, Farmington, CT, USA
e-mail: coll@uchc.edu

© Springer International Publishing AG 2018
M. Wasserman, J. Riopelle (eds.), *Primary Care for Older Adults*,
DOI 10.1007/978-3-319-61329-1_16

younger working residents, a nation with a high number of seniors will have significant difficulty funding and providing healthcare and community services for its seniors.

There will come a time when the baby boom generation has passed into history. It is not clear now what the demographics of the United States will look like when that happens. Mortality rates, birth rates, and immigration will all play a role. There is the possibility that aging and associated mortality will be altered significantly through genetic manipulation, a process which has already been used to significantly extend life expectancy in lower life forms.

The Senior Care Workforce

Senior care workforce issues can be further subdivided into supply and education.

Supply

Historically, adult primary care in the United States has been provided by internal medicine and family medicine practitioners. The majority of primary care for seniors will continue to be provided by internal medicine and family medicine providers. These practitioners are mostly physicians, though an increasing amount of care is being provided by nurse practitioners and physician assistants. There is a current and a projected worsening of primary care availability (https://www.aamc.org/download/458082/data/2016_complexities_of_supply_and_demand_projections.pdf). Factors contributing to this shortage include the increase in the population of the United States, an expansion in the availability of health insurance for low-income Americans related to changes implemented by the Affordable Care Act, an increase in the duration of physician visits [3], and a relatively modest increase in both new medical schools and in class size in existing schools.

Geriatricians also provide primary care for older patients. However, geriatrics is a distinct medical discipline with a distinct knowledge base and approach to patient care. It is more than internal medicine or family medicine for older patients. Just like cardiologists have a particular expertise in the medical care of patients with complex cardiac conditions, geriatricians have a particular expertise in the medical care of older patients with complex age-associated conditions.

There is a current shortage of geriatrics-trained providers, and the number of geriatrics providers is falling, even though the need for their services is increasing. Because their patients are frail and have multiple chronic medical conditions, a full-time clinical geriatrician can provide primary care for approximately 700 patients, less than half the number of patients a typical family physician or general internist would have in their practice. Even if geriatricians were to limit their patient panel to those 90 or older, there would not be enough of them to provide care for all current Americans who are that old.

The benefits of ensuring an adequate supply of primary care providers are being increasingly recognized by payers of healthcare, including government agencies.

Access to primary healthcare providers has been shown to lead to better medical outcomes for Medicare beneficiaries [4]. Because they help improve care and because of a projected shortage, there have been a variety of efforts to increase the number of primary care providers in the United States. To date, these efforts been largely unsuccessful. There will be renewed efforts to increase the number of primary care providers. Three issues will determine their success: changes in how graduate medical education is funded, better reimbursement for primary care providers and better working conditions with less bureaucratic duties, and more direct patient care opportunities.

In the United States, graduate medical education is funded primarily by Medicare, the federal health insurance program for older Americans. Almost all of this funding goes to teaching hospitals which have historically emphasized and promoted the training of physician specialists. The federal government has capped the number of training positions they will pay for. Hospitals are reluctant to develop new training programs for primary care because they do not have well-established community-based training sites and because they may have to reduce the number of specialist trainees. If the supply of primary care physicians is to increase, this will need to change (https://www.ncbi.nlm.nih.gov/books/NBK248022/#sec_000098). Medicare has supported the training of nurses only to a limited degree. There have been recent efforts to rectify this through the funding of several nurse education demonstration projects (http://www.aacn.nche.edu/government-affairs/ian/2015/September-2015.pdf). More funding needs to be directed toward teaching programs that are community based and which emphasize the training of primary care providers (http://www.nationalacademies.org/hmd/~/media/Files/Report%20Files/2014/GME/GME-RB.pdf). More funding needs to be directed toward the education of APRNs and PAs who are planning to follow a career in primary care. As Medicare is held more accountable for the money it spends on the training of the future healthcare workforce and as Medicare and other health insurance program seek to promote the education of a healthcare workforce which better meets the needs of older Americans, these funding changes will occur.

In the face of the demographic imperative and an impending workforce crisis, geriatrics is beginning to reconsider the role it should play in the provision of clinical services for older patients [5]. Instead of providing clinical care for a small number of older Americans, it has been recommended that geriatrics concentrate on research, education, and policy development as a means of promoting high-quality care for all older Americans. Geriatricians will still provide primary care, but will do so almost exclusively as a means of teaching other providers geriatrics skills and as a laboratory for determining ideal care for seniors.

Education

Assuming efforts to increase the supply of primary care providers in the future are successful, it will be critical that these providers are trained to deliver high-quality geriatrics care [6]. Current primary care providers feel ill equipped to meet the needs of their older patients [7]. With few exceptions, all healthcare providers need to be trained to meet the needs of older patients. Exposure to the principles of high-quality geriatrics practices need to be introduced early in the process of training healthcare providers. For those who ultimately choose a career in primary care, this training needs to be more extensive. Teaching experiences need to be available across all medical care settings including the patient's home, nursing homes, assisted living, hospice, post-acute care, primary care offices, and acute care settings. For medical trainees in the United States, the scope of their training is determined by the Accreditation Council for Graduate Medical Education (ACGME). The current ACGME requirements regarding geriatrics training for both family physicians and internists will need to be expanded. The ACGME must seek input from geriatricians regarding the adoption and implementation of training requirements that will prepare the future physician workforce to meet the complex medical needs of older patients. Primary care APRNs and PAs will also be required to have extensive training in the management of the complex medical needs of older patients. Geriatricians and geriatrics APRNs and PAs will play an important role in teaching the new generation of primary care providers.

Innovation

As the funding of healthcare has evolved and as technology has improved, we are beginning to see examples of innovation in terms of the way care is delivered, where it is delivered, who is providing that care, how that care is being documented, and how it is being paid for. Several innovative models of care have been described in earlier chapters of this book.

Technology will play an increasingly important role in the delivery of healthcare in the future. We are in the very early stages of using electronic health records (EHR). Healthcare providers are EHR pioneers and our current EHRs are like Conestoga wagons; they get us to where we want to go, but it is slow and uncomfortable. We can now fly safely across the United States in a few hours; someday our EHRs will fly too. In the future, while seeing a patient or shortly after seeing a patient, the healthcare provider will speak instructions into the EHR. "Arrange a follow-up appointment for Mrs. Smith with me in three months. Book a cardiology consult for the evaluation of a systolic murmur. Arrange for a CBC and a basic metabolic panel to be done this afternoon. Provide Mrs. Smith with some information on exercise and a heart healthy diet and follow up with her every two weeks for the next two months to see if she has any questions. Let her know the results of her lab work when it is available. Check in on her BP measurements and weight which are being streamed to you every time they are done and let me know if her systolic BP is above 150 or her weight is above 160. Bill this visit as a 99214 and add a charge for an EKG. Find the appropriate diagnosis for each charge in other segments of my dictated note. Copy everything to Dr. Richard Jones and her home health care nurse."

Current EHRs are built to meet the needs of fee-for-service medicine and are billing centric. Future EHRs will need to be more care centric. The Medicare and CHIP Reauthorization Act of 2015 (MACRA) is encouraging and assisting medical providers who bill Medicare for services to move from fee-for-service care to value-based care. The quality and cost of care provided will affect Medicare payments. EHRs produce a lot of data. Data will need to be presented to providers, patients, and payer in a manner which facilitates high-quality, coordinated, cost-effective care.

Robots and artificial intelligence (AI) will play an important role in the future of primary care for seniors (http://www.altfutures.org/pubs/pc2025/IAF-PrimaryCare2025Scenarios.pdf). Human contact with a healthcare provider will always be an important part of healthcare delivery. But given the projected shortage of primary care providers and the increasing medical costs associated with an aging population, this human contact will need to be supplemented by robotic assistants who have built in AI. A robotic medical assistant who witnesses a healthcare provider's interaction with a patient will eventually be able to generate a summary of the visit and determine a list of orders such as those listed above without requiring specific instructions from the provider. They will be able to collect preliminary information from the patient before a visit, respond to patient enquiries by phone, text or email the patient or their caregiver, and room the patients when they arrive at the office. Robotic assistants will also be able to manage many of the chronic care management (CCM) tasks which are so important for the care of older patients. Reimbursement for CCM, currently based on time human members of the office team spend on CCM, will need to adjust to this new reality.

Non-face-to-face care will become more and more common as providers and their patients are linked to each other remotely. Telemedicine, e-consults, and robotic assistants will all provide care and monitor medical conditions which currently require a face-to-face visit with the provider. These technologic innovations can improve access, lower costs, and facilitate the provision of geriatrics care by non-geriatrics providers. They can also compensate in part for the fact that many rural parts of the United States have difficulty attracting healthcare providers, including geriatrics providers to live and work there. Acute Care for the Elderly (ACE) Tracker and the provision of e-geriatrics consults has been demonstrated to be an effective way of providing geriatrics expertise remotely for rural hospitals who do not have a geriatrics provider on staff [8]. The ability to routinely search not just hospital records but also nursing home, home care, and outpatient records and identify patients who could benefit from an e-geriatrics consult will increase.

Patients will increasing rely on AI to help diagnose and treat their illnesses and medical concerns. There will be pressure to broaden the patient's independent ability, based on the recommendations of AI, to order tests and treatments. Disease prevention and health promotion recommendations will also be provided by AI. The patient will be able to go to their local pharmacy for a broad range of immunizations and present themselves for a mammogram or screening blood work based on AI recommendations. The PCP will be able to monitor many of these interactions and may be asked to provide assessments, guidance, and recommendations. Even though many patients will have difficulty finding a primary care provider who is willing and available to coordinate their care, primary care providers will be concerned about laws and regulations which broaden the scope of practice and the delegation of responsibilities which previously required a medical license.

Funding

Most medical cares for older patients, including primary care services, are paid for by federal and or state agencies, including Medicare, Medicaid, and the Veterans Administration. These publicly funded government agencies will have difficulty meeting the increasing costs of providing services for a growing number of seniors. Though costs per Medicare beneficiary have increased in recent years at a slower rate than the rate of inflation, overall Medicare expenditures will increase in the future as the number of beneficiaries increase. Medicare beneficiaries will increase by one-third from 54 million to 72 million between 2014 and 2124 [9]. There will be a permanent sense of crisis regarding the fiscal viability of publicly funded healthcare. There will be increasing pressure to shift Medicare costs onto the beneficiary and or to insist that beneficiaries enroll in a Medicare Advantage plan or a similar capitated plan, where the payer's exposure to increasing costs is limited.

Primary care expenditures are a relatively small percentage of overall healthcare expenditures, somewhere between 6 and 8% [10]. There is good evidence that overall healthcare costs are reduced and the quality of care provided is improved when there is a higher percentage of primary care providers providing care [11].

Because of such evidence, Medicare and Medicare Advantage plans in particular will promote the use of PCPs to manage the patient's care across the spectrum of care. This will be at odds with the workforce concerns noted above, but with better reimbursement for PCPs, more physicians, nurses, and PAs will choose to follow a career in primary care. Funders will look to PCPs and their AI and data analytics tools to manage the healthcare needs of the most complex and most costly patients.

Medicare has been clear that it wants to move toward a value-based payment system and away from fee-for-service care [12]. The success of this effort remains to be seen, and both providers and patients will need to be convinced that these changes are in their best interests if it is to succeed. Bundled payments for specific conditions and interventions will become more commons. This will drive disparate healthcare providers to join together and coordinate care in a quality-sensitive, cost-sensitive manner. There will be a continued consolidation of healthcare systems, and these healthcare systems will compete with each other to recruit well-qualified primary care providers. They will increasingly recognize the need to hire geriatrics specialists to help them design, operate, and educate providers in systems of care which promote high-quality services for older patients and their family members.

Primary care providers will become increasingly aware of their worth in this value-based payment (VBP) world. More of them will create primary care groups who will seek to manage care within capitated contracts and bundled payments. This will pose both opportunity and risk. These groups will either work closely with or purchase their own home healthcare agencies. They will consider opening PACE programs. They will provide post-acute care services and direct patients from the emergency department to a post-acute care facility where they manage the patients rather than admit the patient to the hospital, where they have little control over the care provided. In this VBP environment, the primary care providers will insist on access to information and test results so that expensive tests and interventions are not unnecessarily being repeated. VBP is designed to shift financial risk from the payer to the provider, and generally speaking, maximum financial return for the provider is balanced by high risk. In healthcare, value is maintaining the quality of care while lowering the cost of care. There are risks for both the patient and the provider if the payments being received do not adequately reflect the projected care needs. Developing quality metrics for discrete medical services such as surgical procedures or hospitalization is difficult, but developing metrics which represent high-quality care for frail older patients with complex medical needs is particularly difficult. Developing risk adjustment measures that are a true reflection of the patient's comorbidities and disability will be important. Mortality following an elective surgical procedure on a healthy 50-year-old is more likely to represent poor quality than the death of a 99-year-old with advanced heart failure, who has been unable to walk for more than 2 years or feed himself for the past 6 months. Geriatricians can assist with the design of programs that incorporate risk adjustment into payment calculations.

All primary care providers will see an increasing number of older patients in the future. Their ability to provide access and high-quality geriatrics care will depend on their education, the way their practices are organized, and the way they are paid. Though the demand will be significant, with sufficient foresight and planning, the needs can be met.

References

1. May AM, Struijk EA, Fransen HP, Onland-Moret NC, et al. The impact of a healthy lifestyle on disability-adjusted life years: a prospective cohort study. BMC Med. 2015;13:39.
2. Freedman VA, Wolf DA, Spillman BC. Disability-free life expectancy over 30 years: a growing female disadvantage in the US population. Am J Public Health. 2016;106:1079–85.
3. Shaw MK, Davis SA, Fleischer AB, Feldman SR. The duration of physician office visits in the United States, 1993–2010. Am J Manag Care. 2014;20(10):820–6.
4. Chiang CH, Stukel TA, Flood AB, Goodman DC. Primary care physician workforce and Medicare beneficiaries' health outcomes. JAMA. 2011;305(20):2096–105.
5. Tinetti M. Mainstream or Extinction: Can Defining Who We Are Save Geriatrics. J Am Geriatr Soc. 2016;64:1400–4.
6. Boult C, Counsell SR, Leipzig RM, Berenson RA. The urgency of preparing primary care physicians to care for older people with chronic illnesses. Health Aff. 2010;29(5):811–8.
7. Adams WL, Mc Ilvain HE, Lacy NL, Magsi H, Crabtree BF, Yenny SK, et al. Primary care for elderly people: why do doctors find it so hard? Gerontologist. 2002;42(6):835–42.
8. Malone M, Vollbrecht M, Stephenson J, Burke L, Pagel P, Goodwin JS. Acute Care for Elders (ACE) tracker and e-geriatrician: methods to disseminate ACE concepts to hospitals with no geriatricians on staff. J Am Geriatr Soc. 2010;58(1):161–7.
9. U.S. Congressional Budget Office. Updated Budget 2014–2024, April 14, 2014.
10. Phillips RL, Bazemore A. Primary care and why it matters for US health system reform. Health Aff. 2010;29(5):806–10.
11. Kravet SJ, Shore AD, Miller R, Green GB, Wright SM. Health care utilization and the proportion of primary care physicians. Am J Med. 2008;121(2):142–8.
12. Burwell SM. Setting value-based payment goals — HHS efforts to improve U.S. health care. N Engl J Med. 2015;372:897–9.

© Springer International Publishing AG 2018
M. Wasserman, J. Riopelle (eds.), *Primary Care for Older Adults*,
DOI 10.1007/978-3-319-61329-1

Made in the USA
Monee, IL
07 July 2026

56546125R00145